A·N·N·U·A·L E·D·I·T·I·O·N·S

Nutrition

Thirteenth Edition

01/02

S0-DOO-208

EDITOR

Dorothy J. Klimis-Zacas
University of Maine, Orono

Dorothy Klimis-Zacas is associate professor of clinical nutrition at the University of Maine and cooperating professor of nutrition and dietetics at Harokopio University, Athens, Greece. She teaches undergraduate and graduate classes in nutrition and its relation to health and disease for students of dietetics, nurses, and physicians.

Her current research interests relate to basic investigations in the area of trace mineral nutrition and its role in the development of atherosclerosis and to applied investigations that utilize nutritional interventions to reduce cardiovascular disease risk in adolescents both in the United States and in the Mediterranean region.

A Ph.D. and Fullbright Fellow, Dr. Klimis-Zacas is the author of numerous research articles and the editor of two books, *Manganese in Health and Disease* and *Nutritional Concerns for Women*. She is a member of Sigma Delta Epsilon, The American Society of Nutritional Sciences, The International Atherosclerosis Society, The American Dietetic Association, The Society for Nutrition Education, and The American Heart Association.

McGraw-Hill/Dushkin
530 Old Whitfield Street, Guilford, Connecticut 06437

Visit us on the Internet
http://www.dushkin.com

Credits

1. Trends Today and Tomorrow
Unit photo—© Sweet By & By/Cindy Brown.
2. Nutrients
Unit photo—© 2001 by PhotoDisc, Inc.
3. Through the Life Span: Diet and Disease
Unit photo—Dushkin/McGraw-Hill photo.
4. Fat and Weight Control
Unit photo—© 2001 by Cleo Freelance Photography.
5. Food Safety
Unit photo—© Sweet By & By/Cindy Brown.
6. Health Claims
Unit photo—© Sweet By & By/Cindy Brown.
7. World Hunger and Malnutrition
Unit photo—WHO photo by M. Jacot.

Copyright

Cataloging in Publication Data
Main entry under title: Annual Editions: Nutrition. 2001/2002.
　　1. Nutrition—Periodicals. 2. Diet—Periodicals. I. Klimis-Zacas, Dorothy J., *comp.* II. Title: Nutrition.
ISBN 0–07–243305–1　　　613.2′.05　　　91–641611　　　ISSN 1055–6990

Thirteenth Edition

Cover image © 2001 by PhotoDisc, Inc.

Printed in the United States of America　　　1234567890BAHBAH54321　　　Printed on Recycled Paper iii

To the Reader

In publishing ANNUAL EDITIONS we recognize the enormous role played by the magazines, newspapers, and journals of the public press in providing current, first-rate educational information in a broad spectrum of interest areas. Many of these articles are appropriate for students, researchers, and professionals seeking accurate, current material to help bridge the gap between principles and theories and the real world. These articles, however, become more useful for study when those of lasting value are carefully collected, organized, indexed, and reproduced in a low-cost format, which provides easy and permanent access when the material is needed. That is the role played by ANNUAL EDITIONS.

Since nutrition is an evolving science, it necessitates updating *Annual Editions: Nutrition* annually to keep up with the plethora of topics and controversies raised in the field. The main goal of this anthology is to provide the reader with up-to-date information by presenting current topics of information based on scientific evidence. *Annual Editions: Nutrition* also presents controversial topics in a balanced and unbiased manner. Where appropriate, international perspectives are presented. We hope that the reader will develop critical thinking and be empowered to ask questions and seek answers.

Consumers are thoroughly confused with the food choices that they have to make when they walk into a supermarket or visit a restaurant. Additionally, there is conflicting information on several nutrition topics that appear on the news, popular magazines, scientific journals, and over the Internet. "Nutrition experts" and "health advisors" seem to sprout everywhere. We are at the parapet not only of a revolution in information technology but also of nutritional research. Information is distributed at a very fast pace, across continents, and without consideration of country borders. Thus, informing the consumer regularly with reliable and current nutrition information is the duty of the professional.

Annual Editions: Nutrition 01/02 is to be used as a companion to a standard nutrition text so that it may update, expand, or emphasize certain topics that are covered in the text or present a totally new topic not covered in a standard text.

To accomplish this, *Annual Editions: Nutrition 01/02* is composed of seven units that review current knowledge and controversies in the area of nutrition. The first unit describes current trends in the field of nutrition in the United States and the rest of the world, including the new nutrient requirements for the United States. Units two, three, and four include topics that focus on nutrients and their relationship to health and disease, the changing nutrient needs and concerns through the life cycle, and weight control. Unit five focuses on food safety and covers topics on health claims, including subjects about which consumers are misinformed and are thus vulnerable to quackery. Finally, unit seven focuses on world hunger and malnutrition, including environmental sustainability and biotechnology. A *topic guide* will assist the reader in finding other articles on a given subject and *World Wide Web* sites will help in further exploring a particular topic.

Your input is most valuable to improving this anthology, which we update yearly. We would appreciate your comments and suggestions as you review the current edition.

Dorothy Klimis-Zacas
Editor

Contents

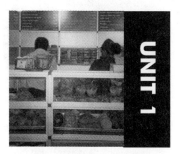

UNIT 1

Trends Today and Tomorrow

Eight articles examine the eating patterns of people today. Some of the topics considered include nutrients in our diet, eating trends, portion size and servings, and eating lunch in restaurants.

The concepts in bold italics are developed in the article. For further expansion please refer to the Topic Guide, the Glossary, and the Index.

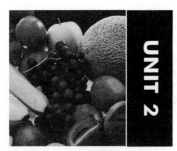

UNIT 2

Nutrients

Nine articles discuss the importance of nutrients and fiber in our diet. Topics include dietary standards, fats, carbohydrates, vitamins, supplements, and minerals.

The concepts in bold italics are developed in the article. For further expansion please refer to the Topic Guide, the Glossary, and the Index.

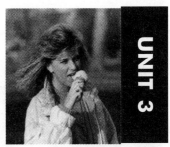

UNIT 3

Through the Life Span: Diet and Disease

Nine articles examine our health as it is affected by diet throughout our lives. Some topics include the links between diet and disease, cholesterol, food allergies, and nutrition for the elderly.

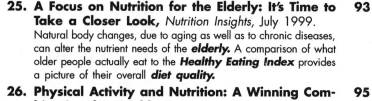

Overview   **100**

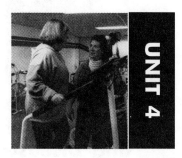

UNIT 4

Fat and Weight Control

Nine articles examine weight management. Topics include the relationship between dieting and exercise, the effects of various diet plans, and the importance of portion control.

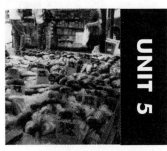

UNIT 5

Food Safety

Eight articles discuss the safety of
food. Topics include food-borne
illness, pesticide residues, naturally
occurring toxins, and avoiding
cross-contamination in the home.

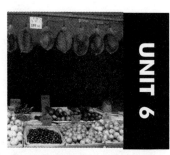

UNIT 6

Health Claims

Eight articles examine some of the health claims made by today's "specialists." Topics include quacks, fad diets, and nutrition myths and misinformation.

The concepts in bold italics are developed in the article. For further expansion please refer to the Topic Guide, the Glossary, and the Index.

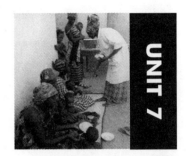

UNIT 7

World Hunger and Malnutrition

Six articles discuss the world's
food supply. Topics include global
malnutrition, nutrition and infection,
agriculture, and biotechnology
and the world's food supply.

The concepts in bold italics are developed in the article. For further expansion please refer to the Topic Guide, the Glossary, and the Index.

Topic Guide

This topic guide suggests how the selections in this book relate to the subjects covered in your course.

The Web icon (◉) under the topic articles easily identifies the relevant Web sites, which are numbered and annotated on the next two pages. By linking the articles and the Web sites by topic, this ANNUAL EDITIONS reader becomes a powerful learning and research tool.

2

3

● AE: Nutrition

The following World Wide Web sites have been carefully researched and selected to support the articles found in this reader. The sites are cross-referenced by number and the Web icon (●) in the topic guide. In addition, it is possible to link directly to these Web sites through our DUSHKIN ONLINE support site at *http://www.dushkin.com/online/*.

The following sites were available at the time of publication. Visit our Web site—we update DUSHKIN ONLINE regularly to reflect any changes.

General Sources

1. American Dietetic Association
http://www.eatright.org
This consumer link to nutrition and health includes resources, news, marketplace, search for a dietician, government information, and a gateway to related sites. The site includes a tip of the day and special features.

2. The Blonz Guide to Nutrition
http://www.blonz.com
The categories in this valuable site report news in the fields of nutrition, food science, foods, fitness, and health. There is also a selection of search engines and links.

3. CSPI: Center for Science in the Public Interest
http://www.cspinet.org
CSPI is a nonprofit education and advocacy organization that is committed to improving the safety and nutritional quality of our food supply. CSPI publishes the *Nutrition Action Healthletter*, which has monthly information about food.

4. Institute of Food Technologists
http://www.ift.org
This site of the Society for Food Science and Technology is full of important information and news about every aspect of the food products that come to market.

5. International Food Information Council Foundation
http://ificinfo.health.org
IFIC's purpose is to be the link between science and communications by offering the latest scientific information on food safety, nutrition, and health in a form that is understandable and useful for opinion leaders and consumers to access.

6. U.S. National Institutes of Health
http://www.nih.gov
Consult this site for links to extensive health information and scientific resources. Comprised of 24 separate institutes, centers, and divisions, the NIH is one of eight health agencies of the Public Health Service, which, in turn, is part of the U.S. Department of Health and Human Services.

Trends Today and Tomorrow

7. Food Science and Human Nutrition Extension
http://www.exnet.iastate.edu/Pages/families/fshn/
This extensive Iowa State University site links to latest news and reports, consumer publications, food safety information, and many other useful nutrition-related sites.

8. Food Surveys Research Group
http://www.barc.usda.gov/bhnrc/foodsurvey/home.htm
Visit this site of the Beltsville Human Nutrition Research Center Food Surveys research group first, and then click on USDA to keep up with nutritional news and information.

9. U.S. Food and Drug Administration
http://www.fda.gov/default.htm
This is the home page of the FDA, which describes itself as the United States' "foremost consumer protection agency." Visit this site and its links to learn about food safety, food and nutrition labeling, and other topics of importance.

Nutrients

10. Dole 5 A Day: Nutrition, Fruits & Vegetables
http://www.dole5aday.com
The Dole Food Company, a founding member of the National 5 A Day for Better Health Program, offers this site to entice children into taking an interest in proper nutrition.

11. Food and Nutrition Information Center
http://www.nal.usda.gov/fnic/
Use this site to find dietary and nutrition information provided by various USDA agencies and to find links to food and nutrition resources on the Internet.

12. Nutrient Data Laboratory
http://www.nal.usda.gov/fnic/foodcomp/
Information about the USDA Nutrient Database can be found on this site. Search here for answers to FAQs, a glossary of terms, facts about food composition, and useful links.

13. NutritionalSupplements.com
http://www.nutritionalsupplements.com
This source provides unbiased information about nutritional supplements and prescription drugs, submitted by consumers with no vested interest in the products.

14. U.S. National Library of Medicine
http://www.nlm.nih.gov
This site permits you to search databases and electronic information sources such as MEDLINE, learn about research projects, and keep up on nutrition-related news.

Through the Life Span: Diet and Disease

15. American Cancer Society
http://www.cancer.org/frames.html
Open this site and its various links to learn the concerns and lifestyle advice of the American Cancer Society. It provides information on alternative therapies, tobacco, other Web resources, and more.

16. American Heart Association
http://www.americanheart.org
The AHA offers this site to provide the most comprehensive information on heart disease and stroke as well as late-breaking news. The site presents facts on warning signs, a reference guide, and explanations of diseases and treatments.

17. The Food Allergy Network
http://www.foodallergy.org
The Food Allergy Network site, which welcomes consumers, health professionals, and reporters, includes product alerts and updates, information about food allergies, daily tips, and links to other sites.

18. Go Ask Alice! from Columbia University Health Services

http://www.goaskalice.columbia.edu

This interactive site provides discussion and insight into a number of issues of interest to college-age people and those younger and older. Many questions about physical and emotional well-being, fitness and nutrition, and alcohol, nicotine, and other drugs are answered.

19. Heinz Infant & Toddler Nutrition

http://www.heinzbaby.com

An educational section full of nutritional information and meal-planning guides for parents and caregivers as well as articles and reviews by leading pediatricians and nutritionists can be found on this page.

20. LaLeche League International

http://www.lalecheleague.org

Important information to mothers who are contemplating breast feeding can be accessed at this Web site. Links to other sites are also possible.

21. Nutrition for Kids: 24 Carrot Press

http://www.nutritionforkids.com

This Web site of 24 Carrot Press publishes material that takes a positive, fun approach to the more serious issues that affect children, including poor eating habits, obesity, and inactivity. Their site includes How to Teach Nutrition to Kids, Activity Guide, stickers, *Feeding Kids Newsletter*, and links.

22. Vegetarian Resource Group

http://www.vrg.org

The VRG offers information on everything of interest to vegans, vegetarians, and others.

Fat and Weight Control

23. American Anorexia Bulimia Association

http://www.aabainc.org/home.html

The AABA is a nonprofit organization of concerned people dedicated to the prevention and treatment of eating disorders. It offers many services, including help lines, referral networks, school outreach, support groups, and prevention programs.

24. Calorie Control Council

http://www.caloriecontrol.org

The Calorie Control Council's Web site offers information on cutting calories, achieving and maintaining healthy weight, and for low-calorie, reduced-fat foods and beverages.

25. Eating Disorders: Body Image Betrayal

http://www.geocities.com/HotSprings/5704/edlist.htm

This extensive collection of links leads to information on compulsive eating, bulimia, anorexia, and other disorders.

26. Shape Up America!

http://www.shapeup.org

At the Shape Up America! Web site you will find the latest information about safe weight management, healthy eating, and physical fitness. Links include Support Center, Cyberkitchen, Media Center, Fitness Center, and BMI Center.

Food Safety

27. Centers for Disease Control and Prevention

http://www.cdc.gov

The CDC offers this home page, from which you can obtain information about travelers' health, data related to disease control and prevention, general nutritional and health information, publications, and more.

28. FDA Center for Food Safety and Applied Nutrition

http://vm.cfsan.fda.gov

It is possible to access everything you might want to know about food safety and what government agencies are doing to ensure it from this Web site.

29. Food Safety Information from North Carolina

http://www.ces.ncsu.edu/depts/foodsci/agentinfo/

This site from the Cooperative Extension Service at North Carolina State University has a database designed to promote food safety education via the Internet.

30. Food Safety Project

http://www.exnet.iastate.edu/Pages/families/fs/

FSP's site contains food safety lessons, 10 steps to a safe kitchen, consumer control points, and food law.

31. USDA Food Safety and Inspection Service

http://www.fsis.usda.gov

The FSIS, part of the U.S. Department of Agriculture, is the government agency "responsible for ensuring that the nation's commercial supply of meat, poultry, and egg products is safe, wholesome, and correctly labeled and packaged."

Health Claims

32. Federal Trade Commission: Diet, Health & Fitness

http://www.ftc.gov/bcp/menu-health.htm

This site of the FTC on the Web offers consumer education rules and acts that include a wide range of subjects, from buying exercise equipment to virtual health "treatments."

33. National Council Against Health Fraud

http://www.ncahf.org

The NCAHF does business as the National Council for Reliable Health Information. At its Web page it offers links to other related sites, including Dr. Terry Polevoy's "Healthwatcher Net."

34. QuackWatch

http://www.quackwatch.com

Quackwatch Inc., a nonprofit corporation, provides this guide to examine health fraud. Data for intelligent decision making on health topics are also presented.

World Hunger and Malnutrition

35. Population Reference Bureau

http://www.prb.org

A key source for global population information, this is a good place to pursue data on nutrition problems worldwide.

36. World Health Organization

http://www.who.ch

This home page of the World Health Organization will provide you with links to a wealth of statistical and analytical information about health and nutrition around the world.

37. WWW Virtual Library: Demography & Population Studies

http://demography.anu.edu.au/VirtualLibrary/

A multitude of important links to information about global poverty and hunger can be found here.

We highly recommend that you review our Web site for expanded information and our other product lines. We are continually updating and adding links to our Web site in order to offer you the most usable and useful information that will support and expand the value of your Annual Editions. You can reach us at: *http://www.dushkin. com/annualeditions/*.

Unit Selections

1. **The Changing American Diet,** Bonnie Liebman
2. **Healthy Lifestyles for Healthy Americans: Report on USDA's Year 2000 Behavioral Nutrition Roundtable,** Eileen Kennedy and Susan E. Offutt
3. **Nutrient Requirements Get a Makeover: The Evolution of the Recommended Dietary Allowances,** *Food Insight*
4. **Picture This! Communicating Nutrition Around the World,** *Food Insight*
5. **Food Portions and Servings: How Do They Differ?** *Nutrition Insights*
6. **A Reality Check for the Lunch-On-the-Run Crowd,** *Tufts University Health & Nutrition Letter*
7. **The 100 Healthiest Foods,** Janis Jibrin
8. **Supermarket Psych-Out,** *Tufts University Health & Nutrition Letter*

Key Points to Consider

❖ What new food trends are affecting the diet of the American population?

❖ Is the philosophical change that has occurred with the changes from RDA to DRIs a good one? Defend your answer.

❖ What sort of similarities are there among the diets in communities around the world?

❖ How do serving sizes differ from portion sizes?

❖ What foods make up a diet that prevents illness?

❖ What sort of techniques do marketers use to influence your food-buying decisions?

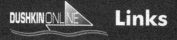 **Links**   **www.dushkin.com/online/**

These sites are annotated on pages 4 and 5.

Consumers worldwide are bombarded daily with messages about nutrients and health. They are presented with "new" food products at the supermarket and in restaurants and it is up to them to distill the sometimes controversial reports and make their own decisions. The first unit describes current trends and developments in the field of nutrition for the new millennium, reports on how the American diet is evolving and on the nature of the "new" dietary guidelines and dietary allowances, explains differences about food portions and servings, and addresses the paradox of nutrition knowledge and eating behavior. Communicating global concepts about nutrition through food guides that have been adopted for different cultures makes the reader aware of the commonalities and interrelatedness of different cultures. New advances in research and the role of nutrients in health and disease have enabled the food industry to develop functional foods whose safety and role in health is questioned. Finally, the reader will be able to read about the foods that are powerhouses of vitamins, minerals, and phytochemicals and be aided in the attempt to make wise food selections.

The first article describes how Americans are still drinking more soft drinks and eating more sugar, sweeteners, and cheese than in the past. On the positive end, they are moving slowly toward cutting down on beef and are eating more fruits and vegetables. Still, most chicken that is consumed is fried in partially hydrogenated fat.

In the second article, the results of a meeting of a panel of experts at a workshop sponsored by the U.S.D.A. is discussed. Attempts to find answers to the elusive question of why, since our knowledge of nutrition has increased, we do not seem to change our eating behavior are explored. The economic, psychosocial, and physiological factors that influence food choices and activity levels are described. Social marketing interventions as well as interventions at the community and individual levels are discussed as part of the solution.

A historical timeline for the evolution of the Recommended Dietary Allowances (RDAs) used until recently and their conversion to the presently used DRIs (Dietary Reference Intakes) is presented in the following article. This change is a result of the necessity of emphasizing prevention of chronic disease rather than an emphasis on deficiencies and the increasing use of supplements without asking for professional advice.

Communicating nutrition information and guidance around the world is discussed in the next article, which makes it clear that nutrition messages travel far and fast and that different countries use pictorial presentations to communicate similar themes of dietary guidance.

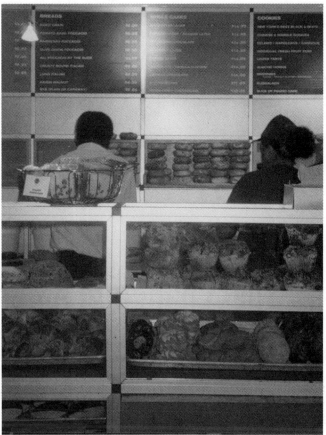

Even though there is diversity, the common message is balance, variety, and moderation in food choices.

Large portions of food are the norm in many eateries. The incidence of obesity in the United States is on the rise and consumers are thoroughly confused about food guide pyramid servings, food label servings, and food portions. The fifth article explains the differences and offers guidance to educators to help consumers understand the concept of servings and portions. The public is not aware that using quick eateries may increase not only the amount that they are eating, but also their fat and calorie intake. The sixth article will help consumers make healthy food choices in many of the fast food establishments that they frequent.

Improved technologies in nutrition research over the last decade have unraveled the content and role of different phytochemicals and other nutrient and nonnutrient components that are primarily found in fruits and vegetables. The seventh article presents 100 nutrient-packed foods that help protect against degenerative disease. The author encourages readers to use the list when shopping.

The last article of the unit reveals some of the secrets that supermarkets use to influence the consumer's buying decisions. Colors, shapes, and sizes are carefully designed to increase purchases. You can be ready, though, with some countertricks of your own.

The Changing American Diet

By Bonnie Liebman

It's report card time again. And once again, the American Diet failed to make the honor roll.

Every few years, we take a peek at changes in what the nation eats. Since 1910, the U.S. Department of Agriculture has kept track of how much meat, potatoes, milk, sugar, and other foods leave the nation's warehouses each year. The numbers overestimate what we actually swallow, but they're valid for year-to-year comparisons.

Our grades rate both what we eat and—more importantly—how we've changed what we eat over the last few decades. So, for example, even though we're still drinking too much whole milk, milk got a B+ because we're gradually shifting to low-fat.

This year isn't a disaster, but it's nothing to write home about either. First, there are the bad trends, like more soft drinks, more sweeteners, and more cheese. Then you've got good trends that are moving ever so slowly, like less beef, less shortening, and more fruits and vegetables. And don't forget the ambiguous trends, like more flour (much of which goes

into pastries), more potatoes (that end up as french fries), and more chicken (can you say KFC?).

Get with it, America. Let's see some improvement by your next report card . . . or no dessert for a year.

SWEETENERS: F

The sky's the limit. Sweeteners (that includes table sugar, corn syrup, and dextrose) keep smashing their previous records. Soft drinks are driving sugar consumption higher, but swelling servings of cookies, ice cream, and other sweets—especially in restaurants—deserve some of the blame.

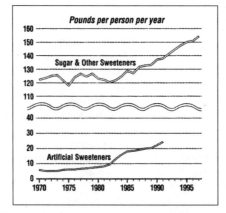

MEAT, POULTRY, & FISH: C+

The average American consumed 195 pounds of meat, poultry, and fish in 1998. That's 18 pounds more than in 1970. It's also more than ever before.

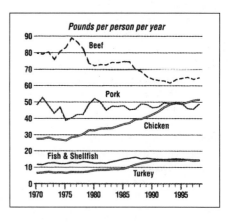

Chicken accounts for most of the rise: it has nearly doubled since 1970, while beef has fallen by about 20 percent. That's good news, given the link between red meat and heart disease and colon and prostate cancer.

But things could be better. We still eat 115 pounds of red meat (beef, pork, veal, and lamb) each year, compared to 80 pounds of poultry and fish. What's more, much of that

The information for this article was compiled by Ingrid Von Tuinen.

chicken is fried in unhealthy partially hydrogenated shortening. And more animal foods leave less room for fruits, vegetables, beans, and other plant foods that may cut the risk of cancer and heart disease.

BEVERAGES: F

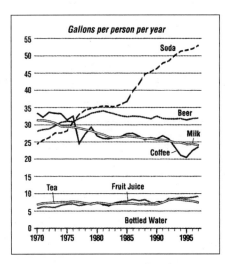

Gallons per person per year

Soon we'll need a magnifying glass to see any line but soda. Add the eight gallons a year of "fruit drinks" like Sunny Delight and Fruitopia (which are little more than sugar-water) to the 53 gallons of carbonated soft drinks and the total dwarfs milk, (real) fruit juice, and bottled water combined. When will it end? When Americans are drinking all soft drinks all the time?

EGGS: B

Egg consumption is down about 20 percent since 1970—and 40 percent since its 1945 high. It's too early to tell whether the modest increase since

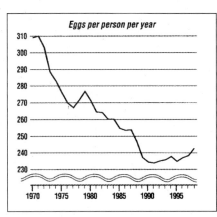

Eggs per person per year

1995 will continue. If so, you can probably blame the egg industry's misleading "eggs-don't-raise-cholesterol" ad campaign. No matter how you cook them, 243 egg yolks a year are still too many.

FLOUR, GRAINS, & BEANS: B-

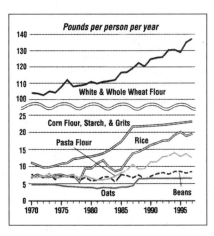

Pounds per person per year

We're still eating only two-thirds as much as our grandparents ate in 1910. But at 200 pounds per person per year, total flour and grains are almost 50 percent higher than in 1970. That means more bread, pasta, cereal, rice, oats, pizza crusts—you name it. The difference is that they probably ate more whole-wheat bread, oatmeal, and Wheatena, while we're eating more doughnuts, brownies, and Cinnabons.

FRUITS & VEGETABLES: A-

Gimme five! Fresh fruits and vegetables are up. Better yet, fruits other than wine grapes and vegetables other than potatoes are up. Now, if we could just pick up the pace, we might hit not only five, but eight-to-ten servings of fruits and vegetables a day. And it wouldn't hurt to make a few substitutions, especially for all those frozen potatoes, which are likely to end up french fried in partially hydro-

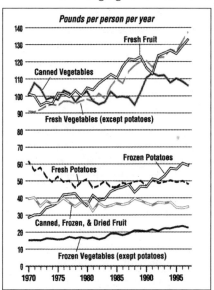

Pounds per person per year

genated, *trans*-fat-laden shortening. Sweet potatoes anyone?

ADDED FATS & OILS: C+

At 66 pounds per person per year, we're still eating 25 percent more

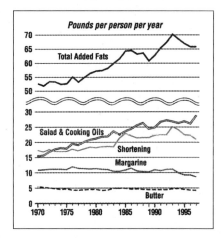

Pounds per person per year

added fats and oils than we did in 1970. But the trends are promising: The total has drifted down from its 1993 peak. What's more, individual fats are moving—however slowly—in the right direction. Margarine, shortening, and butter are all down from their peaks, while salad and cooking oils are up.

MILK: B+

The good news: Whole and reduced-fat (2%) milk continue to fall, while

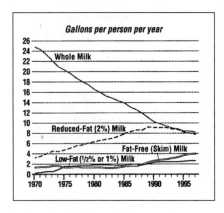

Gallons per person per year

low-fat (1%) and fat-free (skim) continue to creep up. The bad news: The fattier milks still outweigh the lower-fats by well over two-to-one. What's more, total milk consumption contin-

ues its three-decade slide. Make no bones about it, soft drinks are taking over. If the soda industry has its way, kids will be pouring Coke over their Count Chocula.

DAIRY PRODUCTS: D+

We're eating two and a half times more cheese than we did in 1970—28 pounds per person per year. That's a lot of pizza, nachos, and cheeseburgers . . . and a lot of coronary by-passes, angioplasties, and heart attacks. Cheese is now neck-and-neck with ground beef as the largest source of saturated fat in the average person's diet.

In the frozen dairy department, the changes are minor. Regular ice cream still leads the pack at 16 pounds per year, with low-fat ice cream at 8 pounds.

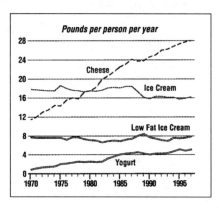

Pounds per person per year

HEALTHY LIFESTYLES FOR HEALTHY AMERICANS: REPORT ON USDA'S YEAR 2000 BEHAVIORAL NUTRITION ROUNDTABLE

In January 2000, the Research, Education, and Economics (REE) mission area of the U.S. Department of Agriculture (USDA) sponsored a round table in New Orleans to address behavioral nutrition. The impetus for the round table was a question recently asked by Agriculture Secretary Glickman. "Why, when we have a greater base of understanding about diet and nutrition than ever before, is obesity on the rise? There isn't an adult American with a pulse that doesn't know, for example, about the dangers of high cholesterol. And yet, we can't seem to convert increased nutrition information into changes in behavior." Participants, representing such diverse fields as economics, nutrition, public health, medicine, psychology, neuroendocrinology, and marketing research, discussed the determinants of food choices and activity levels and identified research needs, gaps, and priorities related to improving consumer eating behavior and activity levels. Highlights of the discussions, chaired by Dr. Eileen Kennedy, are summarized in this article.

Eileen Kennedy, DSc, RD, and Susan E. Offutt, PhD

Dr. Eileen Kennedy is the Deputy Under Secretary for Research, Education, and Economics in the USDA. She provides leadership in shaping and managing the USDA's broad research, education, and extension programs in production agriculture, food safety, nutrition, conservation, and the environment. She was previously the first Executive Director of the USDA's Center for Nutrition Policy and Promotion. She has represented the U.S. on international policy committees and is currently a member of the Advisory Group on Nutrition for the United Nations (U.N.). She serves on a number of boards and committees of the U.N., the National Academy of Sciences, and other profession-related organizations. Her research has been reported extensively in national and international scientific journals.

> ***Many participants also agreed that* Healthy Lifestyles for Healthy Americans *is a universal slogan that encapsulates the preponderance of scientific evidence on the self-determinants of some health outcomes.***

Susan E. Offutt is Administrator of the USDA's Economic Research Service, an agency that provides economic and other social science information and analysis for public and private decisions on agriculture, food, natural resources, and rural America. Prior to that, Susan was the Executive Director of the National Research Council's Board on Agriculture, which conducts studies on a range of topics in agricultural science. Susan has also served as chief of the agriculture branch at the Office of Management and Budget. She was professor from 1982–1987 at the University of Illinois. Her B.S. degree is from Allegheny College (1976) and her M.S. (1980) and Ph.D. (1982) are from Cornell University.

Participants at the round table agreed that America faces a health crisis unlike any in its history. The crisis does not center on a particular disease but is the product of our behavior. We simply eat too much and exercise too little. This results in an increasingly overweight population that is suffering needlessly from excessive rates of heart disease, some cancers, and diabetes. Many participants also agreed that *Healthy Lifestyles for Healthy Americans* is a universal slogan that encapsulates the preponderance of scientific evidence on the self-determinants of some health outcomes. There was broad agreement that even though genetic factors play an important role in the development of obesity, factors such as the physical environment and human behavior drive the pronounced growth in

From *Nutrition Today*, May/June 2000, pp. 84-88. © 2000 by Williams & Wilkins. Reprinted by permission.

There was also unanimous agreement among participants that healthy people are more productive at work and play, more satisfied with their personal lives, and more capable of achieving their goals and aspirations then those who are not healthy.

prevalence of obesity. Changes in the physical environment include communities with sidewalks, amenities, and architectural designs that encourage physical mobility and safety. The human behavior dimension includes a vast array of everyday choices that have potential health implications—what and how much to eat; whether to engage in risky behaviors, such as smoking or excessive alcohol consumption; how much or how little to exercise; and whether to seek preventive medical care—these can be changed and controlled by individuals. Furthermore, the choices made can have a profound influence on health, in both morbidity and longevity. There was also unanimous agreement among participants that healthy people are more productive at work and play, more satisfied with their personal lives, and more capable of achieving their goals and aspirations than those who are not healthy. *Healthy Lifestyles for Healthy Americans* as a goal translates into a nation that is prosperous and is capable of focusing its energies on educational attainment, enhanced medical care, and other worthy goals. These are precisely the reasons for the keen interest by the United States Department of Agriculture (USDA) and other Federal agencies in promoting better nutrition and activity levels and other healthy choices in behaviors.

The round table focused on what we know about nutrition- and exercise-related behaviors and interventions. The goals of the discussions were to identify and summarize what we know and do not know about food choice and physical activity behaviors and how to make the best use of research to improve the effectiveness of interventions.

WHAT WE KNOW

The round table focused on what we know about nutrition- and exercise-related behaviors and interventions. The goals of the discussions were to identify and summarize what we know and do not know about food choice and physical activity behaviors and how to make the best use of research to improve the effectiveness of interventions. The focus was on three fundamental questions: What are the determinants of eating and activity behaviors? How can behavior be modified? How can effective interventions be designed to change behavior? To accomplish these goals, the round table was organized around four sessions: Economic Factors Influencing Food Choices and Activity Levels, Psychosocial Factors Influencing Food Choices and Activity Levels, Social Marketing Interventions, and Interventions on the Community, Group, and Individual Levels.

These environmental-type changes, and certainly not changes in genetics, lie behind increases in obesity and overweight observed over the past two decades.

Participants agreed that many factors influencing eating and physical activity have changed during the past 20 years, especially the types and prices of available foods, technological advances, time pressures, attitudes and knowledge about health and diets, demographics of the population, availability of convenience and fast foods, and family and social structures. These environmental-type changes, and certainly not changes in genetics, lie behind increases in obesity and overweight observed during the past two decades. Furthermore, these increases in obesity are a worldwide phenomena. Consumers are increasingly confused about what is a nutritious diet and what levels of physical activity are necessary to sustain a healthy body. Furthermore, the increasing awareness among consumers of the health dangers associated with obesity and the lack of practical tools to address the problem result in unintended consequences and stress and anxiety over food and weight, even among young children. On the other hand, Americans tend to favor the short-run benefits of consumption and to discount the long-run health benefits. This preference for immediate satisfaction is graphically illustrated by the low savings rates and high credit card balances in this country.

Participants identified an urgent need for effective interventions that center on a clear understanding of factors that motivate people to make desired changes, on positive reinforcement and long-term support, and on environmental changes. Multidisciplinary research teams are key to defining and refining the underlying research necessary to make progress in the fight against poor diets and inactivity.

From the economist's perspective, people may eat unhealthy diets because future health is a lower priority than current taste and convenience.

ECONOMIC FACTORS INFLUENCING FOOD CHOICES AND ACTIVITY LEVELS

Economic models are grounded in the notion that food choices, eating patterns, and activity levels are decisions made by consumers on a daily basis. These are influenced by the prices, time, income, and the human capital environment as well as by intertemporal decisions regarding tradeoffs between current satisfaction and future health production. Behavior viewed as irrational on the surface may in fact be quite rational when all the costs and benefits are considered. From the economist's perspective, people may eat unhealthy diets because future health is a lower priority than current taste and convenience. In addition, eating is an integral part of our family and social lives and can also be an inexpensive source of immediate pleasure.

The economic perspective also argues for a broader outcome variable, such as health, or healthy lifestyles, rather than merely nutrition or weight status as the focus.

The economic perspective also argues for a broader outcome variable, such as health or healthy lifestyles, rather than merely nutrition or weight status as the focus. Participants raised issues about the influence of food prices on consumption behavior and the role of food taxes and subsidies on consumption tradeoffs, income distribution, and price responses among different population subgroups. The impacts of the information environment, in particular food labeling and advertising, on food availability and food choices was thought to be little understood. The same was said for the effects of age and cohort effects on consumption. The impact on food choices, diet quality, and inactivity levels due to higher incomes and education levels, changes in labor-force participation, increased nutrition knowledge, and greater availability of convenience and fast foods all deserve additional research. Food access, participation in government pro-

grams, and budget constraints are areas affecting the nation's poor, which present many challenging research opportunities. Collaborations between economists and other scientists may provide insights often overlooked by a single discipline working in isolation.

PHYSIOLOGICAL AND PSYCHOSOCIAL FACTORS INFLUENCING FOOD CHOICES AND ACTIVITY LEVELS

Food choices, eating patterns, and activity levels are also influenced by a host of physiological, psychological, and cultural factors. The sensitivity of our taste buds, our emotional state, the day of the week, foods eaten in childhood, cultural differences in what is perceived as a "healthy" weight, and advice received from family, friends, and health professionals all influence behaviors.

Genetics may play a role in what we choose to eat, and this, in turn, may affect gene expression. There is still much we do not know about how physiological factors influence food choices. The possibility that individuals may exhibit innate preferences for certain foods, for energy-dense diets, and for variety in consumption would make it more difficult to sustain certain dietary changes during the long run. These may require different approaches as well as long-term reinforcement and support. Changes in dietary patterns among pregnant women, differences in postpartum weight retention, and the formation of food preferences may also be influenced by physiological factors. Research is needed on whether the disease burden associated with childhood obesity is greater than that of adult obesity and on the impact of neonatal interactions on risk for chronic disease.

Although people eat partly as a biological necessity, they mostly eat for pleasure. This, of course, complicates analysis tremendously.

Although people eat partly as a biological necessity, they mostly eat for pleasure. This, of course, complicates analysis tremendously. There was a clear mandate for additional research on psychosocial correlates, such as parent-child feeding interactions, the impact of maternal and individual emotional well-being, food as a source of pleasure, habitual behavior, food in the social environment, and self-gratification. In addition, technological advances, such as the microwave, and shifts in food practices associated with increased female labor-force participation and the proliferation of fast-food restaurants have shifted the control of food away from parents and may also have affected activity levels. There is a need to understand the impact of such shifts on food choices and diet quality. Understanding cultural differences in the perception of food and the different roles that food plays within a culture is increasingly important as the nation becomes more diverse. Research is also needed to evaluate whether it is possible to build on positive behavioral changes, such as those that occur during pregnancy, and make them more permanent. These issues are many and varied. Until we invest in understanding the many psychosocial factors that influence eating and inactivity, progress toward achievement of healthier life styles will be slow.

> *The private sector has enormous experience in selling both food and weight-loss products, and the principles of success in these arenas must be understood.*

Large variations in day-to-day individual food intakes and physical activity levels result in imprecise measurements that affect analysis and conclusions. There was a clear expression that technical advances may facilitate the collection of better data in the near future. In addition, there is a need for longitudinal data and studies that would make it possible for researchers to study causality as well as usual patterns of change. Cross-sectional studies present daunting research challenges in separating causality from correlation.

SOCIAL MARKETING INTERVENTIONS

The private sector has enormous experience in selling both food and weight loss products, and the principles of success in these arenas must be understood. The discussion focused on the lessons we call learn from the private sector that can be applied to the public provision of nutrition information.

> *A "one-size-fits-all" message may not be effective.*

Two clear messages emerged: (1) we cannot underestimate the importance of understanding the target audience, and (2) it is impossible to sell consumers a product they do not want. Because food choices are strongly affected by emotions, it is particularly important to identify the target audience's "archetype" or "the logic of their emotions." What are the target audience's perceived needs and aspirations, and what motivates them to buy a product or to change behavior? For example, many women are motivated to lose weight to feel less tired,

while men expect a measurable health benefit, such as a reduction in their blood cholesterol level. In addition, it is important to understand the target audience's habits and practices. Attempts to modify diet and inactivity patterns need to start with the consumer's baseline knowledge and emotions, in order to address the perceived needs and identify the benefits that are valued by the target audience. The tone of the message is also important. Consumers desire relevant guidance but refuse to be told what to do or buy. To that end, researchers need to consider why some social marketing interventions succeed where others have failed.

A "one-size-fits-all" message may not be effective. Federal guidance is based on national averages, and the target population may differ considerably from "average." Successful messages will most likely need to be adapted in order to address better the target population's needs and practices. Private and public partnerships, in both the research and marketing arenas, merge different expertise and likely improve the success of interventions.

> *There is little disagreement that prevention and intervention priorities are affected by political will, knowledge, and social strategies.*

INTERVENTIONS IN THE COMMUNITY, GROUP, AND INDIVIDUAL LEVELS

There is little disagreement that prevention and intervention priorities are affected by political will, knowledge, and social strategies. The discussion focused on two components of social strategies, preventive services, and structural interventions. Weight-loss programs may be viewed as preventive services in that they prevent additional weight gain. There was agreement on the need to educate better the medical community, schools, employers, and community agencies so that they can play an important role in addressing the obesity problem. Although physician advice seems to be associated with increased efforts to lose weight, it is not clear how many doctors believe they can be effective or how they share knowledge with their patients. Similarly, schools and after-school programs can be effective providers of information and useful peer pressure, such as in TV-turnoff campaigns.

Structural interventions are those incorporating groups not traditionally associated with the health community. This group includes urban planners, transportation departments, parks and recreation units, developers, and employers. The objective is to remove structural barriers that prevent or hinder physical activities, such as a lack of sidewalks, congested roadways, and unsafe neighborhoods and streets.

There was consensus that emphasis should be placed on small behavioral changes with a strong focus on motivating factors. Current research indicates that if people have realistic expectations about weight loss or healthy diets they tend to be more successful. Understanding how these expectations are formed is critical. For example, it is widely known that consumers are more likely to be successful in achieving weight loss than in maintaining weight loss. Unrealistic expectations about the amount of weight loss that may be achieved or the need for sustained behavioral changes to maintain the weight loss may be involved in the low success rate of weight reduction efforts. However, more research is also needed to understand whether physiological factors are involved and the role of physical activity in maintaining weight loss.

There was also consensus that localized and personal interventions appear to be more effective in modifying behaviors than national efforts. Research is needed to understand how to adapt successful small-scale behavioral interventions to a larger scale.

Research efforts to understand why some segments of the population follow a diet consistent with dietary guidelines is needed. It is critical to understand why these people succeed. What can be learned from their behavior that might apply to others? What strategies do these individuals use, and can those strategies be easily adapted by others?

WHERE DO WE GO FROM HERE?

This round table helped define the agenda for the May 2000 National Nutrition Summit at which the Secretaries of Agriculture and Health and Human Services launched the Behavioral Nutrition Initiative. For example, the round table made it clear that a successful research program must be multidisciplinary in scope, reach across both public and private institutions, target a mix of short-term and longitudinal research, and incorporate innovative pilot studies. Research projects under the initiative address many of the topics and problems discussed in this article and help us to think beyond convention, bring new researchers to the table, and make research more timely and relevant.

One of the objectives of the initiative is to encourage multidisciplinary research that will make *Healthy Lifestyles for Healthy Americans* a reality. To accomplish these objectives, the USDA will use a variety of mechanisms, including a large extramural research grant program and the redirection of intramural research priorities.

These are exciting times. The success of this new initiative depends on the sharing of ideas, embracing the contributions of all professions, developing a synergism among researchers, and focusing our energies on a common goal: a healthy well-nourished America.

Nutrient Requirements Get a Makeover:

The Evolution of the Recommended Dietary Allowances

Ever wonder how much of the essential vitamins and minerals, like folate, vitamin A or calcium, you really need to eat every day to be healthy? For more than 50 years, the Food and Nutrition Board of the National Academy of Sciences has been reviewing nutrition research and defining nutrient requirements for healthy people. Until recently, one set of nutrient intake levels reigned supreme: the Recommended Dietary Allowances or RDA.

History of the RDAs

When the RDAs were created in 1941, their primary goal was to pre-

vent diseases caused by nutrient deficiencies. They were originally intended to evaluate and plan for the nutritional adequacy of *groups,* for example, the armed forces and children in school lunch programs, rather than to determine *individuals'* nutrient needs.

But, because the RDAs were essentially the only nutrient values available, they began to be used in ways other than the intended use. Health professionals often used RDAs to size-up the diets of their individual patients or clients. Statistically speaking, RDAs would prevent deficiency diseases in 97 percent of a population,

but there was no scientific basis that RDAs would meet the needs of a single person.

It was evident that the RDAs were not addressing individual needs, and new science needed to be included. Therefore, the Food and Nutrition Board sought to redefine nutrient requirements and develop specific nutrient recommendations for individuals, as well as for groups. Along with these changes, concepts such as tolerable upper intakes and adequate intakes emerged to better meet individuals' needs.

Further, the new RDAs were set with prevention of chronic disease in mind. Sandra Schlicker, Ph.D., Senior Staff Officer with the Food and Nutrition Board, explained that the new RDAs will still prevent nutrient deficiencies, but they are now set with an additional purpose. "For the first time, the RDAs are no longer focused only on preventing deficiency diseases such as scurvy or beriberi. Now they are also aimed at reducing the risk of diet-related chronic conditions such as heart disease, diabetes, hypertension and osteoporosis."

How RDAs became DRIs

In 1993, the Food and Nutrition Board put the RDA revision process into motion by holding a symposium and asking for scientific and public comment on how the RDAs should be revised. Utilizing feedback from

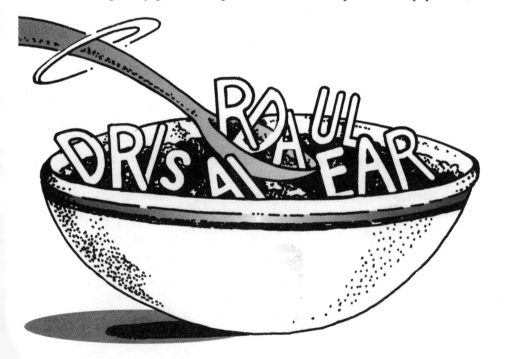

From *Food Insight,* September/October 1998, pp. 1, 4-5. Reprinted with permission from the International Food Information Council Foundation.

RDA/DRI Time Line

1941: First edition of the Recommended Dietary Allowances (RDAs) published.

1941-1989: RDAs periodically updated and revised based on cumulative scientific data. 10th edition published in 1989.

1993: The Food and Nutrition Board (FNB) held symposium, "Should the Recommended Dietary Allowances Be Revised?" Based on comments and suggestions from this meeting, FNB proposed changes to the development process of RDAs.

1995: The Dietary Reference Intake (DRI) Committee announced that seven expert nutrient group panels would review major nutrients, vitamins, minerals, antioxidants, electrolytes, and other food components.

this conference and other sources, the Food and Nutrition Board developed an ambitious framework for revamping the old RDAs: rather than having a single group of scientists revise the existing set of RDAs, they had expert panels review nutrient categories in much more detail than had ever been done before.

Not only did the definition of RDAs change, but three new values were also created: the Estimated Average Requirement (EAR), the Adequate Intake (AI), and the Tolerable Upper Intake Level (UL). All four values are collectively known as Dietary Reference Intakes or DRIs.

The Food and Nutrition Board partnered with Health Canada, the Canadian government agency responsible for nutrition policy, and the two groups jointly appointed a Dietary Reference Intakes (DRI) Committee. Seven expert panels and two subcom-

mittees assisted the DRI Committee. All members of the DRI Committee, the expert panels and the subcommittees are leaders in their fields of nutrition and food science.

The first report of the DRI Committee was released in 1997 and focused on calcium, vitamin D, phosphorus, magnesium and fluoride. The second report on thiamin, riboflavin, niacin, vitamin B6, folate, vitamin B12, pantothenic acid, biotin and choline was released in Spring 1998. Future reports will be published in the next few years. (See timeline for estimated report release dates.)

Extending the RDA Family: Meet the New Members

As a result of the DRI Committee's work to meet individuals' nutrient needs and incorporate current nutrition science, there are now four nutri-

ent requirement values—the RDA, Estimated Average Requirement (EAR), Adequate Intake (AI), and Tolerable Upper Intake Level (UL). The new RDAs are based on Estimated Average Requirements. The Estimated Average Requirement is the amount of a nutrient that will meet the needs of at least 50 percent of healthy people and is typically based on strong research evidence.

However, sometimes an Estimated Average Requirement cannot be accurately determined for a nutrient (e.g., vitamin D, fluoride, pantothenic acid) because the available scientific research is not conclusive. If this is the case, an Adequate Intake is estimated. Although Adequate Intakes are less precise than RDAs, they are still intended to meet or exceed the nutritive needs of nearly all healthy people.

There is more that is new to the nutrient value family. Tolerable Upper Intake Levels for some vitamins and minerals have been established for the first time. The Tolerable Upper Intake Level is the highest amount of a nutrient that can be safely consumed on a daily basis. Past editions of the RDAs have addressed toxicity levels of certain vitamins and minerals but have never clearly defined safe upper intake levels. At this time, Tolerable Upper Intake Levels cannot be established for all nutrients because of incomplete scientific information.

Appropriate Uses of the DRIs

DRIs—the compilation of RDAs, Estimated Average Requirements, Adequate Intakes, and the Tolerable Upper Intake Levels—can be used to evaluate or plan diets for individuals as well as groups. Practitioners who

DEFINITIONS

Dietary Reference Intakes (DRIs): The new standards for nutrient recommendations that can be used to plan and assess diets for healthy people. Think of Dietary Reference Intakes as the umbrella term that includes the following values:

- *Estimated Average Requirement (EAR):* A nutrient intake value that is estimated to meet the requirement of half the healthy individuals in a group. It is used to assess nutritional adequacy of intakes of population groups. In addition, EARs are used to calculate RDAs.

- *Recommended Dietary Allowance (RDA):* This value is a goal for individuals, and is based upon the EAR. It is the daily dietary intake level that is sufficient to meet the nutrient requirement of 97–98% of all healthy individuals in a group. If an EAR cannot be set, no RDA value can be proposed.

- *Adequate Intake (AI):* This is used when a RDA cannot be determined. A recommended daily intake level based on an observed or experimentally determined approximation of nutrient intake for a group (or groups) of healthy people.

- *Tolerable Upper Intake Level (UL):* The highest level of daily nutrient intake that is likely to pose no risks of adverse heath effects to almost all individuals in the general population. As intake increases above the UL, the risk of adverse effects increases.

1997: First DRI report issued on calcium, phosphorus, magnesium, vitamin D, and fluoride.

1998: Second DRI report issued on thiamin, riboflavin, niacin, vitamin B6, folate, vitamin B12, pantothenic acid, biotin, and choline.

1999: Estimated release date of report on vitamins C and E, beta carotene, and other selected antioxidants.

2000-2003: Estimated release dates for reports on trace elements (e.g., selenium, zinc), vitamins A and K; electrolytes and fluids; energy and macronutrients; and other food components (e.g., phytoestrogens, fiber, and phytochemicals found in foods such as garlic or tea).

work with individual clients should use the new RDAs and Adequate Intakes as goals for optimal intake. People who eat less than the RDA/Adequate Intakes or exceed the Tolerable Upper Intake Level for a particular nutrient may be at nutritional risk. However, clinical, biochemical and or anthropometric data are required to accurately assess an individual's nutritional status. For groups, the Estimated Average Requirement can be used to set goals for nutrient intake and to measure the prevalence of poor nutrient intake.

To help practitioners and others learn how to use the new DRIs in their work settings, the Food and Nutrition Board appointed a Uses and Interpretations Subcommittee to develop a "user's manual." Committee chair Suzanne Murphy, Ph.D., R.D., Adjunct Associate Professor of Nutrition at the University of California at Davis, believes that the guide will help health professionals, nutrition policy planners, and others use the DRIs to their full advantage. "The process of developing the DRIs has been very thorough and represents a huge step forward for assessing the nutrient requirements of Americans. Now we want to make sure that health professionals and others know how to correctly use these new numbers." Dr. Murphy's goal is that the manual, which will be published within a few years, "be practical and easy to read. We hope that nutrition professionals and policy makers will be able to use it as a first reference before using the DRIs."

DIETARY REFERENCE INTAKES:
Selected Recommended Levels for Individual Intakes

Nutrient	Old RDA or ESADDI[1] (ages 25–50 yrs) Male	Female	New RDA or AI[2] (31 to 50 yrs) Male	Female
Calcium (mg)	800	800	1,000*	1,000*
Phosphorus (mg)	800	800	700	700
Magnesium (mg)	350	280	420	320
Vitamin D (µg)[3]	5	5	5*	5*
Fluoride (µg)	1.5-4.0§	1.5-4.0§	4*	3*
Thiamin (mg)	1.5	1.1	1.2	1.1
Riboflavin (mg)	1.7	1.3	1.3	1.1
Niacin (mg)	19	15	16	14
Vitamin B6 (mg)	2.0	1.6	1.3	1.3
Folate (µg)	200	180	400	400
Vitamin B12 (µg)	2.0	2.0	2.4	2.4
Pantothenic Acid (mg)	4-7§	4-7§	5*	5*
Biotin (µg)	30-100§	30-100§	30*	30*
Choline (µg)	not determined	not determined	550*	425*

(mg=milligrams µg=micrograms)

[1] RDAs and Estimated Safe and Adequate Daily Dietary Intake (ESADDI) published by the Food and Nutrition Board in 1989.
[2] RDA and Adequate Intake (AI) values from the 1997 and 1998 DRI reports.
[3] Vitamin D as cholecalciferol = 400 IU of vitamin D.
§ ESADDI value.
*AI value.

For More Information

Updates on the DRI process are available on the National Academy of Sciences web site (www2.nas.edu/fnb). The site features information about the committee, expert panels and subcommittees. The DRI reports on calcium and the B vitamins can also be accessed. To order copies of the reports, call the National Academy Press at 800-624-6242.

PICTURE THIS!

Communicating Nutrition Around the World

What picture comes to mind when you think of a healthful diet? The U.S. Departments of Agriculture (USDA) and Health and Human Services hope you think of their Food Guide Pyramid. Since 1992, the Pyramid has served as a visual adaptation of the *U.S. Dietary Guidelines for Americans,* the seven basic dietary recommendations to promote wellness and prevent chronic disease. Today, the Pyramid can be seen not only in nutrition education materials for children and adults, but also on grocery bags, food packages and in the media.

Food guides, such as the USDA's Food Guide Pyramid, are tools used to communicate complex scientific information in a consumer-friendly way. For the most part, government agencies use graphic depictions to communicate dietary guidance messages that provide population-wide recommendations for eating to promote health.

A previous issue of *Food Insight* (March/April 1998) featured various countries' dietary guidelines and noted how cultural norms influence the guidelines. This issue will highlight the evolution of the American food guide as well as visual depictions of dietary guidance used around the world.

A Photographic History

Food guides are not new educational tools. The first United States food guide was developed in 1916 by the USDA and consisted of five food groups—milk and meat; cereals; vegetables and fruits; fats and fat foods; and sugars and sugar foods. By the 1940s, the food guide listed *ten* food groups, including water and eggs. Vegetables and fruits were split into three individual groups—leafy green and yellow vegetables; citrus, tomato and cabbage; and other vegetables and fruits. Ten food groups were difficult for consumers to remember, so these groups were trimmed to *four* food groups by the late 1950s.

Previous versions of the United States food guide were tools used to promote a diet containing essential vitamins and minerals. School children were often the educational target for the simple illustrations used to depict the optimal diet. One of the most familiar food guides of the past is the "Basic Four," containing four food groups—milk, fruit and vegetable, bread and cereal and meat groups—which was used for nearly 25 years. The emphasis of the "Basic Four" food guide was to help Americans get a foundation diet, meaning, it was intended to meet only a portion of caloric and nutrient needs.

After the publication of the first *Dietary Guidelines for Americans* in 1980, work began on a new food guide graphic to reflect the latest science on diet and health. In addition to a review of existing research, government agencies conducted extensive quantitative and qualitative research with American consumers to ensure the resulting graphic communicated key dietary guideline concepts. The pyramid design proved most useful in graphically communicating the intended messages across various socioeconomic groups.

No single adaptation of the pyramid graphic can depict all of the eating practices of the diverse American populace. However, because of the simplicity and

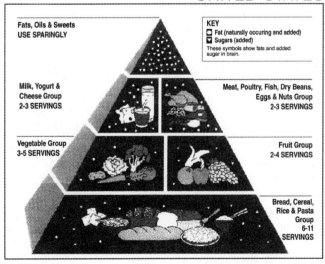

UNITED STATES

From *Food Insight,* January/February 1999, pp. 1, 4-5. © 1999 by the International Food Information Council Foundation, and *Food Insight*. Reprinted by permission.

Food guides, such as the USDA's Food Guide Pyramid, are tools used to communicate complex scientific information in a consumer-friendly way.

understandability of the pyramid shape, the U.S. Food Guide Pyramid can be translated to reflect the customs of numerous ethnic and cultural groups within the United States. The pyramid concept has been adapted to Asian, Mexican, vegetarian and Mediterranean diets by various organizations. For instance, to better serve their state population, the Washington State Department of Health created materials using the pyramid shape to depict diets for Russians, Southeast Asians and Native Americans. The pyramid concept has also been adapted to communicate other health-promoting activities. For example, a physical activity pyramid, developed by a private organization, promotes ways to stay active in everyday life and a "life balance" pyramid by the same group offers ideas to build and maintain emotional well-being.

Pictures From Around the World

The use of the pyramid has been very successful in the United States. The pyramid shape appears to easily convey the concept of variety and the relative amounts to eat of the various food groups. However, because of cultural differences in communicating symbolism and other cultural norms, the pyramid is not necessarily the graphic of choice

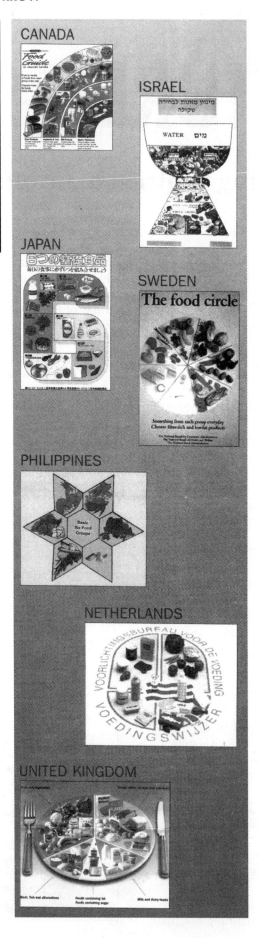

for food guides worldwide. No single graphic can portray the dietary guidelines of various countries around the world. Rainbows, circles, pyramids, and even a chalice are used to represent the "optimal" diet. The different graphics used reflect cultural norms and symbols as well as the emphasis of the dietary guidelines of each country. In developed countries, food guides tend to promote a diet that prevents chronic disease. In developing countries, however, the goal of the food guide is to promote a diet that provides nutrients to safeguard against malnutrition.

Yet, despite the different pictorial representations, different countries communicate similar themes. Food guide graphics from countries as diverse as Italy and South Africa convey a common message—balance, variety and moderation in food choices. While the number of food groups displayed in the graphics varies from country to country, most guides attempt to illustrate the food groups' optimal proportion of the total diet, as does the U.S. Food Guide Pyramid. For instance, based on the *Dietary Guidelines for Americans,* grains should comprise the largest proportion of the diet. Therefore, grains are depicted at the base of the Pyramid—the largest part of the pyramid shape. Breads and grains, fruits, vegetables, dairy foods and meats are included in all the various guides.

The wheel or dinner plate design is a popular graphic that represents the total diet, with each section depicting a food group and its relative proportion to the total diet. This design is used in the United Kingdom, Germany and Norway, among other countries. Many of food guide graphics used are unique to their respective countries. Japan depicts its "optimal" diet through the use of the numeral six as the basis of its food guide to remind consumers of the six food categories. The

The primary role of food guides, whether in the United States or around the world, is to communicate an optimal diet for overall health of the population.

Japanese government has since developed new dietary guidelines. However the same food guide is still used by many as a reference since a new food guide has not been developed.

Canada's Food Guide to Healthy Eating is a four-banded rainbow, with each color representing one of its four food groups. The rainbow shows that all food groups are important but different amounts are needed from each group. The larger outer arcs of the rainbow are the grain products and fruits and vegetables. According to Canada's dietary guidelines, these foods should make up a larger part of a healthy eating plan. Similarly, the smaller inner arcs make up the milk products and meat and meat alternatives that should make up a smaller amount of a healthy eating plan.

Many of the food guides around the world emphasize the bread, cereals and grain foods as the largest part of the diet. Israel's chalice graphic illustrates the importance of water for overall health by placing "water" at the top and largest section of the chalice. Israel has one of few food guides that characterize water as a principal part of the diet.

South Africa's food guide graphic contains the least number of food groups and organizes foods in a unique way—according to the foods' "function" in the body. Group 1 contains "Energy Food," and includes margarine, grains, porridge and maize. The second group is entitled "Body Building Food" and includes chicken, beans, milk and eggs. The third group is "Protective Food," to protect your body from illness and includes cabbage, carrots, pineapples and spinach.

A Picture Paints a Thousand Words

You've undoubtedly heard the phrase "a picture paints a thousand words" numerous times. Nutrition education has long proven this idiom to ring true through the use of food models and pictures to depict such things as portion sizes. Likewise, symbols such as a heart, checkmark or apple are often used on restaurant menus to denote choices that meet specific nutrition or health guidelines.

The primary role of food guides, whether in the United States or around the world, is to communicate an optimal diet for overall health of the population. Whether a star, a chalice, a square or a pyramid graphic is used, all are meant to improve quality of life and nutritional well-being in a simplified and understandable way.

FOOD PORTIONS AND SERVINGS
How Do They Differ?

Consumers appear to be confused about serving sizes—what they mean and how to use them. Complicating the problem are large portions of food that are becoming the norm in many eating establishments, which differ from the servings in the Food Guide Pyramid (FGP) and on the Nutrition Facts Label on food packaging. For example, a large deli bagel might weigh 6 ounces (about 6 FGP servings of bread) while the ½ medium bagel listed on the Food Guide Pyramid weighs 1 ounce (about 1 serving of bread). With so much variation in portions of foods, it's easy for consumers to become confused about what serving sizes mean and how to use them.

What's a Food Guide Pyramid Serving?

The Food Guide Pyramid serving is a unit of measure used to describe the total amount of foods recommended daily from each of the food groups. Criteria for selecting the serving sizes are identified in the box. Larger portions count as more than one serving; smaller portions count as partial servings. The Pyramid shows a range of servings for each of the five major food groups. The number of servings an individual requires depends on how many calories he or she needs. For example, the Pyramid suggests 6 to 11 servings of grain products each day. An individual consuming 1600 calories would eat 6 servings of grains while an individual consuming 2800 calories would need 11 servings of grains. Additional information on what counts as one food guide serving unit and the suggested number of servings for various calorie levels is reported in *The Food Guide Pyramid (1)*.

What's a Food Label Serving?

A food label serving is a specific amount of food that contains the quantity of nutrients listed on the Nutrition Facts Label. The 1990 Nutrition Labeling and Education Act (NLEA) specified reference serving amounts for almost 200 product categories to be used on labels. To make food label servings consumer-friendly, the

---

Serving Sizes in the Food Guide Pyramid are based on four criteria (2,3):

1. Amount of foods from a food group typically reported in surveys as consumed on one eating occasion;

2. Amount of foods that provide a comparable amount of key nutrients from that food group, for example, the amount of cheese that provides the same amount of calcium as 1 cup fluid milk;

3. Amount of foods recognized by most consumers (e.g., household measures) or that can be easily multiplied or divided to describe a quantity of food actually consumed (portion);

4. Amount traditionally used in previous food guides to describe servings.

---

serving sizes are expressed in household measures, such as cups, ounces, or pieces, as well as grams, and generally reflect the amount an individual might reasonably consume each eating occasion.

Food Label vs. Food Guide Pyramid Serving Sizes—How Do They Differ?

For many food items, the serving size in the Food Guide Pyramid and on the food label are the same (e.g., ½ cup canned fruit or vegetables). However, some serving sizes differ because the Pyramid and the food label serve different purposes. The Pyramid describes serving units for each food group (e.g., ½ chopped or cooked vegetables and 1 cup raw leafy vegetables) so that they will be easy to remember and help consumers select a healthful diet. The food label serving unit is specific for each product category and designed to help consumers compare nutrient informa-

Amounts of foods reported at each occasion,[1] 50th percentile, by age and gender

Food	FGP[2] serving sizes	20–39 years Men	20–39 years Women	40–59 years Men	40–59 years Women	60+ years Men	60+ years Women
		Number of FGP serving sizes					
Apples, raw	1 medium	1.0	1.0	1.0	1.0	0.9	0.9
Orange juice	¾ cup	1.3	1.3	1.3	1.1	1.1	1.0
String beans, cooked	½ cup	1.5	1.0	1.0	1.0	1.4	1.0
Broccoli, cooked	½ cup	1.3	1.0	1.6	1.3	0.8	1.1
Fluid milk	1 cup	1.0	0.9	1.0	0.7	0.8	0.7
Cheese[3]	1-½ oz	0.7	0.6	0.7	0.7	0.7	0.7
White bread	1 slice	2.0	1.8	1.9	1.7	1.8	1.5
Rice, cooked	½ cup	1.7	1.5	1.6	1.3	1.4	1.2
RTE cereals	1 oz	2.1	1.5	1.8	1.3	1.7	1.2
Pasta, cooked	½ cup	2.2	1.5	2.0	1.5	1.7	1.5
Muffins	1 oz (approx.)	2.3	1.9	2.1	1.8	2.0	2.0
		Number of 1-ounce meat equivalents[4]					
Beef steak, cooked	1 oz	5.7	4.9	5.3	4.3	4.9	3.8
Ham, cured cooked	1 oz	1.9	1.5	2.0	1.6	2.0	1.9
Eggs, fried	1 large	1.8	1.4	1.8	1.0	1.6	0.9
Dry beans, cooked	½ cup	1.9	1.0	1.5	1.0	1.3	1.0

[1]Data calculated from CSFII 1989–91, NFS Report No. 91-3.
[2]FGP (Food Guide Pyramid).
[3]Includes all cheeses, other than cream or cottage, regardless of fat content.
[4]Serving sizes of meats and meat alternates are listed in 1-ounce equivalents because serving amounts vary by type of food (steak, roast, ground meat, beans, eggs, or peanut butter). The Food Guide Pyramid suggests 2 to 3 servings of meat or meat alternates for a total of 5 to 7 ounces each day.

tion on a number of food products within a category. The food label serving units cover mixed dishes (e.g., frozen entrees) as well as simple items (e.g., canned fruits). Pyramid serving units are primarily for simple food items, such as fruits, vegetables, and plain grain products.

Additionally, the Pyramid serving size specifies the amount of food that provides a designated amount of key nutrients from that food group; for example, ¾ cup fruit juice and 1 cup milk. Some food label product categories such as "beverages" specify the same serving size (1 cup), regardless of the food group in which the beverage (fruit juice, milk, or soda) belongs.

In both cases—the Food Guide Pyramid and the food label—the "serving size" is a unit of measure and may not be the portion of food an individual actually eats at one occasion.

What's a Portion?

A "portion" can be thought of as the amount of a specific food an individual eats for dinner, snack, or other eating occasion. Portions, of course, can be bigger or smaller than the servings listed in the Food Guide Pyramid or on a food label. Many factors affect food portions, such as the individual's age, gender, activity level, and appetite and where and when the food is obtained and eaten.

How Do Food Guide Pyramid Serving Sizes Compare With Portions Typically Reported?

Recently, the Center for Nutrition Policy and Promotion (CNPP) reviewed data on quantities of some foods com-

Amounts of selected foods reported per eating occasion,[1] 50th percentile, by age and sex

Food	FGP[2] serving sizes	20–39 years		40–59 years		60+ years	
		Men	Women	Men	Women	Men	Women
		Number of FGP serving sizes					
Apples, raw	1 medium	1.0	1.0	1.0	1.0	0.9	0.9
Orange juice	¾ cup	1.3	1.3	1.3	1.1	1.1	1.0
String beans, ck	½ cup	1.5	1.0	1.0	1.0	1.4	1.0
Broccoli, ck	½ cup	1.3	1.0	1.6	1.3	0.8	1.1
Fluid milk	½ cup	1.0	0.9	1.0	0.7	0.8	0.7
Chesse	1-½ cup	0.7	0.6	0.7	0.7	0.7	0.7
White bread	1 slice	2.0	1.8	1.9	1.7	1.8	1.5
Rice, ck	½ cup	1.7	1.5	1.6	1.3	1.4	1.2
RTE cereals	1 oz	2.1	1.5	1.8	1.3	1.7	1.2
Pasta, cooked	½ cup	2.2	1.5	2.0	1.5	1.7	1.5
Muffins	~1 oz	2.3	1.9	2.1	1.8	2.0	2.0
Crackers	6–8 crax	1.0	0.8	0.9	0.7	0.7	0.6
		Number of 1 ounce meat equivalents[3]					
Beef, ground	1 oz	2.5	2.0	2.5	2.1	2.8	2.3
Beef steak	1 oz	5.7	4.9	5.3	4.3	4.9	3.8
Pork, chops, rst	1 oz	3.8	3.0	3.6	2.8	2.8	2.4
Ham	1 oz	1.9	1.5	2.0	1.6	2.0	1.9
Eggs, fried	1 large	1.8	1.4	1.8	1.0	1.6	0.9
Dry beans, ck	½ cup	1.9	1.0	1.5	1.0	1.3	1.0
Peanut butter	2 Tbsp	0.9	0.6	0.9	0.5	0.8	0.5

[1]Data calculated from CSFII 1989–91, NFS Report No. 91-3.
[2]FGP (Food Guide Pyramid).
[3]Serving sizes of meats and meat alternates are listed in 1-ounce equivalents because serving amounts vary by type of food (steak, roast, ground meat, beans, eggs, peanut butter). The Food Guide Pyramid suggests 2 to 3 servings of meat or meat alternates for a total of 5 to 7 ounces per day.

monly eaten in the United States that individuals reported consuming at each eating occasion in the USDA 1989–91 Continuing Survey of Food Intakes by Individuals (CSFII) (4). The table presents typical amounts of selected foods expressed in food guide serving units, that were consumed by three age groups of adult men and women. Results are similar to data on typical portion sizes obtained from a study using the USDA 1977–78 Nationwide Food Consumption Survey (5). Consistent with their greater calorie need, men's portion sizes (number of food guide servings at each eating occasion) are larger than those for women; for both genders, portion sizes decrease with age, especially for foods such as meats and grain products.

What Is the Challenge for the Grain Products?

As in the earlier study (5), individuals' typical portion sizes for grain products in the 1989–91 CSFII equaled 1½ to 2 food guide serving units, for example, 2 slices of bread or a cup of cooked pasta. However, the Food Guide Pyramid retains the grain serving size units of 1 slice of bread or ½ cup of cooked pasta, etc., used in previous food guides, in part because the serving units are familiar and easy to use. This may have caused some confusion among consumers who are unaware of the specified serving unit—they may either perceive 6 to 11 servings of grain products suggested by the Pyramid to be far more than can be eaten or may alternatively interpret this as permission to consume more than they should of these foods, often with added fats and sugars. However, changing the *serving unit* to the more typically reported 2 slices of bread or 1 cup of cooked pasta would *reduce* the *number* of servings suggested by the Pyramid to 3 to 5 and might give an appearance of a conflict with the Dietary Guideline to include plenty of grain products in the diet.

How Can Educators Help?

Educators can help consumers better understand the concepts of servings and portions by:

- *Explaining that Food Guide Pyramid servings are units of measure that are easy to use and understand. They are not prescribed portions to eat as a meal or snack.*
- *Explaining that the number of servings suggested in the Food Guide Pyramid are related to the caloric needs of the individual—the higher the caloric needs, the higher the suggested number of servings.*
- *Providing tips on how to visually estimate serving sizes.*
- *Explaining why Food Guide Pyramid servings and food label servings differ.*

- *Explaining how serving sizes differ from portion sizes.*
- *Showing individuals how to evaluate their diets to determine if changes are needed to achieve a healthful diet. One way to evaluate an individual's diet is to total the number of Food Guide Pyramid servings eaten daily and compare them—based on caloric need—with the number of servings suggested by the Food Guide Pyramid.*

References

1 U.S. Department of Agriculture. 1996. *The Food Guide Pyramid.* Home and Garden Bulletin No. 252.

2 Cronin, F.J., Shaw, A.M., Krebs-Smith, S.M., Marsland, P.M., and Light, L. 1987. Developing a food guidance system to implement the dietary guidelines. *J. Nutr. Educ.* 19:281–302.

3 Welsh, S.O., Davis, C., and Shaw, A. 1993. *USDA's Food Guide: Background and Development, USDA.* Miscellaneous Publication No. 1514.

4 Krebs-Smith, S.M., Guenther, P.M., Cook, A., Thompson, F.E., Cucinelli, J., and Udler, J. 1997. *Foods Commonly Eaten in the United States: Quantities Consumed Per Eating Occasion and in a Day, 1989–91.* USDA ARS NFS Report No. 91-3.

5 Krebs-Smith, S.M., and Smiciklas-Wright, H. 1985. Typical serving sizes: Implications for food guidance. *J. Am. Diet. Assoc.* 85:1139–1141.

Authors: Myrtle Hogbin, R.D., Nutritionist; Anne Shaw, Ph.D., Nutritionist; Rajen S. Anand, Ph.D., Executive Director, Center for Nutrition Policy and Promotion, USDA.

A Reality Check for the Lunch-On-the-Run Crowd

Quick lunches from popular eateries can pack more calories and fat than you think—but we identified healthful options, too

YOU NEED TO EAT at your desk today because you're in the middle of a big project. But you still want to choose a healthful meal, so you run out for a slice of Stuffed Vegetable Pizza from Sbarro. After all, it has the word "vegetable" in it, so you figure you're doing okay, right?

Or you need a shopping break at the mall and decide to get a Steak Fajita Salad at Chili's. True, steak can be fatty, but there are only a few thin slices, and it is a salad after all.

Well, we sent the pizza and salad to a laboratory for nutrition analysis, and guess what?

Just a single stuffed pizza slice contains 674 calories, with 28 grams of fat and 11 grams of saturated fat—half the saturated fat that someone on a 2,000-calorie diet should be averaging daily. And **alas, the salad isn't rabbit feed. A serving, which comes with dressing and guacamole, con-**

Filling in the Numbers that Popular Eateries Sometimes Leave Out

MANY EATERIES THAT OFFER quick lunches do not provide nutrition information. Thus, it can be hard to tell whether the slice of pizza, salad, or other dish that might seem like a perfectly reasonable fit in your diet really is.

Even shops that do provide the numbers don't always make them terribly accessible. Chili's, for instance, will provide calorie and fat information on any item you want if you call the company. But obviously most people are not going to do that before running out for a bite.

Following is the nutrition lowdown on some popular lunch items. Those marked with a check (✔) fit easily into a healthful diet.

Au Bon Pain[*] Au Bon Pain supplies nutrition information readily. You can either pick up a brochure with a partial listing from one of its outlets, check the company's Web site at http://www.aubonpain.com/, or call (800) 825-5227.

	Calories	Fat[1] (grams)	Sat Fat[2] (grams)	Comments
Country Ham Sandwich (with mustard, not mayonnaise)	410	9	NA	Round out the sandwich nutritiously with lettuce, tomato, and alfalfa sprouts.
Fields and Feta Sandwich	560	17	NA	The cheese and dressing add the calories and fat here.
Provolene Cheese Sandwich	560	24	NA	The 3 oz of cheese contains 300 calories and 22 fat grams. You might want to take out some cheese and snack on it later.
✔Tomato Florentine Soup (medium)	90	2	NA	Round out this soup with a bagel (350 calories, 1 gram of fat), and a slice of cheese.
✔Vegetarian Chili (medium)	220	4	NA	Have it with the chain's Garden Salad (160 calories) and a small yogurt. An excellent choice.

Bruegger's Bagels[*] Pick up nutrition information at your Bruegger's outlet. If it's not available, call the Burlington, VT, headquarters-(802) 660-4020-to have a brochure mailed.

✔Chicken Salad Sandwich	430	11	2	A perfectly good fit into your healthful day.
✔Deli-Style Ham Sandwich	400	7	1	Another good fit; honey cured ham, sliced tomatoes, leaf lettuce, and mustard.
✔Hummus Sandwich	450	10	1	Ask your sandwich preparer to add in some lettuce and tomato.
Leonardo da Veggie Sandwich	420	11	6	This offering, with light herb garlic cream cheese, meunster cheese, and raw vegetables, makes an okay lunch, even though it's a bit high in saturated fat. End the meal with a fresh fruit.
✔Marcello Minestrone Soup	70	1	0	Enjoy with any Bruegger's sandwich.

cont. following page

From the *Tufts University Health & Nutrition Letter*, September 1999, pp. 4-5. © 1999 by Tufts University Health & Nutrition Letter. Reprinted by permission.

Chili's For nutrition information, call (800) 983-4637.

	Calories	Fat[1] (grams)	Sat Fat[2] (grams)	Comments
Chili (bowl, not cup)[†4]	496	22	9	It's on the high side for fat, but rounded out with a small House Salad (go easy on the dressing), it makes a reasonable meal.
Classic Nachos[*]	902	50	NA	The menu calls it a "starter". But nutrition-wise, this dish, with fried nacho chips, cheese, guacamole, and sour cream, is no appetizer.
Grilled Chicken Pasta[*]	1,629	93	NA	Yes, you read the numbers correctly.
Guiltless Grill Pita[*]	597	9	NA	Low-fat Southwest dressing helps limit the fat tally.
Guiltless Veggie Pasta[*]	680	13	NA	Fairly moderate fat count but rather high in calories. Save some for another meal, or split it with your dining partner and order a small House Salad.
Steak Fajita Salad[†4]	813	48	11	Unless your dinner is going to be a bowl of soup, cup of yogurt, or other light meal, you might want to pass on this or split it in half.
Veggie and Smoked Cheese Quesadillas[*]	879	47	NA	The sour cream and pico de gallo (diced tomato with olive oil and spices) add a lot of calories. Don't be misled by the word "veggie."

Panda Express[†] You can order a brochure from this Chinese take-out chain by calling (800) 877-8988. But the serving sizes you actually purchase may weigh more—and contain significantly more calories—than what the brochure says. According to our lab analysis, the Fried Rice and Orange Flavored Chicken combined have about 500 more calories than the brochure indicates they do.

	Calories	Fat (grams)	Sat Fat (grams)	Comments
Fried Rice	614	24	5	These three items together add up to more than 1,400 calories, 63 grams of fat, and 13 grams of saturated fat. And it's not the biggest lunch you can get. The fried rice and egg rolls are considered side dishes (the egg rolls are smallish), but you can get three "sides" instead of two.
Orange Flavored Chicken	596	30	6	
2 Egg Rolls	198	9	2	

Pizzeria Uno[†] Pizzeria Uno does not offer nutrition information.

	Calories	Fat (grams)	Sat Fat (grams)	Comments
Pasta Ceasar Salad	867	42	9	Caeser salad dressing tends to be quite high in fat. No matter what restaurant you eat in, do not assume that a Caeser salad is an even nutritional swap for a traditional garden salad.

Sbarro[†] Sbarro did not offer information when we went to press.

	Calories	Fat (grams)	Sat Fat (grams)	Comments
✔ Low-Fat Vegetable Pizza (one slice)	445	9	3	While a slice of this pizza isn't low in calories, it is reasonably low in fat, particularly saturated fat. Finish it off with a fruit, and you've had a nutritious meal with room left for an ample dinner. It's easy to get fooled by the word "vegetable," but any pizza that's double-crusted is sure to come with plenty of calories and fat. Those crusts fairly glisten with oil.
Stuffed Vegetable Pizza (one slice)	674	28	11	

Subway[*] Subway offers extensive nutrition information. Pick up a brochure at a Subway outlet, order one by calling (800) 888-4848, or find the numbers online at www.subway.com (*Note:* Values below do not include add-ons of cheese or condiments.)

	Calories	Fat (grams)	Sat Fat (grams)	Comments
Classic Italian BMT 6" Super Sub (BMT = Biggest, Meatiest, Tastiest)	668	39	14	"Super" at Subway can mean an abundance of calories and fat; meat portions are doubled. (The Classic Italian contains bologna, ham, pepperoni, and salami.)
Classic Italian BMT 6" Cold Sandwich	450	21	8	Not an easy fit into a healthful diet, but much easier than a "Super" Classic Italian.
✔ Deli Style Bologna Sandwich	293	10	3	Add mayonnaise, cheese, or the olive oil "blend," and calories and fat start to shoot up.
Meatball 6" Hot Sandwich	413	15	6	If your meatball sandwich at Subway isn't "Super", it won't be too hard on your diet.
✔ 6" Subway Club Sub	304	5	2	Eat it with one of Subway's Veggie Delight salads, and you'll even have room for one of the chain's 2-oz cookies (at about 200 calories each).
✔ Steak & Cheese Wrap	353	9	4	Have it with a fruit salad in the afternoon.

[*] Nutrition information supplied by the company
[†] Nutrition information via lab analysis commissioned by the *Tufts Health & Nutrition Letter.*
[1] Someone following a 2,000-calorie diet should average a maximum of 66 grams of fat a day. [2]Someone following a 2,000-calorie diet should average a maximum of 22 grams of saturated fat a day. [3] Not available.
[4] Our calorie count for Chili's bowl of Chili was 7 percent lower than the figure the chain provided; our calorie count for the Steak Fajita Salad, 15 percent higher

tains 813 calories and 48 grams of fat, 11 of them saturated.

Would you have chosen differently had you been aware of the numbers? A new study says yes. Researchers supported by the National Cancer Institute surveyed thousands of people who had been provided with calorie, fat, and other nutrition information about foods available at the work site—either in cafeterias or vending machines. They then compared them with thousands of others who had not been given nutrition information about the foods offered at work. The upshot: the informed lunch eaters showed greater improvement in eating habits over a three-year period. Armed with nutrition facts and, in many cases, more healthful lunch options than they had had previously, they ate less fat and more fiber, in part because of an increase in fruit and vegetable consumption.

The study was part of the National Cancer Institute's Working Well Project, which has involved more than 100 work sites and 18,000 employees around the country. The institute wants to get people to eat more healthfully during the work day as a way of reducing cancer risk.

It would be great if everyone had the opportunity to choose healthful meals at lunchtime. But it can be hard. One reason is that many popular eateries do not provide nutrition information; federal law does not require it. Furthermore, in the quest to eat more healthfully, the midday meal can get short shrift. It's often the least well-planned, as many people literally run out the door in the morning. Then, too, it's easy to rationalize that it's just a slice of pizza or a salad—especially when your favorite restaurant chain doesn't provide any nutrition numbers.

To close some of the gaps that might be separating you from more healthful lunches, we sent more than a half dozen dishes from popular chains to a laboratory for nutrition analysis. We also looked at nutrition information that a number of eateries provide themselves. The chart, (on the preceeding pages) gives the lowdown on many of the 100-plus dishes we surveyed. Those items we've marked with a check ([check]) can fit easily into a healthful eating plan. They have no more than 500 calories, no more than 12 grams of total fat, and fewer than 6 grams of saturated fat.

the 100 healthiest foods

By Janis Jibrin, R.D.

JANIS JIBRIN, R.D., is a writer living in Washington. Her latest book is *The Unofficial Guide to Dieting Safely* (Macmillan, 1998).

In the fast-paced world of nutrition research, it seems like a hot discovery hits the news every week. So we asked prominent scientists doing groundbreaking work on how edibles stave off illness to pin down the 100 most nutrient-packed foods. To make our list, a food had to be very rich in at least one vitamin, mineral or other compound known to protect against cancer, heart disease or other diseases. Be supermarket smart and use this list as your shopping list. Your body will be glad you did!

The Best of Everything

food	fat/calorie breakdown	body benefits
(FRUITS)		
1. Apples	1 medium apple: 81 calories, 0 g fat	An apple's 3 g of fiber help you meet your fiber goal of 20 g. to 30 g daily. High-fiber diets can lower heart disease risk.
2. Apricots	3 apricots: 51 calories, 0 g fat	A good source of beta-carotene (which is converted to vitamin A by the body), providing the equivalent of 35% of the RDA for vitamin A.
3. Bananas	1 medium: 105 calories, 0 g fat	Bananas are a great source of potassium, which plays a key role in heart health and muscle function. Plus each one has 2 g of fiber.
4. Blackberries	1 cup: 74 calories, 0 g fat	This fruit boasts a whopping 10 g of fiber in a single cup.
5. Blueberries	1 cup: 81 calories, 0 g fat	Blueberries help prevent and treat bladder infections by making it hard for bacteria to stick to urinary tract walls.
6. Cantaloupe	1 cup, cubed: 84 calories, 1 g fat	An antioxidant double whammy, with 68 mg of vitamin C and enough beta-carotene to cover 65% of your daily vitamin A quota.
7. Cherries	1 cup: 84 calories, 1 g fat	A good source of perillyl alcohol, which helps prevent cancer in animals. Heart-protective anthocyanins give cherries their color.
8. Cranberry juice	1 cup: 144 calories, 0 g fat	Fights bladder infections the same way blueberries do.
9. Grapefruits	½ fruit: 39 calories, 0 g fat	A good source of vitamin C and a compound called naringenin, which helps suppress tumors in animals.

Continued

From *American Health,* May 1999, pp. 87-91. © 1999 by Janis Jibrin. Reprinted by permission.

10. Purple grapes and juice	1 cup seedless: 113 calories, 9 g fat	Offer three heart-guarding compounds: flavonoids, anthocyanins and resveratrol. (Sorry, green grapes are not rich in them.)
11. Kiwi fruit	1 medium kiwi: 46 calories, 0 g fat	Just one little fruit packs a mean vitamin-C punch (74 mg) and an impressive 2.8 g fiber.
12. Mangoes	1 mango: 135 calories, 1 g fat	A single mango has enough beta-carotene to cover your RDA for vitamin A while racking up 57 mg of vitamin C.
13. Oranges	1 orange: 61 calories, 0 g fat	One orange provides an impressive 50 g to 70 g of vitamin C, 40 mcg of folic acid and 52 mg of calcium.
14. Orange juice	1 cup: 112 calories, 0 g fat	One of the richest sources of folic acid: A cup provides one-quarter of the 400 mcg RDA for folic acid and boasts 96 mg of vitamin C.
15. Calcium-enriched orange juice	1 cup (from concentrate): 112 calories, 0 g fat	Drinking this beverage is a healthful way to make a 300- to 350-mg dent in your daily 1,500-mg calcium requirement.
16. Papayas	1 cup, cubbed: 55 calories, 0 g fat	Loaded with vitamin C (86 mg per cup), a healthy dose of fiber (2.5 g) and a sprinkling of beta-carotene and calcium.
17. Prunes	$\frac{1}{3}$ cup, stewed: 87 calories, 0 g fat	Prunes famed laxative effect is no mystery: There are 5 g of fiber (both soluble and insoluble) in just $\frac{1}{3}$ cup.
18. Raspberries	1 cup: 60 calories, 0 g fat	Teeming with 8 g of fiber per cup, they also boast vitamin C, ellagic acid and anthocyanins.
19. Red grapefruit	$\frac{1}{2}$ fruit: 37 calories, 0 g fat	All the goodies of white grapefruit and more: They provide up to 100% of RDA for vitamin A and are also high in lycopene.
20. Strawberries	1 cup, sliced: 50 calories, 0 g fat	Strawberries have high levels of ellagic acid and anthocyanins, and are rich in vitamin C (95 mg per cup) and fiber (3.8 g per cup).

(VEGETABLES)

21. Artichokes	1 medium: 60 calories, 0 g fat	In addition to their high fiber content (6 g), artichokes contain a flavonoid that has been shown to reduce skin cancer in animals.
22. Arugula	1 cup: 5 calories, 0 g fat	A cruciferous (cabbage family) veggie, this tangy green contains cancer-preventative compounds such as isothiocyanates.
23. Avocado	$\frac{1}{2}$ avocado: 170 calories, 13 g fat	Yes, they're high in fat, but fortunately half of it's the heart-healthy monounsaturated variety. And they're a good source of vitamin E.
24. Beets	$\frac{1}{2}$ cup, sliced: 37 calories, 0 g fat	Beta-cyanin, which gives beets their reddish-purple color, is a disease-fighting antioxidant.
25. Bok choy	1 cup, cooked: 20 calories, 0 g fat	This staple of Chinese cuisine contains isothiocyanates, plus lots of calcium (158 mg per cup) and vitamin C (44 mg per cup).
26. Broccoli	1 cup, cooked: 44 calories, 0 g fat	This superfood is loaded with sulphoraphane. Then there's the 72 mg of calcium, 78 mcg of folic acid and all the vitamin C.
27. Broccoli sprouts	$\frac{1}{2}$ cup: 10 calories, 0 g fat	As protective as broccoli is, these little sprouts may be even better. They're sprouting up in health food stores and supermarkets.
28. Brussel sprouts	$\frac{1}{2}$ cup cooked: 30 calories, 0 g fat	Along with good-for-you isothiocyanates and indoles, these vegetables give you an impressive 48 mg of vitamin C.
29. Cabbage	1 cup raw, chopped: 22 calories, 0 g fat	The indoles in cabbage help make it a cancer fighter. For a healthy coleslaw, top shredded raw cabbage with lowfat dressing.

Continued

30. Cauliflower	1 cup, raw: 24 calories, 0 g fat	Another great source of indoles; plus it's high in fiber (2.5 g per cup) and vitamin C (72 mg per cup).
31. Carrots	1 medium: 26 calories, 0 g fat	A stellar source of beta-carotene. One carrot contains twice the RDA for vitamin A. Cooked carrots are even healthier than raw.
32. Celery	2 medium stalks: 13 calories, 0 g fat	Celery doesn't get much hype, but it's got the goods—namely phthalides, compounds that lower blood pressure and cholesterol.
33. Garlic	1 clove: 5 calories, 0 g fat	Raw, cooked or granulated: all forms contain cholesterol-fighting organosulfur compounds.
34. Green beans	1 cup, cooked: 43 calories, 0 g fat	Green beans carry a variety of antioxidant carotenoids, including beta-carotene, lutein and zeaxanthin.
35. Green pepper	1 medium: 32 calories, 0 g fat	One of the more vitamin C-rich vegetables—66 mg per pepper—and it's got a little capsaicin, too (see peppers, below).
36. to 39. Greens (Collard, kale, mustard, turnip)	1 cup, cooked: 29 to 49 calories, 0 to 1 g fat	These greens are packed with disease fighters: lutein, zeaxanthin, and isothiocyanates and 93 to 226 mg of calcium per cup.
40. Onions	½ cup, chopped: 30 calories, 0 g fat	They're important suppliers of the same heart-healthy organosulphur compounds that are found in garlic.
41. Peas	½ cup, cooked: 67 calories, 0 g fat	A good source of the carotenoids lutein and zeaxanthin—both of which help protect against age-related eye disease.
42. Peppers (hot)	1 pepper: 18 calories, 0 g fat	Their phytochemical claim to fame is capsaicin, which helps short-circuit the cancer process.
43. Potato (white)	1 7-oz. potato: 220 calories, 0 g fat	Don't peel it, and you get a generous 5 g of fiber, 43% of the day's vitamin C requirement and a major dose of potassium.
44. Pumpkin	½ cup, canned: 41 calories, 0 g fat	Gives you three times the RDA for vitamin A and 3.5 g of fiber. Use canned pumpkin to make pumpkin bread, risotto and soup.
45. Radishes	4 radishes: 4 calories 0 g fat	The beginning of the bite is cool, but soon things get hot; chewing activates the veggies' indoles and isothiocyanates.
46. Romaine and other dark lettuce	2 cups, shredded: 18 calories, 0 g fat.	The darker the green, the more carotenoids. These lettuces are also high in folic acid: There's 40% of the RDA in 2 cups of romaine.
47. Red peppers (sweet)	1 pepper: 32 calories, 0 g fat	An improved version of the already top-notch green pepper, with twice its vitamin C content and a day's supply of vitamin A.
48. Seaweed	1 cup: 32 calories, 0 g fat	Seaweed is carotenoid- and calcium-rich and has a delicate taste.
49. Spinach	1 cup, cooked: 41 calories, 0 g fat	Offers enough beta-carotene to surpass the RDA for vitamin A, a ton of lutein and more than half the RDA for folic acid.
50. Squash (winter types, butternut)	1 cup, cooked: 82 calories, 0 g fat	Not only does a cup equip you with three day's worth of vitamin A but it fulfills nearly 10% of your daily calcium needs.
51. Tomatoes	1 tomato: 26 calories, 0 g fat	Technically considered a fruit, tomatoes are loaded with cancer-fighting lycopene and are great sources of vitamin C.
52. Turnips	1 cup, cooked, cubed: 32 calories, 0 g fat	Neglected members of the cruciferous family, turnips provide both indoles and isothiocyanates and 3 g fiber.

Continued

53. Watercress	2 cups: 8 calories, 0 g fat	One of its compounds detoxifies a major carcinogen in tobacco and as such may help prevent lung cancer. Also contains carotenoids.
54. Yams and sweet potatoes	½ cup, mashed: 103 calories, 0 g fat	They win the carotenoid prize, with astonishing levels amounting to six times the RDA for vitamin A.

(TEA, HERBS & SPICES)

55. Chives	1 tbsp.: 1 calorie, 0 g fat	A member of the same family as garlic, chives contain cholesterol-lowering organosulfides.
56. Cinnamon	½ tsp.: 3 calories, 0 g fat	Recent research found that ¼ tsp. to 1 tsp. of cinnamon daily improves insulin function and, in turn, blood-sugar control.
57. Ginger	5 1-in. slices: 8 calories, 0 g fat	Helps quell nausea and may reduce joint inflammation in diseases such as rheumatoid arthritis.
58. Horseradish	1 tsp. prepared horseradish: 2 calories, 0 g fat	Whether it's fresh, jarred or in the sharp green wasabi served with sushi, horseradish is infused with anticancer isothiocyanates.
59. Mint	2 tbsp.: 5 calories, 0 g fat	Spearmint, the type normally found in the fresh herb section of your grocery, is rich in covone, an antioxidant and anticarcinogen.
60. Mustard	½ tsp. mustard seed: 8 calories, 0 g fat	Both prepared yellow mustard and mustard seed contain health-protective isothiocyanates.
61. Parsley	2 tbsp., chopped: 3 calories, 0 g fat	Parsley is a great source of several carotenoids: beta-carotene, lutein and zeaxanthin. Try it in tabbouleh.
62. Rosemary	½ tsp., dried or 1 tsp., fresh: 1 calorie, 0 g fat	Test-tube studies found that carnosol, a compound in rosemary, thwarts the action of carcinogens.
63. Sage	½ tsp., ground: 1 calorie, 0 g fat	Contains a variety of moneterpenes, substances that prevent the spread and progression of tumors.
64. Tea (black or green)	1 cup: 2 calories, 0 g fat	Tea (regular and decaf) and its antioxidant catechins are linked to reduced heart-disease risk. Tea may also help inhibit cancer.
65. Turmeric (used in curry spice)	½ tsp.: 4 calories, 0 g fat	This spice gets its yellow color from compounds called curcumins, which have reduced the size of tumors in animals 50%.

(BEANS & SOY)

66. Beans (kidney, black, navy)	1 cup, cooked: 220 to 270 calories, 0 g fat	A super rich fiber source, ranging from 6 g to 16 g per cup, depending on the variety. Also high in iron.
67. Soy milk	1 cup: 81 calories, 4 g fat	A cup has 20 mg to 25 mg of health-promoting isoflavones.
68. Soy protein isolate powder	1 oz.: 95 calories, 1 g fat	Studies show that it takes 25 g of soy protein daily (the amount in just 1¼ oz. to 3 oz. of the powder, depending on the brand) to get a 10% drop in cholesterol. Try blending it in a smoothie.
69. Tofu	½ cup: 97 calories, 6 g fat	A rich source of isoflavones. Studies indicate that 90 mg of isoflavones daily improves bone density; ½ cup of tofu has 30 g.
70. Textured vegetable protein	½ cup, rehydrated: 60 calories, 0 g fat	This is the stuff that mimics meat in vegetarian chili. TVP is one of the richest sources of isoflavones, at 40 mg per ½ cup.

(DAIRY)

71. Cheese (full fat)	1 oz.: 70 to 110 calories, 6 g to 9 g fat	One ounce packs 210 mg of calcium and a dose of conjugated linoleic acid (CLA). It's high in saturated fat; eat with lowfat foods.

Continued

72. Skim milk	1 cup: 90 calories, 0 g fat	Our calcium lifeline at 300 mg per cup, and one of the few dietary sources of vitamin D, which is vital to calcium metabolism.
73. Yogurt (plain lowfat or nonfat)	1 cut lowfat: 150 calories, 3.5 g fat	Those friendly bacteria (called probiotics) in yogurt help boost immunity and prevent yeast infections.

(MEAT)

74. Beef	3 oz., cooked: 150 to 280 calories, 5 g to 20 g fat	Beef is a good source of both CLA and iron, but since it's also high in saturated fat, have it no more than three times a week.
75. Chicken (without skin)	3 oz., cooked: 162 calories, 6 g fat	Remove the skin and you've got an excellent, lowfat source of protein. And 3 oz. provides 38% of the RDA for the B vitamin niacin.
76. Lamb	3 oz., cooked, trimmed of fat: 175 calories, 8 g fat	Lamb, like beef, is also a good source of CLA. Ditto beef's saturated fat warning and weekly consumption recommendation.
77. Lean pork	3 oz., cooked, trimmed of fat: 140 calories, 4 g fat	Fat-trimmed pork tenderloin has one-third less fat than even lean beef. And it boasts 71% of the RDA for thiamine.

(SEAFOOD)

78. Fatty fish (salmon, mackerel)	3 oz., cooked, 155 to 225 calories, 5 g to 15 g fat	The richest source of the heart-protective omega-3 fatty acids DHA and EPA, considered the most potent.
79. Other fish	3 oz., cooked: about 100 calories, 1 g fat	Omega-3s comprise the little bit of fat found in fish, plus fish are a good source of selenium, which is essential for immunity.
80. Lobster	3 oz., cooked: 122 calories, 2 g fat	Try lemon juice instead of butter and you've got a virtually fat-free way to meet your daily selenium and copper requirements.
81. Mussels	3 oz., cooked: 146 calories, 4 g fat	Mussels have two to three times as much iron as a burger, and completely cover you for selenium.
82. Oysters, Eastern	6 medium, steamed (1½ oz.): 58 calories, 2 g fat	Just six oysters give you nearly five times the RDA for zinc, which is critical for immune function.

(NUTS, SEEDS & OILS)

83. Almonds	½ oz. (11 nuts): 83 calories, 7 g fat	A recent study showed that a daily 3½-oz. serving of almonds can lower LDL cholesterol 14%.
84. Brazil nuts	½ oz. (3 to 4 nuts): 93 calories, 9g fat	Just three to four nuts deliver an astronomical 420 mcg of selenium, eight times the recommended daily amount.
85. Peanut butter	2 tbsp.: 200 calories, 16 g fat	Eating five ounces of nuts weekly reduces heart-disease risk. Buy peanut butter without partially hydrogenated oils.
86. Sunflower seeds	¼ cup: 205 calories, 18 g fat	One of the richest sources of vitamin E (besides oils), with an impressive 6 IUs in just ¼ cup.
87. Tahini	1 tbsp.: 89 calories, 8 g fat	Amazingly, 1 tbsp. of the stuff has got 64 mg of calcium, 1.3 mg of iron and nearly one mg of zinc. And it's a good source of protein.
88. Walnuts	1 oz. (14 halves): 182 calories, 17 g fat	Walnuts are exceptionally rich in an omega-3 fatty acid called alpha-linolenic acid, which helps protect against heart disease.
89. Canola oil	1 tbsp.: 124 calories, 14 g fat	The only cooking oil that's rich in the two healthiest fats: monounsaturated and omega-3s. It's a good all-purpose oil.

Continued

90. Flaxseed oil	1 tbsp.: 124 calories, 14 g fat	It's rich in the vegetarian form of omega-3 fatty acids. Mix with balsamic vinegar for a tasty salad dressing.
91. Olive oil	1 tbsp.: 120 calories, 14 g fat	Besides its extremely high monounsaturated fat content, olive oil also contains a heart-healthy compound called squalene.

(GRAINS)

92. Barley	½ cup, cooked: 97 calories, 0 g fat	Barley is a great source of a soluble fiber called beta-glucan (also found in oats, below), which helps lower blood cholesterol.
93. Bran cereal	Varies by brand. ½ cup: 80 calories, 1 g fat	The easiest way to make inroads into that 20- to 30-g fiber recommendation. These cereals range from 2 g to 9 g of fiber per serving.
94. Flaxseed	1 tbsp. seeds: 60 calories, 4 g fat	One of the richest sources of health-protective lignans and a good source of omega-3 fatty acids.
95. Oats and oat bran	1 cup: 88 calories, 2 g fat	Studies show that a cup of cooked oat bran or 1½ cups oatmeal daily lowers cholesterol 5%.
96. Rye crackers	1 4½" x 2½" cracker (.5 oz.): 37 calories, 0 g fat	Rye crackers are one of the few foods containing rye bran. The bran has lignans and 2.5 g of fiber per ½ oz. of crackers.
97. Wheat germ	¼ cup wheat germ: 103 calorie, 4 g fat	Wheat germ is rich in fiber, provides your daily selenium dose and is one of the few foods rich in vitamin E (7 IU of E per ¼ cup).
98. Whole grains such as bulgar	1 cup, cooked: 150 to 220 calories, 0 g to 2 g fat	Besides the lignans and vitamins, these grains supply complex carbs that mete out a slow, even supply of energy all day long.
99. 100% whole wheat bread	2 slices: 138 calories, 2 g fat	Each slice of 100% whole wheat bread has 1.5 g of fiber, plus other nutrients. Forget regular "wheat" bread.
100. Whole wheat pasta	1 cup, cooked: 174 calories, 1 g fat	It's got all the nutrients of whole wheat bread, and it's a great source of selenium as well.

SOURCES: David Kritchevsky, PhD., professor emeritus of biochemistry, University of Pennsylvania; Clare Hasler, Ph.D., executive director of the functional foods for health program, University of Illinois, Champaign-Urbana; John Weisburger, M.D., Senior Member, American Health Foundation, Valhalla, NY; Gary Beecher, Ph.D., scientist, USDA Human Nutrition Research Center, Beltsville, MD; Paul La Chance, Ph.D., executive director, Nutraceuticals Institute at Rutgers University, New Brunswick, NJ; Mark Messina, Ph.D., associate professor of nutrition, Loma Linda College, Loma Linda, CA; Jed Fahey, faculty research associate, John Hopkins School of Medicine, Baltimore.

A GLOSSARY OF HEALTHY-FOOD TERMS

ANTHOCYANINS: Plant pigments that help protect you from heart disease.

ANTIOXIDANT: A substance that prevents harmful molecules called free radicals from damaging DNA. Free radicals may be a cause of cancer, heart disease and other chronic diseases.

CAROTENOIDS: Antioxidant plant pigments that are converted to vitamin A by the body. There are several types: beta-carotene, a major plant source of vitamin A, which lowers the risk for heart disease and cancer; lutein and zeaxanthin, which are linked to a reduced risk of age-related macular degeneration, a major cause of vision loss and blindness in older adults; lycopene, linked with a lower risk of heart attack and cancer.

CONJUGATED LINOLEIC ACID: Beef, lamb and full-fat cheeses are rich in CLA, which halts tumor formation in animals.

ELLAGIC ACID: A plant compound that detoxifies and traps carcinogens.

FLAVONOIDS: Plant compounds that deter cancer in a number of ways.

FOLIC ACID: B vitamin that helps prevent birth defects and lower levels of homocysteine, an amino acid linked to heart disease.

INDOLES: Compounds that help fight cancer.

ISOFLAVONES: Compounds that act as weak estrogens (phytoestrogens). Eating 90 mg of isoflavones daily can improve bone density.

ISOTHIOCYANATES: Compounds, including sulphoraphane, that protect against cancer.

LIGNANS: Phytoestrogens that help prevent cancer.

MONOUNSATURATED FAT: The heart-healthiest type of fat.

OMEGA-3 FATTY ACIDS: A type of fat that reduces the risk factors for heart disease.

ORGANOSULFIDES: Substances that help lower cholesterol.

PHYTOESTROGENS: Compounds that are structurally similar to human estrogen. One difference: They do not promote breast and endometrial cancer. In fact, they help protect against these cancers, while providing many of the same heart-and bone-protective effects as human estrogen.

Supermarket Psych-Out

REMEMBER THE AD for Sheba cat food, the one in which the woman with the luxurious voice feeds her luxuriously furry feline from a tin that has large black lettering and a picture of a black cat? Well, it's no accident that the tin has all that black on it.

There was a time when black had a "no-frills association," explains Mona Doyle, president of The Consumer Network, a Philadelphia firm that conducts research on consumer perceptions. "It would have looked doleful" to people shopping for food products," she says. But today, she points out, black has become "a symbol of quality—a status connotation, elegant." In other words, it's associated in people's minds with high-class, expensive goods (a relevant point, since Sheba costs more than twice as much as several other brands).

Color is "a very powerful tool," notes Eric Johnson, head of Research Studies for the Chicago-based Institute for Color Research, which collects scientific information about the human response to color. A customer spends only the briefest amount of time at the supermarket deciding which products and which brands to buy, and the colors food manufacturers use to package their products are chosen with a great deal of care to sway you in what are sometimes split-second decisions.

But color is not all that's used to influence you at what marketers call the "point of purchase." The shape of a food package is meant to entice, too, as are (of course) various price promotions. Here's a look at color, shape, and a couple of other tricks of the trade that companies use to send silent messages to you when you're making choices about which products to buy.

The color of your purchases

There has been "a longstanding understanding in industry that if you want to sell a product, package it in red and white," says The Consumer Network's Ms. Doyle. Think of Campbell's soup, Carnation Instant Breakfast, and Marlboro cigarettes, to name just a few red-and-white-packaged items. But the color field has been thrown open, so to speak. Take a look.

Red Red stimulates feelings of arousal and appetite. Indeed, the Institute for Color Research's Mr. Johnson explains that when the eye sees red, the pituitary gland sends out signals that make the heart beat faster, the blood pressure increase, and the muscles tense—all physiologic changes that can lead to the consummation of a purchase. (No wonder so many foods have red on their packaging.)

Red is also considered a "warm and inviting color," says Paul Brefka, a Boston-area product designer. You'll often see at least some red on boxes of pasta, he says. It evokes shared, hearty Italian meals.

Green "Thirty years ago, green was barf color," Ms. Doyle remarks. But then it "became associated with the environment, and that meant pro-health. It has morphed 180 degrees." Just how much green's reputation has come around has been underscored in a study conducted by Brian Wansink, PhD. The director of the University of Illinois Food & Brand Lab, which looks at how consumers make pur-

chasing decisions at the point of sale, Dr. Wansink did a covert color switch on a popular sweet treat. He put O'Henry candy bars, normally found in yellow wrappers, into green ones. When the bars were seen in green, consumers said they had fewer calories, more protein, and fewer calories from fat than when they were in their usual packaging.

Green's effect is probably why Hershey's reduced-fat Sweet Escapes candy bars have green on their wrappers, just as Healthy Choice frozen dinners are packaged in largely-green boxes. Decaffeinated coffee tends to come wrapped in green, too, while regular coffee often comes in "robust" red.

White By itself, white suggests reduced calories. Sales of sugar-free Canada Dry Ginger Ale increased when its labels incorporated more white, Dr. Wansink says. Silver also means fewer calories. A bottle of Diet Coke is mostly silver; a bottle of regular Coke, mostly red.

Yellow Yellow is the fastest color that the brain processes, Mr. Johnson explains. Thus, he says, it's an "attention getter." There's also "a mythic thing about yellow being a happy color," he notes. For those reasons, it's not surprising that yellow is a very common color in supermarkets, appearing on everything from boxes of Cheerios to Domino Sugar to Triscuit wafers to Hellmann's mayonnaise.

Orange In sociologic studies, Mr. Johnson says, orange indicates affordability. It suggests, "I'm easy, I'm cheap," perhaps because it's not considered a classy color. But its suggestion of accessibility and affordability make it a good color for such "Everyman" products as Arm & Hammer Baking Soda, Burger King meals, and Stouffer's frozen entrees.

Brown Rich browns indicate "roasted" or "baked" says Mr. Johnson, which is why you'll often see brown as a background color on things like bags and boxes of gravy and cake mixes. Brown also suggests rich flavor—a reason it often appears on cans of coffee.

Blue You won't find a preponderance of foods packaged in blue. People generally want the colors on their boxes, bottles, and cans to reflect what's inside. Mr. Johnson puts it this way: "Human beings require congruency of color in order to buy the goods. People will not buy baked beans in a purple can. Beans are not purple."

Interestingly, that is not so for children, who think incongruously colored foods and food packages are "fun." That's why there has been, for instance, blue Kool-Aid, blue popcorn, and blue candies.

The shape of things to come ... into your home

Most instant coffee comes in cylindrical jars—but not Taster's Choice. It's packaged in a deep square jar. The reason: Nestle, Taster's Choice's maker, felt it would provide more of an image of a "hefty" taste if presented that way—a sort of antidote to people's assumption that freeze-dried coffee crystals can't pack a hearty flavor.

Nestle, of course, is not the only company that pays careful attention to the shape of its packaging. "Shape is probably the hottest tactic in differentiating brands," says Jim Peters, editor-in-chief of *BrandPackaging* magazine. Ms. Doyle agrees that package shape has become an extremely important marketing tool.

Just think about the "sensuous, literally provocative shapes of today's packages," she says, giving ice cream containers as an example. They used to be "brick-like," she says—utilitarian. Now, they're "more hand-friendly, sensuous," she notes—round, oval, trapezoidal. It's thought that be-

cause ice cream is an indulgence product, she explains, it "should have an indulgent look and feel."

Even dishwashing detergent containers are "tactile, designed for the hand" today, she says. They all have "silhouette shapes—it's easy to look at them as a female form. They have a waist line. They're easy to hold." Which goes to show, she says, that "we're no longer Puritan in many ways."

Bigger seen as better

Consumers often go for the larger size of a product at the supermarket. One reason, of course, is that bigger is generally seen as cheaper on a per-ounce basis. In addition, a larger container is thought to last longer, saving the shopper from having to schlep back to the supermarket as quickly to restock. Neither is necessarily the case.

On a recent trip to the grocery store, we found that a 40-ounce jar of Heinz Tomato Ketchup, at $2.49, cost 6.2 cents an ounce, whereas the smaller, 28-ounce bottle, at $1.49, was only 5.3 cents an ounce. It was a similar story with some cereals. A 24-ounce box of Kellogg's Corn Flakes cost 12.5 cents an ounce, but the littler, 18-ounce box came to just 11.9 cents an ounce.

That happens about 10 percent of the time, Dr. Wansink says. The way around it is simple. Simply check "unit prices" listed on supermarket shelves, which list the price by the pound next to the price for a particular-size container. That way, you can be certain that the size you take is the best buy that day. (Prices and deals change frequently from shopping trip to shopping trip.)

As for the bigger-package-lasts-longer tack, the reason it might not work is that people tend to take bigger portions from bigger containers. Dr. Wansink made the discovery when he asked 98 women in New Hampshire and Vermont to take enough spaghetti from a box to make dinner for two. When they took spaghetti from a 1-pound box, they averaged 234 strands each. When they took it from a larger, 2-pound box

on a separate occasion, they averaged 302 strands each—a 29 percent increase (and a 105-calorie difference per serving).

The same thing happened with cooking oil. The women poured 3.5 ounces into a pan when they poured it from a 16-ounce bottle; 4.3 ounces from a 32-ounce bottle (a difference of 192 calories).

All packaged foods list serving sizes on the Nutrition Facts panel. But, says Dr. Wansink, "few people appear to read them."

"Limit: 2 per customer" and other messages by the numbers

Sometimes it's not the package itself that does the enticing but the sign above it. A limit on how many boxes or bottles the shopper is allowed to take can be particularly effective, as Dr. Wansink demonstrated when he experimented with signs for displays of canned soup in a Sioux City, Iowa, grocery store. When consumers saw soup for 79 cents a can with no limit on how many they could purchase, they typically bought three to four cans. But when the display was changed to limit the purchase to 12 cans, they purchased as many as seven cans each, increasing sales by 112 percent.

Ironically, when supermarkets set a limit like that, they often are not trying to get consumers to buy more of a particular product; they simply are trying to make sure people don't buy too much of it. Such products are frequently loss leaders—items that are marked down so much the store loses money on them in an effort to lead people in so they will end up doing the rest of their shopping there.

"Limit" signs are not the only kind to get people to buy more of a product. Even a sign that says "4 cans for $4" as opposed to "1 can for $1" makes people buy more, Dr. Wansink explains, because it "anchors" people to a higher number. When he manipulated supermarket signs to give prices for multiple units of an item instead of the price for a single package, sales increased 32 percent in 12 out of 13 categories, including cookies, frozen dinners, and soft drinks.

Straightforward suggestions to buy a certain amount, as in "Buy 18 Snickers Bars for Your Freezer," also make people buy more than twice as much as when a sign simply says, "Buy Snickers Bars for Your Freezer." When Dr. Wansink put up a sign for Snickers Bars in a Philadelphia convenience store that did not include any suggestions on how many bars people should buy, they tended to buy one each. But when the sign suggested to people that they buy 18, they bought an average of three.

"People say, 'I'm not going to buy 18!'" Dr. Wansink explains. But they're still influenced to buy more than they would otherwise. Even signs stamped on cartons that say things like "Shipped to stores in boxes of 28 units" make people buy more, Dr. Wansink says.

Fortunately, he points out, the numbers game is very easy to get around. All you have to do is write quantities next to the items on your grocery list. That anchors you to a number of your own choosing before you even walk inside the store.

Unit Selections

Key Points to Consider

❖ Check out several labels from foods containing fats and oils that you eat frequently. Can you tell how much trans fat each contains? Determine the percentage of your average daily calories that is contributed by total fat and saturated fat. What do your calculations tell you about potential health risks?

❖ Are some nutrients more important than others in maintaining health? Support your answers.

❖ What are the best ways to supplement your diet with vitamins and minerals?

❖ What kind of interactions do some drugs have on foods?

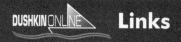 **Links** **www.dushkin.com/online/**

These sites are annotated on pages 4 and 5.

This unit focuses on the most recent advances that have been reported on nutrients and their role in health and disease. With the onset and development of new technologies in the area of nutrition, the plethora of information on the role of certain nutrients, and the speed with which information is printed and disseminated, even the professional has a very hard time keeping up with the data. The media reports any sensational, even erroneous data, which confuses the public and creates many misunderstandings. Preliminary reports have to undergo rigorous testing in animal models and clinical trials before they are accepted and implemented by the scientific community.

Additionally, how individuals will respond to dietary changes will depend on their genetic make-up along with other environmental factors. Thus, the National Academy of Science has a difficult task in trying to establish exact amounts of nutrients that will cover the requirements but not create toxicity in the long run for the majority of the population.

The articles of this unit have been selected to present current knowledge about nutrients resulting from state-of-the-art research and controversies brewing at the present time. Articles related to nutrient function and their effects on chronic disease such as cardiovascular disease, cancer, and osteoporosis are included. A topic that has serious implications for health, which is not given enough attention, is that of drug/nutrient interactions. Unfortunately many unnecessary deaths or organ malfunctions occur because of these interactions. It seems that the consumer is not aware of or educated about these potential life-threatening effects. Increased awareness, especially among the elderly and low-literacy individuals, will ensure prevention.

The section of the population that has syndrome X has the problem that too many carbohydrates may predispose them to heart disease. The first article in this unit points out that the proliferation of low-fat products that have even more calories than the original product due to added sweeteners worsens syndrome X. Focusing on reducing fat and increasing carbohydrate intake may not be desirable for this particular population. Another area of perennial controversy concerns fats and the types of fat. Americans have focused on single ingredients, attempting to exclude them from food. This has resulted in the proliferation of low-fat products that are not necessarily low in calories. Trans fatty acids that arise from food processing, which convert liquid oils to solid margarines, are as harmful to heart health as saturated fat. Since no labeling exists for fried foods, baked goods, and food purchased in restaurants, the consumer should avoid them, using instead soft or semi-liquid margarine or olive oil, thus limiting trans fat from the diet.

Osteoporosis is a debilitating disease whose incidence is steadily increasing worldwide as the population is getting older and pollution gets worse in major cities around the world. The second article

points out that the National Academy of Sciences has released new and higher recommendations to promote bone health and guard against osteoporosis.

The importance of vitamins is of great interest to consumers since vitamins have been touted to cure and/or prevent disease. It is also the favorite area of many quacks and nutritional salespeople. Recent research about vitamins provides insights into their functions, but also alerts the consumer to be careful of megadosing, since vitamins may have pharmacological effects. The fascinating history and discovery of vitamins that caused clear-cut dietary deficiencies in North America when absent is presented by Kenneth Carpenter in the third article, and the role of food processing as a source of precipitating vitamin deficiencies along with benefits is described. One common fear among aging Americans and baby boomers is memory loss. This has resulted in the increased intake of vitamin supplements. Evidence on the role of B complex vitamins and vitamin E, K, and C on brain function and memory is still sketchy and far from conclusive. Americans in large numbers are taking supplements either to bolster their diet or protect against chronic disease, but they are not aware of when, how, and in what form the vitamins should be taken. They are also unaware of vitamin and mineral interactions that may either enhance or limit the absorption of their supplements. Practical advice offered by professionals is very important to increase consumer awareness and dispel many myths perpetuated from unreliable sources, as the next article points out.

The next two articles discuss Vitamin D and folic acid. Even though research suggests that lack of vitamin D may lower risk of breast and colon cancer, vitamin D is crucial for strong bones. Since vitamin D is found in low amounts in the diet, exposure to sunlight becomes a pivotal factor for enhancing a person's vitamin D supply. Geographical area, skin type, and age are factors that may enhance or diminish the synthesis of Vitamin D. Folic acid has been known to prevent heart disease and birth defects, and, most recently, research has been pointing to its possible role in reducing cancer risk. Since high levels of folic acid taken as supplements may mask vitamin B12 deficiency, consumers are advised to eat food sources high in this vitamin.

Finally, both professionals and consumers are not paying attention to the area of drug/nutrient interactions. This area becomes especially important among the elderly and people with chronic diseases who take a large number of different kinds of medications, as it may bring about primary or secondary nutrient deficiencies and lead to malnutrition. Potentially detrimental effects on body systems and compromising a person's nutritional status as well as death may result from such interactions. Educating the public as to the health problems that may be precipitated by interactions of different categories of drugs and food is crucial to public health, as the last article in this unit points out.

Nutrients

Should You Be Eating *More* Fat and *Fewer* Carbohydrates?

If you have a condition called syndrome X, too many carbohydrates could prove bad for your heart

YOU'VE CUT OUT some of the saturated fat found in foods like burgers, whole milk, and cakes and cookies and now fill up on more high-carbohydrate fare like bread and pasta. But rather than going for an extra helping of spaghetti, would you be doing your heart better by having a little extra fatty salad dressing instead? Or a handful of fatty nuts instead of a bagel? As bizarre as it may sound, it goes right to the heart of a fierce debate raging between nutrition and heart disease experts entrenched in opposing camps.

On one hand are those who argue that while the mono- and polyunsaturated fats in foods like salad dressing and nuts don't raise "bad" LDL-cholesterol in the blood the way that saturated fats do, people should still be limiting them. The reason, they say, is that unsaturated fats, just like saturated ones, supply more than twice as many calories as carbohydrates. And that, in turn, contributes to overweight, which in itself raises blood cholesterol and increases the risk for heart disease.

But **those who argue in favor of poly- and monounsaturated fats over starchy foods and other high-carbohydrate choices say that in an estimated 25 percent of the population, piling on carbohydrates lowers "good" HDL-cholesterol.** It also raises triglycerides (fats in the blood that are now thought to raise heart disease risk on their own); renders LDL-cholesterol even more harmful by making the LDL particles smaller and heavier (and therefore more likely to harm arteries); increases the risk for high blood pressure; and makes the blood more likely to form obstructive clots.

The cluster of problems is known as syndrome X, a term coined in 1988 by Stanford University researcher Gerald Reaven, MD. It occurs in people who are hyperinsulinemic, that is, who secrete too much of the hormone insulin. Carbohydrate-rich foods cause the highest spikes in their insulin levels. That's because after carbohydrates are eaten and broken down into blood sugar, or glucose, insulin is needed to get the glucose out of the bloodstream and into all the body's tissues, where it's used as fuel.

In the 75 percent of the population who aren't hyperinsulinemic, eating a lot of carbohydrate isn't a problem. Their bodies' tissues are insulin-sensitive, meaning they "allow" blood sugar to enter even with the secretion of relatively small amounts of insulin. But in those afflicted with hyperinsulinemia, the pancreas must secrete large amounts of insulin to move sugar out of the blood. The more insulin secreted, the worse the untoward effects. (In some people, hyperinsulinemia is a precursor to diabetes.)

Consider a study on a small group of postmenopausal women with an average age of 66 who appeared to be hyperinsulinemic. For three weeks, Dr. Reaven and colleagues put them on an eating plan that contained 60 percent of calories as carbohydrate and 25 percent as fat. For another three weeks, they ate a diet containing only 40 percent of calories as carbohydrate and 45 percent as fat (protein remained constant at 15 percent of total calories). Both diets had the same number of calories.

For the higher-fat diet, the researchers trimmed the women's carbohydrates and upped their fat consumption by serving them, for instance, peanut butter at breakfast rather than bread. The women also received a little more margarine and salad dressing and a little less potato at dinner.

The result: on the higher-fat regimen, they ended up with an average triglyceride level of just 114 milligrams per deciliter of blood. (Research suggests that the closer to 100 the triglyceride level, the better for the heart. Levels below 100 are ideal.) But they had a significantly higher level of 174 on the diet that was higher in carbohydrates. The higher-fat diet also allowed the women to maintain better "good" HDL-cholesterol levels. But presumably because neither diet had much in the way of saturated fat, "bad" LDL-cholesterol levels did not differ from one eating plan to the other.

From the *Tufts University Health & Nutrition Letter,* February 1999, pp. 1, 4-5. © 1999 by Tufts University Health & Nutrition Letter. Reprinted by permission.

Before you start eating more fat . . .

Not all researchers are convinced that higher-fat regimens should be recommended for the public at large. They argue that **while people who are *fed* a high-fat diet don't have to worry about overdoing it on calories, men and women *on their own* can easily go calorically overboard** on a high-fat diet—and become overweight—because of the fact that fat has nine calories per gram and carbohydrate, only four. And overweight people, in addition to having higher levels of LDL-cholesterol than others, are much more prone to being afflicted with syndrome X. In fact, the condition usually doesn't manifest itself in someone unless he or she is overweight. Excess weight indirectly leads to the release of more insulin.

Consider that the women in the study, while not obese, were decidedly overweight. The average weight of a woman who was, say, five feet, four inches tall was 157 pounds. Desirable weight for a woman that height is fewer than 145 pounds.

Ernst Schaefer, MD, a heart disease researcher who heads the Lipid Metabolism Laboratory at Tufts, is one of those who firmly believes that advising people to eschew carbohydrates for fat would end up doing more harm than good. He points to research which shows that when people migrate from countries where the diet is low in fat to the U.S., where the diet tends to be relatively fatty, weight—and heart disease deaths—rise substantially.

Because of evidence like that, Dr. Schaefer believes that Americans should try to lower their *total* fat intake, not just their intake of saturated fat. He acknowledges that lower-fat diets automatically raise the proportion of carbohydrates someone consumes, which could be a problem for people with syndrome X. But, he says, the weight kept off—or taken off—with reduced-fat diets will attenuate the effects of syndrome X much better than eating a high-fat, lower-carbohydrate diet without any attendant weight loss.

As proof, he points out that the traditional Japanese diet is extremely high in carbohydrates, with rice being a staple—yet people who follow it are protected from heart disease, largely because they remain quite thin. In addition, when University of California researcher Dean Ornish, MD, put people on extremely low-fat, low-calorie, high-carbohydrate diets in which fully 70 to 75 percent of calories came from carbohydrate-rich foods, there was actually a reversal in the progression of their heart disease—no doubt due in part to the fact that they lost an average of 22 pounds in a year's time.

Those on the other side of the fence agree with Dr. Schaefer that losing, or keeping off, excess weight mitigates the effects of syndrome X much more powerfully than eating a diet relatively high in mono- and polyunsaturated fats and relatively low in carbohydrates. But, they argue, it is far from proven that eating low-fat foods automatically helps Americans keep trimmer. For instance, **Walter Willett, MD, head of nutrition at the Harvard University School of Public Health, points to the fact that there has been a proliferation of reduced-fat cakes, cookies, ice cream, luncheon meats, salad dressings, and other foods without a national slimming down.** In fact, Americans are only getting heavier.

The reason, at least to some degree, is that Americans have come to equate low-fat with low-calorie, but many of these products have as many—or more—calories than their full-fat counterparts. Worse still, Dr. Willett notes, in many items like reduced-fat cakes and cookies, the calorie count remains high because when fat is taken out, carbohydrates such as sugar and other sweeteners replace it, which only intensifies insulin secretion in people with syndrome X and thereby worsens their condition.

It is not even clear that people who follow a diet with foods *naturally* low in fat, such as fruits, vegetables, and grains, will lose substantial amounts of weight over the long term. Perhaps people just lose weight at first and then the weight loss tapers off. Long-term data do not exist to settle the issue.

All of which begs the question of just what a person is supposed to do. Fortunately, there is actually much more overlap between the two camps than disagreement. But how to proceed depends largely on your own particular situation.

A personalized approach to keeping your heart healthy

Before you make a decision on whether to follow a low-fat diet with lots of carbohydrates or a diet higher in poly- and monounsaturated fats with fewer carbohydrates, **you need to get some results from your physical at the doctor's office.** Your blood pressure will be measured, and the doctor will also withdraw a little of your blood after an overnight fast. From that blood sample a lab can determine your level of LDL-cholesterol, HDL-cholesterol, triglycerides, blood sugar, and insulin. If your blood pressure is fine and your blood levels of these substances are within normal levels, chances are you don't need to worry much about the proportion of fats or carbohydrates you eat.

Here are the normal levels:

- Blood pressure: less than 140/90
- LDL-cholesterol: less than 160 (less than 130 if you already have two other risk factors for heart disease, such as being a male over age 45, a woman over 55, or overweight)
- HDL-cholesterol: at least 35, preferably 60 or higher
- triglycerides: less than 200, preferably less than 100
- blood sugar: less than 110

The more "out of range" you are on LDL-cholesterol (which is not related to syndrome X), the more important it is to cut back on foods high in saturated fat, which include not just burgers and full-fat dairy products like cheese and premium ice cream but also steaks, roasts, doughnuts, cookies, other pastries, and eggs. The doughnuts and other sweets not only have saturated fat, they also often contain substances called trans fatty acids, which are likely to raise LDL-cholesterol just as much as saturated fat does. And the more LDL-cholesterol in your arteries, the more likely they are to become clogged.

People with high LDL-cholesterol should also lose excess weight, if necessary. Extra pounds raise the concentration of LDL particles.

The more "out of range" you are on all the other parameters, the more likely you are to have syndrome X. Syndrome X is not an all-or-nothing condition; it varies by degree, so some people who have it are "off" on certain measurements but not others.

Lifestyle changes specific to syndrome X:

■ If you are overweight, try to lose some excess poundage. Granted, this is easy to say and hard to do, but Stanford's Dr. Reaven estimates that fully 25 percent of the detrimental effects of syndrome X arising from hyperinsulinemia are attributable to overweight. The good news: losing even just 10 to 15 percent of body weight is enough for some people to significantly blunt syndrome X's effects. It makes their tissues more insulin sensitive, thereby requiring less insulin to be secreted. That means that a five-foot, four-inch woman with syndrome X who weighs 157

pounds can substantially improve her health parameters by getting down to 140 pounds; she doesn't need to achieve, say, 120 pounds for highly beneficial results.

Note: Research suggests, but doesn't prove, that it's easier for most people to lose weight on a diet that's high in carbohydrates and relatively low in fat. As long as significant weight loss occurs, a high-carbohydrate diet should not cause further harm to people with syndrome X. But people with syndrome X might not want to go on a very high-carbohydrate, very low-fat diet that has only about 15 percent of calories as fat. Since carbohydrates do cause higher-than-normal spikes in their insulin levels, they should consider a more moderately reduced-fat diet that has at least 20 percent of calories as fat, if not more. Either way, losing weight is more a matter of reducing *calories* by keeping portion sizes moderate rather than simply choosing anything that has a "low-fat" burst on the label.

■ If you're sedentary, engage in some vigorous physical activity, perhaps for 30 minutes a day, three to five times a week. A sedentary lifestyle, just like excess weight, Dr. Reaven says, is responsible for about 25 percent of the effects of syndrome X.

■ If you're already a healthy weight and moderately active and your

blood tests still indicate that you have syndrome X, eat a little less in the way of carbohydrates and a little more poly- and monounsaturated fats. Admittedly, that could be hard to do without weight gain. Just a handful of nuts could contain a couple of hundred calories. A little extra oil in your stir-fry or margarine on your toast could add 100 calories or more here and there, too. Thus, **as you remove carbohydrates from the diet, be sparing with the amount of fats you add back in.**

And try to remove carbohydrates that are high in sugar and relatively low in nutrients, such as cakes, cookies, and the like (including the reduced-fat varieties). *Don't* remove high-carbohydrate vegetables and fruits. "You should have most of your calories from carbohydrates, no matter what kind of diet" you're on, Harvard's Dr. Willett says. And he and others agree that your high-carbohydrate choices should be items that are naturally low in fact, including beans, vegetables, and fruits.

As far as grains, whole grains are better than refined grains like those in pasta, white bread, and white rice, Drs. Schaefer and Willett say. The fiber they contain may help to slow the rush of sugar into the blood during digestion—and consequently blunt the flow of insulin.

Fats: The Good, the Bad, the Trans

THE STORY

Fats are a dietary paradox. We need them for the essential fatty acids that keep cells healthy, and to help regulate important metabolic processes and transport certain vitamins throughout our bodies. But, for healthy hearts and arteries, we're encouraged to restrict fat to no more than 30 percent of our total daily calorie intake—or about 65 grams a day in a 2,000-calorie diet.

Scientists classify the fatty acids that make up the fat in food as saturated, monounsaturated or polyunsaturated, depending on the degree to which the molecules are saturated with hydrogen atoms (see box "Fat Facts"). While most of the fat we eat contains all three types, one usually predominates. Because saturated fat—the primary fat in red meat and many dairy products—raises blood levels of total and LDL (bad) cholesterol, we're advised to consume no more than 10 percent of total calories as saturated fat. At the other extreme, monounsaturated fats—found abundantly in canola and olive oil—are considered good fats because they lower LDL cholesterol without decreasing HDL (good) cholesterol. Polyunsaturated fats lower both LDL and HDL, but they are also a source of omega-3 fatty acids, which have purported heart-protective properties such as preventing blood clots.

Then there's a fourth category—trans fatty acids (TFAs)—commonly found in cooking oil, margarine, shortening and processed foods made with these ingredients. TFAs arise when hydrogen atoms are added to oils containing mono- or polyunsaturated fats. This so-called hydrogenation process converts liquid oils into a more solid form. Makers of packaged foods and fast-food restaurants use hydrogenated oils extensively because they enhance taste and texture and are more stable during frying and other high-temperature food processing. But a new study suggests that food high in trans fats is just as likely to raise LDL cholesterol as food high in saturated fat—a finding that corroborates results from several other recent studies on TFAs.

To further clarify the effect of TFAs on cholesterol, 36 adults with higher-than-normal blood-cholesterol levels went on five consecutive diets for 35 days each that differed only in trans-fat content. As a benchmark, participants also ate a sixth diet consisting of butter-rich foods (high in saturated fat but low in trans fat) for 35 days. Near the end of each 35-day diet, the Tufts University researchers measured the participants' blood-cholesterol levels.

In all the diets, the fat calories equaled the recommended 30 percent of total daily caloric consumption. Of the five TFA diets, the two diets with the lowest TFA content used liquid oil and semiliquid margarine and had less than 0.5 g of TFAs per 100 g of fat. The diet with the most TFAs included stick margarine and contained 20 g of trans fat. The TFA content of the two remaining diets—made from soft margarine and shortening—fell in the middle of that range. Except for water and noncaloric beverages, participants did not eat or drink anything but the food provided, and no one knew who was getting which diet.

When all the results were compared, the average total and LDL cholesterol levels were highest after people consumed the butter, stick-margarine and shortening diets. The liquid-oil, semiliquid-margarine and soft-margarine diets yielded the lowest average total and LDL levels. When compared with the butter diet, LDL levels from the soft-margarine diet averaged 9 percent lower, those from the semiliquid-margarine diet were 11 percent lower and those from the liquid-oil diet were 12 percent lower.

These findings, in the June 24 *New England Journal of Medicine,* seem straightforward, but how should you apply them to daily food choices?

—*The Editors*

THE PHYSICIAN'S PERSPECTIVE

George Blackburn, M.D.
Associate Editor

This study represents really great science, and for people with cholesterol concerns, it corroborates what other similar studies have found: Foods high in trans fat are just as potentially harmful as foods high in saturated fat. The results are especially believable because researchers carefully controlled the people's diets. This approach is far more reliable than the use of food questionnaires, a more common method of studying the effects of nutrients on health. In questionnaire-based studies, people try to remember what they ate and scientists estimate nutrient intake from those recollections.

But despite the tight dietary controls of this study, we can't generalize the findings to all people, because the participants already had higher-than-normal levels of total and LDL cholesterol. People with normal or low cholesterol levels might not respond the same way. Also, the study involved relatively few people and tracked their cholesterol for a short time. Thus, we don't know if the lower cholesterol levels associated with the low trans-fat diets will last

Fat Facts

Type of Fatty Acid	Primary Sources	State at Room Temperature	Effect on Cholesterol
MONOUNSATURATED	Canola* and olive oils; foods made from and prepared in them	Liquid	Lowers LDL; no effect on HDL
POLYUNSATURATED**	Soybean, safflower, corn, and cottonseed oils; foods made from and prepared in them	Liquid	Lowers both LDL and HDL
SATURATED	Animal fat from red meat, whole milk, and butter	Solid	Raises LDL and total cholesterol
TRANS	Partially hydrogenated vegetable oil used in cooking oil, margarine, shortening, and baked and fried foods	Semi-Solid	Raises LDL and total cholesterol

○ = Carbon atom
● = Hydrogen atom

*Many nutritionists consider canola oil the healthiest vegetable oil because it's low in saturated fat, high in monounsaturated fat, and has a moderate level of omega-3 polyunsaturated fat.

**Contain the omega-3 and omega-6 essential fatty acids that the human body can't make on its own.

Chart by Mary Tanner

and eventually translate into healthier hearts. A much larger study of more than 80,000 women two years ago found that those who ate less saturated fat and TFAs and more mono- and polyunsaturated fats substantially reduced their risk of heart disease, but that was a questionnaire-based study.

Even if we assume that trans fats are as unhealthy as saturated fats for most of us, it's not easy to determine how much trans fat we're eating. Food labels don't list trans-fat content. So the best you can do is make ballpark estimates by looking at the ingredient list. Any food that lists par-

tially hydrogenated vegetable oil as one of the first three ingredients is likely to contain a significant amount of trans fat. Unfortunately, "partially" does not tell us how hydrogenated the oil is—and the more hydrogenated the oil, the more TFAs it contains.

Realize, too, that the majority of the TFAs consumed in the U.S. come from baked goods and food purchased in restaurants, the latter of which usually has no labeling whatsoever. So, when dining out, there's no way to assess whether the french fries you are considering with lunch are a less harmful indulgence than an apple-pie dessert.

In the near future, monitoring TFAs in food may become easier. The federal government is currently engaged in an every-five-year review of dietary guidelines and might issue recommendations for trans-fat intake. Of course, new guidelines would be of limited value without more informative labels, and thus the Food and Drug Administration has announced that it will eventually require trans-fat content on food labels.

For now, though, my advice is to place the findings from this new study in the context of generally healthy eating. First, concentrate on making the most of your daily calories that *don't* come from fat by eating a variety of whole foods, including at least five servings of fruit and vegetables a day. **When it comes to fat, stick to the 30 percent/10 percent rule for total and saturated fat, respectively, by cutting back on red meat and dairy products such as butter and whole milk. To control your trans-fat consumption, go easy on food made with hydrogenated vegetable oils and eliminate fried foods altogether. Also, choose soft or semiliquid margarine that lists liquid vegetable oil as the first ingredient and use nonhydrogenated oils for cooking.** With creative use of herbs and spices, it's entirely possible to enjoy satisfying meals that provide the healthy fats while limiting the unhealthy ones.

FOR MORE INFORMATION:

▼*International Food Information Council, 202-296-6547, ificinfo. health.org*

NATIONAL ACADEMY OF SCIENCES INTRODUCES

NEW CALCIUM RECOMMENDATIONS

LUANN SOLIAH, PhD, R.D., CFCS,
Associate Professor and Dietetics Director, Department of Family and Consumer Sciences, Baylor University

ABSTRACT

Osteoporosis is a serious, chronic condition of porous (easily fractured) bones. It develops silently and slowly over time and is directly related to decreased calcium storage in the bones. New calcium recommendations have been published by the National Academy of Sciences. The new guidelines recommend increased calcium intake to prevent bone deterioration. This article reviews these new guidelines, food sources of calcium, and common calcium supplements. Attaining the increased calcium recommendations is possible, but it does require balanced, healthful food choices.

Osteoporosis is a preventable disease of porous, easily fractured bones. It afflicts more than 28 million Americans—most of them women (Wilde, Economos, & Palombo, 1997). Women are most at risk because bone decreases rapidly after menopause. Prevalence of osteoporosis increases with age; however, prevention strategies can begin at any time in one's life. For adults, proper nutrition, balanced meals, and generous calcium intakes are reasonable preventive recommendations. Specifically, the role of calcium nutrition in bone health is well established (National Institutes of Health [NIH], 1994). High calcium intakes have been shown to reduce the loss of bone in postmenopausal women (Dawson-Hughes et al., 1991) and decrease fractures in persons who had fractures previously (Chapuy et al., 1992).

NEW CALCIUM RECOMMENDATIONS

Scientists agree that bone strength later in life depends on how well the bones are developed during youth and that adequate calcium nutrition during the growing years is essential to achieving optimal peak bone mass (National Acad-

For the first time since 1989, the federal government has increased its recommendations for calcium intake.

emy of Sciences [NAS], 1997; NIH, 1994). On the basis of this agreement, the National Academy of Sciences has released a new report that revises calcium requirements for Americans. For the first time since 1989, the federal government has increased its recommendations for calcium intake (NAS, 1997).

The Food and Nutrition Board at the National Academy of Sciences reviewed, adjusted, and increased the recommendations for calcium because of new research findings. The new recommendations are called Dietary Reference Intakes (DRI), and they expand the scope and application of the former Rec-

ommended Dietary Allowances (RDAs; National Research Council [NCR], 1989; see also NAS, 1997). The new DRIs provide two sets of measures for each nutrient: Adequate Intakes (similar to RDAs) and Tolerable Upper Intake Levels (maximum nutrient intake guidelines; NAS, 1997; "Higher Levels of Calcium," 1997). The concept of the DRIs extends the RDA goal of avoiding nutrient deficiency. DRIs quantify the relationship between a nutrient and the risk for disease (e.g., calcium intake and osteoporosis prevention). Thus, the new DRIs are designed to reflect the latest research about nutrient requirements based on optimizing health among all life-stage groups (NAS, 1997; "Higher Levels of Calcium," 1997).

Table 1 illustrates the new (1997) Adequate Intake (AI) calcium recommendations for each life-stage group. AIs are the observed or experimentally set intake by a defined population or subgroup that appears to sustain a defined nutritional status, such as growth rate, normal circulating nutrient values, or other functional indicators of health (NAS, 1997).

The new DRIs (AI) state that adults between the ages of 19 and 50 years should consume 1,000 mg of calcium per day, and all adults older than 50 years should consume 1,200 mg of calcium per day (NAS, 1997). Some authorities suggest even higher levels of calcium (1,500 mg/day) for post-menopausal women who are not receiving estrogen replacement therapy (Gums, 1996; NIH, 1994; Whitney & Rolfes, 1996). These recommendations are considerably higher than the former 1989 RDAs of 800 mg per day for most adults (NRC, 1989). The calcium recommendations were increased because adults lose bone mass as they age and are, therefore, at increased risk for osteoporosis. The government scientists were responding to the mass of accumulated evidence that the need for calcium is high throughout life (Matkovic & Heaney, 1992; NAS, 1997; NIH, 1994). Research evidence from several controlled, randomized trials verified that the 1989 RDA (10th edition) for calcium was too low and understated the true need for maximum bone accretion (Johnston et al., 1992; Lloyd, Andon, & Rollings, 1993; Recker, Davies, & Hinders, 1992).

There is general agreement that consuming the recommended amount of calcium will help protect bones and teeth over a lifetime. Unfortunately, a relatively small percentage of women (20%–50%) consistently meet their daily calcium requirement (Crane, Hub-bard, & Lewis, 1998; Eck, Relyea, & Klesges, 1997; Galvacs, 1997). The challenge is even greater for female adolescents. The new guidelines recommend that adolescents between the ages of 9 and 18 years should receive 1,300 mg of calcium per day (see Table 1). Data from the Continuing Survey of Food Intakes by Individuals (CSFII) indicate that the proportion of female adolescents who regularly consumed the recommended amount of calcium-rich foods was only about 10% (United States Department of Agriculture [USDA], 1988; see also Crane et al., 1998).

In contrast, young boys and men generally obtain more calcium from their diets because they eat more food (Crane et al., 1998; NRC, 1989; Whitney & Rolfes, 1996). They also have a higher reported intake of mean dairy products (beginning at age 2) compared to girls and women of the same age (USDA, 1988).

SOURCES OF CALCIUM

Bone requires several nutrients to develop normally and to maintain itself after growth ceases. The most important nutrients for proper bone development are protein, calcium, phosphorus, vitamin D, vitamin C, vitamin K, and a few trace minerals (Heaney, 1996). The nutrients most likely to be deficient in western nations are calcium and vitamin D (Heaney, 1996; Ryan, Eleazer, & Egbert, 1995). For this reason, food sources of calcium and vitamin D are important to include in the daily diet.

Dairy foods are excellent sources of both calcium and vitamin D. Milk is fortified with vitamin D and is thus the best guarantee that people will meet their daily requirement (Ryan et al., 1995). In addition, with proper exposure to sunlight, ample vitamin D can be synthesized within the body (Ryan et al., 1995).

Milk, cheese, and yogurt are the primary food sources of calcium (NRC, 1989). In addition, these foods provide multiple nutrients (vitamin D, phosphorus, lactose, and calcium), rather than a single nutrient. The presence of vitamin D and lactose increases the absorption of calcium (Heaney, 1996). Also, calcium appears to be used better if accompanied by a reasonable amount of phosphorus (Spencer, Kramer, & Osis, 1988).

Milk contains about 300 mg of calcium per cup. To consistently meet the 1,200 mg calcium guidelines (for adults 51 years of age and older), a person would have to consume approximately four dairy products or the equivalent each day. Examples of calcium-rich foods are shown in Table 2.

Unfortunately, many adults do not like dairy products or cannot comfortably drink milk. Twenty-five percent of U.S. adults are lactose intolerant (Suarez, Savaiano, & Levitt, 1995). Lactose-intolerant adults need information on lower lactose-content dairy foods (e.g., yogurt and cheese), and they need encouragement to drink small amounts of milk (e.g., 4-oz portions) several times each day. They also need education on calcium-fortified foods such as specially formulated fruit juices. High-calcium dairy products (milk and yogurt with added calcium) and calcium-fortified breads are sold at some supermarkets. Calcium-fortified breakfast cereals provide additional calcium. Powdered nonfat milk can be added to soups and casseroles to augment calcium intake.

A variety of other foods also supply calcium (see Table 2). Leafy green vegetables, legumes, sardines, and some homemade breads provide additional calcium. Dark green, leafy vegetables contain a reasonable amount of calcium, but absorption and binding problems occur, so there is little, if any, calcium

Table 1. **Dietary Reference Intakes for Calcium**

LIFE STAGE GROUP	CALCIUM MG/DAY ADEQUATE INTAKE
Infants	
0–6 months	210
6–12 months	270
Children	
1–3 years	500
4–8 years	800
Males/Females	
9–18 years	1,300
19–50 years	1,000
>51 years	1,200

[a] Adequate Intake is the observed or experimentally set intake by a defined population or subgroup that appears to sustain a defined nutritional status, such as growth rate, normal circulating nutrient values, or other functional indicators of health.

Source: National Academy of Sciences–Institute of Medicine (1997). *Dietary Reference Intakes.* Washington, DC: National Academy Press.

Table 2. Food Sources for Calcium [a]

Food	Portion size	Calcium(mg)
Dairy		
Skim milk	1 cup	301
2% milk	1 cup	298
Whole milk	1 cup	290
Swiss cheese	1 oz	272
Yogurt	1/2 cup	207
Cheddar cheese	1 oz	204
Processed cheese	1 oz	174
Vanilla pudding	1/2 cup	139
Ice cream	1/2 cup	86
Cottage cheese	1/2 cup	63
Vegetables		
Broccoli	1/2 cup	36
Spinach	1/2 cup	27
Okra	1/2 cup	27
Green beans	1/2 cup	17
Protein Foods		
Sardines with bones	3 oz	433
Salmon with bones	3 oz	242
Tofu (soybean curd)	1/2 cup	130
Almonds	1/3 cup	129
Breads		
Waffle	7" waffle	191
Biscuits (two)	3" biscuits	134
Pancakes (two)	4" pancakes	68

a   ESHA Research and West Publishing Company (Nutripro Plus) ® (1993). (Macintosh Version 3.0). Salem, OR.

available for the body's uptake (Weaver & Plawecki, 1994). Specifically, oxalates greatly reduce the absorbability of calcium from vegetarian sources (Weaver, Heaney, Proulx, Hinders, & Packard, 1993). Another dilemma to consider is the enormous quantity of green vegetables (15 cups) that would have to be consumed each day to reach the 1,000 to 1,200 mg recommendation.

Consumers need to read food labels to identify the calcium content of canned, frozen, and packaged foods. If possible, one calcium-rich food needs to be consumed at each meal. A balanced diet that includes all food groups is the best assurance of nutrient adequacy.

CALCIUM SUPPLEMENTS

When calcium requirements cannot be consistently met by eating calcium-rich food, a calcium supplement is recommended. During the menopausal years, calcium supplements of 1,000 mg per day may slow, but cannot fully prevent, the inevitable bone loss of aging (Reid, Ames, Evans, Gamble, & Sharpe, 1993). Nevertheless, supplements are frequently used as a part of therapy for osteoporosis prevention as well as osteoporosis treatment.

A number of types and brand names of calcium supplements are available (see Table 3). The "ideal" calcium sup-

plement would have the following characteristics: reasonable size for comfortable swallowing, no unpleasant side effects, quick dissolving action, highly absorbable, affordable, and the appropriate calcium dosage could be easily achieved. In general, these characteristics are difficult to accomplish.

One of the most important factors to consider is how well the body absorbs and uses calcium from various supplements. The elemental calcium content (absorbable quantity) varies from product to product and directly influences the amount required to achieve the recommended guidelines. For example, calcium carbonate has a 40% absorption rate, thus a 1,200-mg dose provides 480 mg calcium (Gums, 1996). In contrast, calcium gluconate only has a 9% absorption rate and thus would require a 5,333-mg dose to provide an equal quantity of calcium (Gums, 1996).

Basically, three major types of calcium supplements are sold (Whitney & Rolfes, 1996). First, there are purified calcium compounds, such as calcium carbonate, citrate, gluconate, lactate, or phosphate. Second, there are mixtures of calcium with other substances, such as calcium with magnesium, aluminum salts, or vitamin D. Finally, there are powdered calcium products such as bone meal, oyster shell, and dolomite. Dolomite is a "natural" calcium compound (from limestone and marble), but it may be contaminated with hazardous toxic minerals such as cadmium, mercury, or lead (Whitney & Rolfes, 1996).

Only proven bioavailable supplements (e.g., chewable or tablets that meet U.S. Pharmacopeia standards for disintegration) are recommended (Packard & Heaney, 1997). A quick and easy household test for dissolving action is to add one calcium tablet to 6 ounces of vinegar. A high-quality product will dissolve within 30 minutes (Whitney & Rolfes, 1996).

Calcium carbonate is one of the most frequently used supplements, but it may not dissolve in the stomach as easily as some of the other calcium compounds, because it requires gastric acid for optimal absorption. In general, calcium carbonate is absorbed best when it is taken with meals and distributed in small doses throughout the day (Packard & Heaney, 1997).

Calcium citrate is an alternative to calcium carbonate and it offers some unique advantages. Calcium citrate does not require gastric acid for absorption, thus it may be taken with or without meals and it does not interfere with the absorption of other nutrients (McKane et al., 1996). In addition, calcium citrate is available in several forms (effervescent liquitabs, caplets, and tablets).

Calcium lactate and calcium gluconate are much less concentrated than either calcium carbonate or calcium citrate, thus much larger doses have to be taken to receive an equivalent amount (see Table 3). The absorption of calcium from antacids (e.g., Tums or Rolaids) or from powdered materials such as oyster shells is poor.

As previously stated, calcium supplements will not cure osteoporosis, but they may decrease the risk. Along with this advantage, taking calcium supplements may present some disadvantages. For example, some calcium compounds may impair iron, magnesium, and zinc absorption (McKane et al., 1996). Some individuals may be at increased risk for urinary tract stones or kidney damage (Gums, 1996). Other considerations include nutrient-drug interactions. An example of a calcium-drug interaction is calcium and tetracycline. The two together may form an insoluble complex that impairs both mineral and drug absorption. To avoid these problems, consumers should disclose and discuss all the medicine and supplements they take with their health care professionals.

As awareness of osteoporosis increases, more people are seeking advice about calcium supplementation. Consumers need to read the labels of the supplements to determine how many tablets they will have to take each day to receive the appropriate amount. The product's cost can be reduced by choosing generic supplements rather than name brand products. Some of the common side effects of calcium supplements include bloating, gas production, constipation, and reduction in stomach acid. Consumers should be prepared to go through a stage of "trial and error" until they find a product that is the most comfortable choice for them.

CONTEMPORARY APPLICATIONS

Experts agree that it is highly desirable to eat a nutritious diet containing rich sources of calcium. Young adults who achieve a higher bone density are less likely to experience health problems as they grow older. In contrast, low calcium uptake by the bones during the growing years makes a person vulnerable to osteoporosis.

Health policy makers for the government have assessed the situation and concluded that Americans need more calcium in their daily diets to delay bone loss and prevent osteoporosis. Food is always the preferred method for providing calcium. Creative menu planning requires effort; but if at least one calcium-rich food or beverage is provided at each meal on a consistent basis, most of the calcium recommendation can be obtained. For those who cannot drink milk or do not like dairy products, several calcium-fortified foods are available, and they should be included in the diet as often as possible. Furthermore, calcium supplements can increase total calcium provision and help achieve at least part of the new NAS recommendations.

For older adults, proper nutrition, regular physical activity, and health education can decrease the risk of osteoporosis and related bone injuries. Family and consumer science professionals employed in home health care agencies, county extension offices, rehabilitation centers, and area agencies for senior citizens should provide information on healthful food choices and calcium supplements for individuals with

Table 3. **Common Calcium Supplements**		
Product	**Source of calcium and mg of elemental calcium/tablet**	**Number of tablets/day to provide about 900–1,000 mg calcium**
Caltrate 600®	carbonate (600 mg)	1.5
Caltrate 600 + Vitamin D®	carbonate (600 mg)	1.5
Os-Cal 500®	carbonate from oyster shell (500 mg)	2
Os-Cal 500 + Vitamin D®	carbonate from oyster shell (500 mg)	2
Posture® (600 mg)	phosphate (600 mg)	1.5
Posture-Vitamin D®	phosphate (600 mg)	1.5
Citracal®	citrate (200 mg)	5
Citracal® + Vitamin D	citrate (315 mg)	3
Citracal Liquitab®	citrate (500 mg)	2
Tums® 500 mg	carbonate from limestone (500 mg)	2
Tums E-X® 300 mg	carbonate from limestone (300 mg)	3.5
Tums Ultra®	carbonate from limestone (400 mg)	2.5
Calcet® + Vitamin D	carbonate, lactate, gluconate (300 mg)	3.5
Fosfree®	carbonate, gluconate, lactate (175 mg)	6

calcium-related concerns. Community outreach programs on osteoporosis should be developed for middle-aged and senior citizens because they have the potential to reach the largest number of people within a community.

All consumers should be made aware that bone building is not a static process. Osteoporosis is a gradual thinning or weakening of the bones that develops over several decades. The value of consistently healthy lifestyle choices is important to reinforce for good consumer compliance and healthy outcomes. Therefore, even though bone loss is an inevitable consequence of older age, broken bones and osteoporosis can be prevented.

References

Chapuy, M., Arlot, M., Duboeuf, F., Brun, J., Crouzet, B., Arnaud, S., Delmas, P., & Meunier, P. (1992). Vitamin D3 and calcium to prevent hip fractures in elderly women. *New England Journal of Medicine, 327,* 1637–1642.

Crane, N. T., Hubbard, V. S., & Lewis, C. J. (1998). National nutrition objectives and the Dietary Guidelines for Americans. *Nutrition Today 33*(2), 49–58.

Dawson-Hughes, B., Dallal, G., Krall, E., Harris, S., Sokoll, L., & Falconer, G. (1991). Effect of vitamin D supplementation on wintertime and overall bone loss in healthy postmenopausal women. *Annals of Internal Medicine, 115,* 505–512.

Eck, L. H., Relyea, G., & Klesges, L. M. (1997). Awareness of nutrient intake adequacy in adult women. *Journal of The American Dietetic Association Abstracts, 97*(9), A–20.

ESHA Research and West Publishing Company [Nutripro Plus] ® (1993). (Macintosh Version 3.0). Salem, OR.

Galvacs, K. G. (1997). Dietary calcium intake and the prevalence of calcium supplement use among well-educated women. *Journal of The American Dietetic Association Abstracts, 97*(9), A–17.

Gums, J. G. (1996). New methods of diagnosis and treatment of osteoporosis. *U.S. Pharmacist, 21*(9), 85–93.

Heaney, R. P. (1996). Bone mass, nutrition, and other lifestyle factors. *Nutrition Reviews, 54*(4), S3–S10.

Higher levels of calcium recommended in the new Dietary Reference Intakes. (1997). *Nutrition Week, 27*(31), 1, 6.

Johnston, C. C., Miller, J. A., Slemenda, C. W., Reister, T. K., Hui, S., Christian, J. C., & Peacock, M. (1992). Calcium supplementation and increases in bone mineral density in children. *New England Journal of Medicine, 327,* 82–87.

Lloyd, T., Andon, M. B., & Rollings, N. (1993). Calcium supplementation and bone mineral density in adolescent girls. *JAMA, 270,* 841–844.

Matkovic, V., & Heaney, R. P. (1992). Calcium balance during human growth: Evidence for threshold behavior. *American Journal of Clinical Nutrition, 55,* 992–996.

McKane, W. R., Khosla, S., Egan, K. S., Robins, S. P., Burritt, M. F., & Riggs, B. L. (1996). Role of calcium in modulating age-related increases in parathyroid function and bone resorption. *Journal of Clinical Endocrinology Metabolism, 81,* 1699–1703.

National Academy of Sciences-Institute of Medicine. (1997). *Dietary Reference Intakes.* Washington, DC: National Academy Press.

National Institutes of Health Consensus Development Conference. (1994). Optimal Calcium Intake. *JAMA, 272,* 1942–1948.

National Research Council-Food and Nutrition Board. (1989). *Recommended Dietary Allowances* (10th ed.). Washington, DC: National Academy Press.

Packard, P. T., & Heaney, R. P. (1997). Medical nutrition therapy for patients with osteoporosis. *Journal of The American Dietetic Association, 97*(4), 414–417.

Recker, R. R., Davies, K. M., & Hinders S. M. (1992). Bone gain in young adult women. *JAMA, 268,* 2403–2408.

Reid, I. R., Ames, R. W., Evans, M. C., Gamble, G. D., & Sharpe, S. (1993). Effect of calcium supplementation on bone loss in postmenopausal women. *New England Journal of Medicine, 328,* 460–464.

Ryan, C., Eleazer, P., & Egbert, J. (1995). Vitamin D in the elderly. *Nutrition Today, 30,* 228–233.

Spencer, H., Kramer, L., & Osis, D. (1988). Do protein and phosphorus cause calcium loss? *Journal of Nutrition, 118,* 657–660.

Suarez, F. L. Savaiano, D. A., & Levitt, M. D. (1995). A comparison of symptoms after the consumption of milk or lactose-hydrolyzed milk by people with self-reported severe lactose intolerance. *New England Journal of Medicine, 333,* 1–4.

United States Department of Agriculture. (1988). *Food Consumption Nationwide Survey* (Continuing Survey of Food Intakes by Individuals [CSFII]; USDA NFCS, CFS2, Rep. No. 86–93).

Weaver, C. M., Heaney, R. P., Proulx, W. R., Hinders, S. M., & Packard, P. T. (1993). Absorbability of calcium from common beans. *Journal of Food Science, 58,* 1401–1403.

Weaver, C. M., & Plawecki, K. L. (1994). Dietary calcium: Adequacy of a vegetarian diet. *American Journal of Clinical Nutrition, 59,* 1238S–1241S.

Whitney, E. N., & Rolfes, S. R. (1996). *Understanding nutrition* (7th ed.). Minneapolis, MN: West Publishing Company.

Wilde, A., Economos, C., & Palombo, R. (1997). Focus group research in the development of an osteoporosis educational program targeting seniors. *Journal of The American Dietetic Association Abstracts, 97*(9), A–86.

VITAMIN DEFICIENCIES IN NORTH AMERICA IN THE 20TH CENTURY

by Kenneth J. Carpenter, PhD, ScD

Kenneth Carpenter, Kellogg Fellow at Harvard and faculty member at Cambridge (U.K.) for 20 years, moved to Berkeley in 1977. He is known for research on the bioavailability of nutrients (lysine and niacin) and documenting the history of nutrition.

Dr. Carpenter's paper was prepared in response to an invitation from the Editor to provide an end-of-the-century review of an aspect of nutrition history in the 1900s.

Three deficiency diseases are discussed. Infantile scurvy resulted from babies being fed sterilized milk (in which the vitamin C had been destroyed) or formulas that lacked the vitamin. Beriberi occurred among Louisiana farmers consuming fried white rice almost exclusively for three months after harvest, and in Newfoundland, it came from a restricted winter diet that included bread baked with baking soda instead of yeast. Pellagra, the major killer, occurred in the South after millers were equipped to make de-germed corn meal. Food processing was in each case the unexpected source of trouble.

Today we think of nutritional problems in North America typically in terms of excesses rather than deficiencies—the problems associated with an ever-ready supply of foods, combined with a much reduced need for the physical labor that would "burn them off" again, in a society where machines do most of the heavy work. Nevertheless, in our century there have been vitamin deficiencies sufficiently severe to cause at least 50,000 deaths.

A problem that was severe in the big cities in the early years of the century was rickets, which we now know can be prevented by providing infants with supplements of vitamin D. However, it now seems more correct to consider rickets as an air pollution disease than a vitamin deficiency[1] because we normally obtain the active material from the sun's ultraviolet radiation of our skin.[2] The change in circumstance that accounted for the appearance of rickets was the smoke from coal-burning fires that absorbed much of the ultra-violet portion of the sunlight in the big industrial cities in the late 19th and early 20th centuries. In addition, low-income urban housing gave mothers less opportunity to expose their babies to fresh air and sun.

> ## The babies of "good" mothers often risked scurvy.

For those reasons I confine my discussion to diseases caused by the more clear-cut dietary deficiencies of vitamin C, thiamin, and niacin, and will then try to draw some general lessons from these unfortunate experiences.

INFANTILE SCURVY

As the 20th century began, cases of infantile scurvy appeared to be on the increase. For example, in successive 5-year periods, the Children's Hospital of Philadelphia saw 21 cases in the first 5 years, then 35 cases, and from 1910–15, 65 cases.[3] Physicians in the United States had first become aware of the condition in the late 1890's, and it was thought that cases had probably been occurring even earlier, but had then been misdiagnosed as acute rheumatism or an unusual form of rickets.

The young children, typically 6–12 months old, appeared to be paralyzed, but really were extremely reluctant to move from a prone position because it hurt them, and they were in pain if touched or moved. Similar cases were being seen in Europe, and there was much debate as to the cause of the disease. It was agreed that breast-

From *Nutrition Today*, November/December 1999, pp. 223-227. © 1999 by Williams & Wilkins. Reprinted by permission.

fed babies were generally immune, and that scurvy attacked babies who were given either one of the newly developed "formulas" or cow's milk. Also, unlike most disorders, it seemed to be at least as much a problem in better off, highly organized households as in the slums. Some pediatricians linked it particularly to the consumption of sterilized milk, and suggested that the heat process promoted chemical reaction in which toxins were formed.[4]

The heat-sterilization of cow's milk was being encouraged by physicians because one of the major causes of death in infants reared in American cities was summer diarrhea. Given the fairly primitive dairying procedures on farms at that time, and in subsequent transport to the consumer, milk samples showed a high bacterial count. As one pediatrician wrote: "It does not seem fair to put into an infant's stomach a food containing thousands of bacteria in each drop . . . of unknown quality and possibly dangerous."[5]

> ## Beriberi was a seasonal disorder in parts of Louisiana and Newfoundland.

Conscientious mothers, reading of the dangers of germs for their baby would, in some cases, reboil even the sterilized milk that they purchased, just to "make quite sure." These precautions undoubtedly had a major effect in reducing infant deaths from infections, but there remained, unfortunately, the risk of an infant fed solely on sterilized milk developing scurvy.

Adult scurvy, the "sailor's disease," had long been known to be preventable by giving fruit juices and/or fresh vegetables but not dried ones. However, with the successes of the germ theory in explaining many diseases and the failure of some overprocessed preparations of lime juice, the accepted idea began to be questioned. One suggestion was that scurvy came from bacterial toxins that remained even after the organisms themselves had been killed. The idea that scurvy was one of the newly termed "vitamin deficiency diseases" was opposed even by E. V. McCollum, the pioneer experimenter who had demonstrated the "fat-soluble A" and "water soluble B" factors. The principal reason was that he could not reproduce scurvy in his rats, and believed it unlikely that mammalian species would differ so drastically in their requirements. In 1918 he told the American Medical Association he thought it more likely that scurvy "is an intestinal intoxication or an autointoxication."[6]

We now know, of course, that "unlikely" as it may be, rats along with most animal species, make their own vitamin C, and we are one of the few who have lost this ability and require it in our diet. It is also understandable that a cow's milk has less vitamin C than breast milk because her calf does not require it. We now know that heat sterilization, particularly in the presence of copper, will destroy most of the vitamin C that is present. It is also thought that households that did not strictly follow "doctor's orders" at the time may have saved their infants' health by holding them at the table and giving them spoonfuls of mashed potato and gravy, which supplied a little extra of the vitamin, from the family meal.[7]

The simple recommended solution was to supplement the infant's food with orange juice, and efforts were made to ensure that mothers knew its importance. However, there are reports from Canada that the problem continued in the 1950s and 1960s. The mothers were typically from the lowest socioeconomic group and had been feeding their infants on nothing but evaporated milk. This, of course, was not a recommended practice but, since it was still being done, the government decided in 1965 to permit the marketing of evaporated milk with added vitamin C.[8]

BERIBERI

This disease has been thought of as a purely Asian problem and associated with the use of rice as a staple food. When it was first investigated by Western physicians in Japan, they were of the opinion, since people of European descent living there were not subject to it, that Westerners were immune for some reason.[9]

However, it is now clear that Westerners are just as subject to beriberi as anyone else when their diet contains too little thiamin. In 1903 it was reported from Louisiana that a group of rice farmers of French descent suffered in the fall each year from what they called "maladie des jambes" (disease of the legs).[10] It appeared some three months after the farmers had sold their harvest to millers and received white rice in part payment. Apparently they fed on "rice fried in bacon fat" three times a day, and little else, until November. It was then time for the traditional slaughtering of farm animals before winter, and the farmers changed their diet to meat, potatoes, and bread. The condition of the sufferers now slowly improved, with the legs taking the longest to recover their strength. Their condition was already identified as beriberi, but the cause was not yet understood.

In 1928, another physician reported that cases of beriberi were still occurring in the rice farming area of Louisiana and that people had discovered that "taking a trip" to an area with a reputation for its healthiness aided recovery.[11] Interestingly, in both Japan and Brazil also, this had been a common piece of physicians' advice, and in both countries sufferers had been sufficiently well off to take that advice. We can now see that the advantage must have come primarily from a change of diet, and I am reminded of Charles Lamb's fable that the pleasure of eating roast pork was discovered when a Chinese peasant's cottage burnt down accidentally and a pig was burned to death; the peasants decided not to waste the meat but still eat it, then finding how much better it was when cooked, they would periodically burn down another cottage with a pig in it before realizing that there was a cheaper way to obtain it. Similarly, where beriberi was a problem, people could have changed their diet without leaving home.

Beriberi had also been occurring for many years under quite different circumstances in Newfoundland. There coastal fisherman living in small "outposts," ie, harbors along the coast that were frozen and isolated during the winter months, had to live for nearly six months on supplies they had purchased in the autumn. These people had limited means and their supplies consisted mainly of white flour and salted fish and meat, margarine, and molasses.[12] The communities typically had no live yeast and, instead, baked their flour with baking powder. It is now known that this would have destroyed much of the thiamin remaining in the white flour. By the end of the winter, beriberi was a common problem. After synthetic thiamin had become available, the Newfoundland government made its addition to white flour compulsory and the problem disappeared.[13]

> ### In the early parts of the 20th century alcoholics were often thiamine deficient

It had long been known that alcoholics in the United States, as elsewhere, could develop a type of polyneuritis that was similar to that seen in cases of beriberi. As early as 1890 one physician who had worked for a time in China wrote that it was impossible to distinguish the two conditions. However, it was not until 1928 that George Shattuck of the Harvard Medical School suggested that alcoholics might truly be suffering from vitamin deficiency.[14] Further studies confirmed that the clinical condition of most alcoholics could be greatly improved, even though they continued their drinking, if they would take vitamin supplements. This was explained by alcoholics typically failing to eat a normal pattern of meals, and also by their reduced ability to absorb thiamin from their intestinal tract.

After white bread and flour began to be enriched with thiamin and other micronutrients from 1940 on, the appearance of neuritis among men living on "skid row" became less common. However, it has been urged both in the United States and Australia that alcoholic drinks should also be fortified with thiamin. A small proportion of alcoholics still develop a form of brain damage called the Wernicke-Korsakoff syndrome, which is incurable and requires the state to care for them for the rest of

> ### Pellagra was thought to be an infectious disease because of its epidemic appearance early in the century

their lives in some type of institution. There is evidence that an improved supply of thiamin to those at risk would prevent the development of this condition. Since long-term care is so expensive, it would actually be an economic advantage to add thiamin to all alcoholic beverages that are marketed.[15] There is opposition to this from both brewers and temperance organizations, the latter being afraid that beer, in particular, would then be touted as a 'health food.'

PELLAGRA

Pellagra was a disease long known in Europe, but it first seemed to burst onto the scene in the southern United States between 1905 and 1915. The condition was said to be characterized by the three "D's"—dermatitis, diarrhea, and dementia. The most noticeable was the horrible dry flaky dermatitis appearing where the skin had been exposed to the sun. For a time it was suspected that this new "infection" had been carried to the states by immigrants from Northern Italy where it had been a problem throughout the 19th century.[16] Then, since doctors and nurses did not seem to "catch it" from contact with patients, alternative explanations were sought.

In the Mediterranean countries it was believed that eating corn was in some way responsible for the disease since pellagra had been unknown before Columbus had brought corn back from the New World and it had gradually come to be adopted as a staple food. In particular, it was thought that moldy corn might be responsible since the disease usually flared up in springtime when the previous year's corn harvest had been in storage for many months. Because of this, the corn being eaten in the South was investigated for molds. Suspicion turned to the increased proportion of corn now being grown in the Midwest and then shipped in bulk to the South, but nothing deleterious was discovered.

Joseph Goldberger and his colleagues in the Public Health Service carried out some deservedly famous studies of the problem from 1914–1918. In one of them, the diets of families in a Carolina mill village were compared. No difference was found in the amount of corn consumed by pellagrous and nonpellagrous families. However, those with cases of pellagra were found to have consumed considerably less milk.[17] It seemed that the families who remained healthy were those that kept a cow. This was ironic because the local public health authorities had been trying to discourage the practice on the ground that cows attracted flies, and flies carried diseases that might even include pellagra. With hindsight we can understand that cow's milk would be protective against pellagra. Although it has only a very low level of niacin, the protective vitamin, it is a rich source of the amino acid tryptophan, which our body can convert to niacin when it is present in relative excess.[18] I refer to niacin as the "main protective vitamin" because many pellagrous diets were also low in riboflavin, and a mix of B vitamins was often found to be more effective in cure than niacin alone.[19]

Changes in processing caused decreases in dietary niacin status.

Goldberger's work did not provide an explanation for pellagra developing into a serious problem between 1905 and 1915. Studies of dietary patterns in the preceding decade had shown no obvious change from a period when the disease was absent. But we can now see that there had been a change. Before that time, corn was stone-ground to give a meal comparable to whole-wheat flour. The problem with stone-grounding was that the germ of the corn contained most of the oil, and this highly unsaturated fat would make traditional corn meal quickly go rancid during storage, which resulted a short shelf-life for traditional cornmeal.

When the Beall degerminator was developed at the beginning of the century and gradually adopted, it allowed millers to both produce a much more stable degermed corn meal and obtain an additional income from the valuable germ that could be processed to yield an attractive oil. Although the germ formed little more than 10% of the grain, it contained some 60% of the tryptophan, so that the residual meal now contained even less than whole corn.[20]

Most of the niacin remained in the de-germed meal, but evidence has proven that as corn matures, most of the niacin forms complexes that are nutritionally unavailable. This would not matter if the remainder of the whole dietary was niacin-rich, and we know that typical Southern diets contained at least as much wheat as corn products. However, the wheat was also in the form of low-extraction white flour prepared in the modern smooth-roller machinery and relatively poor in both tryptophan and "available niacin." The meat in the typical pellagrous diet was also mainly "fat back" from hog carcasses and really a source of fat rather than tryptophan-rich protein.

"Good" mothers in the South often suffered from pellagra.

As a consequence of all these factors, it seems that the de-germing of the corn portion of the diet could have been just enough to have tipped the balance to its being pellagragenic for the most susceptible. We know that women from 20 to 45 years old were the most likely to develop the condition. I suggest that they were the "good mothers" of traditional families who gave what milk there was to their children and most of any meat to their husband, in the belief that a man needed extra protein to do the work required for him to remain the family's "bread winner."[21]

There remains the question as to why their poorer neighbors across the border into Mexico who typically ate much more corn and much less wheat, meat, and milk, did not have a pellagra problem. This puzzle seems to have been ignored by early investigators. One is reminded of Sherlock Holmes' saying "We must consider the behaviour of the dog in the night," then Dr Watson's "But the dog did nothing in the night," and Holmes again: "that is what is so interesting."

One factor certainly was the greater consumption of beans in Mexico, but another at least as important was their method of processing corn to obtain the meal for tortillas. It is now realized that their initial soaking of the mature grains in an alkaline solution of lime (calcium hydroxide), in addition to softening the corn, splits the niacin from its bound form and makes it nutritionally available.[22] This, in combination with the tryptophan of the germ, is adequate to protect the typical consumer, which is why corn has remained the favorite staple in Mexico and Central America for centuries.

In the United States, Joseph Goldberger went on, in the 1920s, to study which food supplements would help prevent the disease in the South. On the basis of tests first using dogs as a model species, and then confirming the results with mental patients, it was found that dried yeast was a powerful preventive. Then, with the Great Depression threatening to make things worse and an estimated 200,000 cases of pellagra, the American Red Cross organized the distribution of brewer's yeast in areas where pellagra was endemic.[23] In part because of this and also, it seems, because of general awareness that pellagra was a form of malnutrition, the death toll began to diminish from more than 7,000 per year in the late 1920s even before the discovery that niacin (nicotinic acid) was the specific pellagra-preventive vitamin.[24] Since the enrichment of cornmeal with niacin began after 1940, and poverty generally decreased in the South, the disease has virtually disappeared.[25]

> *History provides lessons that are worth learning.*

LESSONS TO BE LEARNED

First, the experience of the rice farmers in Louisiana who chose to eat a diet that induced beriberi reminds us that we do not instinctively choose a balanced diet. In this respect, even chickens do better: I have seen them refuse to eat more than one taste of a purified mix from which thiamin had been accidentally omitted. Early commentators could not believe that beriberi was the result of malnutrition because it affected people with ample means to select a diet of their choice. Now we know better.

From the last example of pellagra, we see that the traditional way of doing things can sometimes provide hidden benefits and that discarding them as trivial can have a high cost. Thus one could fancy that if Columbus had brought corn back to Europe with instructions as to how it was traditionally prepared after soaking in lime, the suffering of hundreds of thousands of corn-eaters in Southern Europe could have been prevented.

One also sees how new techniques of food processing that have obvious advantages may also have a downside for which those with responsibilities for food protection should always be on the lookout. Thus the sterilization of milk was an admirable way to reduce the danger of "summer diarrhea" in infants, but the destruction of vitamin C needed to be compensated. Even now there is the question of whether "evaporated milk," which uneducated mothers may still use to feed their infants, should be supplemented with its missing vitamins, particularly when exported to Third World countries.

Again, the polishing of rice and the de-germing of corn produce palatable products with increased shelf-life. The food industry can restore their content of specific micronutrients with enrichment. Some people will prefer to go back to unrefined products—brown rice, whole-wheat flour, etc.—on the grounds that there may be other unrecognized factors lost in processing. Others will count on obtaining these forms from the variety of other foods that they eat.

At least we can see from these examples from here in North America that life-threatening problems may occur with dietaries that pass the conventional standards of the time. On the other hand, we know that with huge, and ever-increasing populations, most have to be provided with foods that can be transported over long distances and stored through some seasons of the year in forms and under conditions that are not "natural" in most senses of the term.

We have to be grateful to the food industries for their technical skills and organization in maintaining a steady year-round supply of palatable foods. Nevertheless, we will still have to be vigilant in the coming century that some developments, admirable in their immediate effect, do not have some quite unexpected and long-term downside, as demonstrated in these examples from the past.

REFERENCES

1. Loomis WR. Rickets. Sci AM 1970;223(6):71–91.
2. Holick MF. The intimate relationship between sun, skin and vitamin D: a new perspective. Bone 1990;7(2):66–69.
3. Gittings JC. Infantile Scurvy. Arch Pediatr 1923;40: 508–518.
4. Carpenter KJ. The History of Scurvy and Vitamin C. New York: Cambridge University Press; 1986.
5. Freeman RG. Should all milk used for infant feeding be heated for the purpose of killing germs. Arch Pediatr 1898;15:509–514.
6. McCollum EV. The "vitamin" hypothesis and the diseases referable to faulty diet. Am Med Assoc J 1918; 71;937–940.
7. Hess AF. Scurvy Past and Present. Philadelphia: JB Lippincott, 1920.
8. Demers P, Fraser D, et al. An epidemiological study of infantile scurvy in Canada. Can Md Assoc J 1965;93: 573–576.
9. Carpenter KJ. Beriberi, White Rice and Vitamin B. Berkeley: University of California Press, in press.
10. Young FF. Beri-beri in Louisiana. Am Med Assoc J 1903;40:11.
11. Scott LC and Herman GR. Beriberi ("malady des jambes") in Louisiana. Am Med Assoc J 1928;90: 2083–2090.
12. Aykroyd WR. Beriberi and other food deficiency diseases in Newfoundland. J Hyg 1930;30:357–386.
13. Aykroyd WR, Jolliffe N et al. Medical resurvey of nutrition in Newfoundland. Can Med Assoc J 1949;60: 329–352.
14. Shattuck GC. The relation of beri-beri to polyneuritis from other causes. AM J Trop Med 1928;8:539–543.
15. Centerwall BS, and Crigin MH. Prevention of the Wernicke-Korsakoff syndrome. N Engl J Med 1978;299:285–289.
16. Carpenter KJ, ed. Pellagra. Stroudsburg, Pa: Hutchinson Ross; 1981.
17. Spics TD, Bean WB, and Ashe WE Recent advances in the treatment of pellagra ad associated deficiencies. Ann Intern Med 1939;12:1830–1844.
18. Goldberger J, Wheeler GA, and Sydenstricker E. A study of the diet of nonpellagrous and pellagrous households in textile mill communities in South Carolina. Am Med Assoc J 1918;71:944–949.
19. Krehl WA. Discovery of the effect of tryptophan on niacin deficiency. Fed Proc 1981;40:1527–1530.
20. Carpenter KJ. Effect of different method of processing maize on its pellagragenic activity. Fed Proc 1980;40: 1531–1535.
21. Carpenter KJ and Lewin WJ. A re-examination of the composition of diets associated with pellagra. J Nutr 1985;115:543–552.
22. Carter EGA, and Carpenter KJ. The available niacin values of foods for rats and their relation to analytical values. J Nutr 1982;112:2091-2103-3.
23. Etheridge E. The Butterfly Caste: A Social History of Pellagra in the South. Westport, CT: Greenwood Press; 1972.
24. Remington RE. The enigma of pellagra. South Med J 1944;37:605–613.
25. Davis JNP. The decline of pellagra in the Southern United States. Lancet 1964;ii:195–196.

Can Taking Vitamins Protect Your Brain?

Memory loss and losing the ability to think straight is a common fear. Many take vitamins in hopes of keeping it from happening. No one questions that certain severe vitamin deficiencies cause neurological problems. But there is no solid proof yet of extra vitamins protecting the brain, although suggestive studies and a theoretical basis for hope have made this an active area of research.

There are two principal ways that vitamins, or lack thereof, affect brain cells. Some vitamins are *antioxidants,* which means they react with, and therefore blunt the deleterious effects of, *oxygen free radicals.* Oxygen free radicals are a very chemically reactive form of oxygen. What makes them reactive is that they have unpaired electrons. This reactivity means that when they encounter DNA or cellular membranes, they cause damage. The antioxidant properties of some vitamins may be especially relevant in the brain because brain cells are particularly vulnerable to the effects of oxygen free radicals. Brain cells have low levels of *glutathione,* an important cellular peptide, which functions as a natural antioxidant. (Peptides are shorter versions of proteins.) Also, the membranes of brain cells are loaded with polyunsaturated fatty acids, and polyunsaturated fatty acid molecules are easily damaged by oxygen free radicals. Brain cells are highly dependent on large amounts of oxygen for energy production, so they are bound to be exposed to more than their fair share of oxygen free radicals.

The other way that some vitamins affect brain cells is by playing a role in several brain cell *metabolic pathways,* complex chains of biochemical reactions that produce energy and sustain life. A missing vitamin can derail an important metabolic pathway.

Here is a summary of some of the evidence for vitamins that may be important to protecting brain cells.

B vitamins

Folate (or folic acid), B_6, and B_{12} are three of the B vitamins that play an important role in the brain. Epidemiologic studies have hinted at their importance because people with low concentrations in their blood or diet have scored lower on memory and nonverbal abstract thinking tests. Infants fed a formula in which B_6 was inadvertently destroyed through heat processing developed convulsions and had abnormal electroencephalograms, which measure electrical activity in the brain. Adults with low B_6 diets have been reported to have some of the same problems.

The B vitamins are not antioxidants. Instead, they figure in several key metabolic pathways. They play a role in the production of S-adenosylmethionine (SAMe), an important brain molecule that is currently being marketed as an all-purpose feel-good pill. Homocysteine also shares a pathway with this trio of B vitamins; if the vitamin concentrations are low (especially folate), then homocysteine levels go up. High homocysteine concentrations in the blood have been implicated as a cause of heart disease and stroke. And several studies have shown an association between high homocysteine levels and Alzheimer's disease and depression. Severe B_{12} deficiencies can lead to breakdown of the protective myelin sheath that surrounds nerves, which causes nerve damage both inside and outside the spinal cord and brain.

Whether it is important or effective to get these B vitamins in amounts above and beyond what a good diet will provide is a big, unanswered question. But there is no question that with a good diet you can get the minimum requirements—and many people aren't meeting even those basic dietary levels. Framingham Heart Study researchers found that of participants in that study aged 67 and older, 30% weren't getting enough folate, 20% weren't getting enough B_6, and 20–25% weren't getting enough B_{12}. Folate (it is called *folate,* a derivative of *foliage,* because it was first found in spinach) is in leafy greens, organ meats, citrus fruits, and whole grains, although there has been a recent push to increase the amount of folate-fortified food. Vitamin B_6 is in meat, poultry, and fish, as well as in grain and dairy products. Vitamin B_{12} is found in appreciable amounts only in animal products, and in greater quantities in meat than in dairy foods. Strict vegetarians, therefore, need to be mindful of B_{12} deficiency. But the more common danger is *atrophic gastritis,* an inflammation of the stomach lining caused by the immune system, which in extreme cases prevents B_{12} absorption. Atrophic gastritis is a common condition among older people. In the Framingham study, 37% of the people over age 80 had it, although those weren't all necessarily extreme cases. A blood test of B_{12} levels can be used to detect whether atrophic gastritis is causing a B_{12} absorption problem.

Vitamin E

Many people already take vitamin E pills in hopes of staving off memory loss and Alzheimer's. Based on what is known about the way vitamin E works in the body, it's not unreasonable to take it. Not only is it a powerful antioxidant, vitamin E is especially active in cell membranes. And because the membranes of brain cells are loaded with polyunsaturated fatty acids, they are prone to oxygen free radical damage.

The research results on the actual use of vitamin E are a mixed bag. An NIH-funded study published in the April 24, 1997, *New England Journal of Medicine* got a great deal of attention because it showed that large amounts of vitamin E (two doses of 1000 IU per day) slowed the progression of Alzheimer's in people classified as having moderate cases of the disease. And a study published in the July 1999 *American Journal of Epidemiology* based on a large national health survey found that as blood levels of vitamin E per unit of cholesterol decreased, so did people's performance on memory tests. On the other hand, plenty of other studies have shown that neither vitamin E intake nor the amount of the vitamin in the blood correlate with better memory or Alzheimer's prevention.

The main sources of vitamin E in the average diet are the vegetable oils—corn, safflower, soybean oil and so forth—and the increasing number of foods—orange juice and breakfast cereal—to which vitamin E has been added. Even with fortified foods, it is virtually impossible to reach the daily intake levels of 1000 IU or more that some studies have hinted might be good for the brain. You have to take vitamin E pills to get to those kinds of intake levels. But be careful: Large doses of vitamin E can interfere with vitamin K, which is important in blood clotting and might also play a role in the brain. Also,

if you take warfarin (Coumadin) then you have to be cautious about taking vitamin E because it interferes with vitamin K metabolism.

Vitamin K

This vitamin is essential for blood clotting. Babies aren't born with the bacteria and liver function necessary to produce vitamin K, so they are given vitamin K shots in the hospital. But vitamin K is found in so many foods that deficiencies in adults are extremely rare. The tragedy of brain-damaged children being born to women taking warfarin, which blocks the action of vitamin K, has raised the possibility of vitamin K playing a role in brain function. Various lines of research suggest that it may be crucial to *nerve growth factors,* highly specific proteins necessary for neurons. Still, the evidence for vitamin K having an effect on the brain is far from conclusive.

Vitamin C

Like vitamin E, vitamin C is an antioxidant. It is also essential to some important enzyme functions that the body needs to make collagen and *norepinephrine,* a key neurotransmitter. Several studies have shown a correlation between vitamin C blood levels and memory performance, although it's a mistake to take correlation to mean cause and effect. A Swiss study published in the June 1997 *Journal of the American Geriatrics Society* found that in a group of 442 study subjects aged 65–94, high blood concentrations of vitamin C and beta-carotene (a form of vitamin A)—but interestingly, not vitamin E—were associated with better memory performance. But, as the authors noted, vitamin C and beta-carotene come in fruits and vegetables, so this could be a more complicated fruit-and-vegetable effect, not vitamin C and beta-carotene by themselves. That same point has been made about vitamin C with respect to cancer prevention and other health claims made on its behalf.

When (and How) to Take Your Vitamin and Mineral Supplements

ERHAPS YOUR DOCTOR has recommended that you take a calcium supplement to help forestall osteoporosis. Or extra folate, either as a hedge against heart disease or to protect against birth defects. Or maybe you're in the habit of taking a daily multivitamin/mineral supplement to bolster a diet that's sometimes not as nutritious as you'd like it to be.

In any case, you may have wondered whether your body is really soaking up whatever nutrients are compressed into that little pill. Should you take it with food or without? Avoid certain beverages, like coffee? And, if you're taking more than one kind of vitamin or mineral, swallow the tablets all at once—or spread them throughout the day?

"There's a lot of mythology out there," says Robert Russell, MD, a gastroenterologist at Tufts. To clear up the confusion, we've spelled out what you need to consider when you're looking to get the most from your vitamin or mineral supplements.

If you take a multivitamin pill . . .

The advice here is straightforward: take your daily multivitamin/mineral supplement with a meal. A full stomach takes longer to empty, allowing more time for muscles there to agitate and break down the tablet at the same time that they shred food. That lets the pill dissolve more thoroughly and, in turn, be absorbed more easily into the system later on. Having food in the stomach may also help reduce the gastric irritation that some people experience with vitamin pills.

It's not necessary to spend a lot of money on a daily multivitamin. **Supplements marked "timed released," in particular, aren't worth the extra expense.** GNC's Women's Ultra Mega, for example, costs $21.99 for a 45-day supply of horse-sized pills claiming "Timed release for around-the-clock impact." But, "timed release' on vitamin products does not mean anything at all," says Srini Srinivasan, PhD, director of the Dietary Supplements Division at the United States Pharmacopeia (USP), a scientific body of experts that sets quality standards for drugs as well as supplements.

That's because there's no need to maintain a precise, constant level of vitamins in body fluids as you would for prescription drugs such as antibiotics. Thus, any standard preparation, like Theragran-M, One-A-Day Maximum, or a pharmacy brand, will do.

However, make sure to look for a designation of USP on the label. That assures you that the product has been lab-tested to disintegrate and dissolve (so that its ingredients can be properly absorbed), and that its potency and purity meet established standards.

If you take single vitamins or minerals . . .

Iron Iron is often a concern for women of childbearing age, who may not get enough of it from food to make up for losses of iron-rich blood during menstruation. Women who take iron supplements (or multivitamin/mineral pills that contain iron), should take them at mealtime, or with a glass of juice. Certain foods, including iron-rich meat, fish, and poultry—and vitamin C-rich juice, fruits, and vegetables—help the body to extract more iron from supplements.

If you're a tea or coffee drinker, however, it's best to avoid those two beverages when taking an iron supplement or eating an iron-rich meal. Substances in coffee called polyphenols can inhibit absorption of iron from plant foods by as much as 40 percent. Tannins, the polyphenols found in tea, can inhibit iron absorption up to 70 percent. Wait about an hour and a half before taking your beverage break.

Another potential iron blocker is the mineral calcium, which has been shown in some lab studies to inhibit iron absorption. If you depend on a multivitamin/mineral supplement to round out your iron intake, you may be concerned, since many multi's include both calcium and iron. But, according to the USP's Dr. Srinivasan, there's probably not enough calcium in any daily multivitamin/mineral preparation to cause a problem. "No single multi will give you large doses of calcium, such as the 1,000 to 1,200 milligrams necessary to meet the RDA," he says. It "would be too big to swallow." Multi's tend to contain only between 100 and 200 milligrams of calcium.

If you are taking an iron-containing multi and a separate calcium supplement, you can avoid potential interactions altogether by taking the pills at different meals. But whether you even need to worry about iron-calcium interactions is controversial. According to James Fleet, PhD, a mineral expert at the University of North Carolina at Greensboro, the interaction is a valid one. But, he says, "Even the best research doesn't necessarily reflect what happens in the real world," where people eat different foods—in different amounts—every day. In other words, as he puts it, "the debate about calcium and iron may simply be a tempest in a teapot."

Indeed, clinical studies by Bess Dawson-Hughes, MD, who heads the Calcium and Bone Metabolism Laboratory at Tufts's USDA Human Nutrition Research Center, have shown that iron status was virtually unchanged in premenopausal women who took 1,000 milligrams of calcium a day for three months. Granted, some studies have shown impaired iron absorption in women who ate high-calcium test meals in a research lab, but Dr. Dawson-Hughes comments that "we didn't see the same problem in real diets."

The bottom line: Combining iron and calcium is not an issue for most people. However, those whose iron is on the low side might choose to play it safe by taking calcium supplements separately from their iron pills—or taking calcium tablets at a relatively low-iron meal, like a meatless lunch.

Calcium If calcium is your priority, as it is for many women trying to forestall brittle bones in their later years, the focus changes from getting enough iron to getting enough calcium.

Calcium carbonate, the most widely available form of calcium (found in Tums and other popular supplements), "is absorbed more consistently" with meals, says Dr. Dawson-Hughes. But the most important thing to remember, especially for those following a high-dose calcium regimen, is to divide the doses. **"If you're taking 1,000 to 1,200 milligrams of calcium a day, you should divide the doses in half, one in the morning, one in the evening, to get the best absorption,"** says Leon Ellenbogen, PhD, adjunct professor at Cornell University Medical College. The body may not be able to absorb larger doses all at once.

Also, it's a good idea in many cases to choose a calcium supplement that contains vitamin D, without which calcium cannot be efficiently absorbed. People who live in northern latitudes (like Boston or Chicago) or otherwise don't get enough sun are at the greatest risk for not getting the 200 to 600 International Units of vitamin D they need each day (vitamin D is manufactured in the skin upon ex-

posure to the sun's rays). They should look for a supplement that has 200 to 400 units of D per 1,000 milligrams of calcium.

It should be noted that a significant portion of the population (an estimated 20 percent of people over 60 and 40 percent of people over 80) cannot absorb some kinds of calcium supplements *unless* they take them at mealtime. These people have a condition called atrophic gastritis, in which they don't secrete enough stomach acid in between meals to break down calcium carbonate.

Most people don't know whether they have atrophic gastritis—it tends to go undiagnosed—but once you're past 60 it doesn't hurt to play it safe and assume you do. Fortunately, there are two ways around it. The obvious one is to take calcium citrate instead of calcium carbonate. It can be absorbed with or between meals, whether or not the stomach secretes enough acid. The drawback is that it's hard to pack enough into a pill: you'd need to take two or three tablets to get the same 500 to 600 milligrams of calcium found in one calcium carbonate tablet. Calcium citrate also trends to be more expensive.

Chelated minerals Available at many health food stores, chelated minerals aren't worth the extra money you'll pay for their promises of superiority. The term "chelated" doesn't mean that a mineral is more absorbable or more available to the body than the unchelated form; it merely describes a type of chemical bond that can occur when a mineral is attached to certain compounds. If a manufacturer claims that a particular chelated formulation has been proven more absorbable in scientific studies, "they're lying," says mineral expert Dr. Fleet. "There are no great studies doing direct comparison" of chelated minerals to other kinds.

The B vitamins The B vitamins—thiamin, niacin, riboflavin, folate, and vitamins B_6 and B_{12}—"are generally very easily absorbed," says Tufts's Dr. Russell. The exception, as with calcium, is for people with atrophic gastritis, who can't absorb enough vitamin B_{12} because they don't have enough acid in their stomach to cleave the vitamin from the protein in food. For that reason, people over 50 should take a supplement with 2.4 micrograms of B_{12} (the RDA) or regularly eat B_{12} fortified cereal—regardless of how much they get from foods such as meat, fish, poultry, or cheese. The B_{12} from supplemental sources is easily absorbed whether or not stomach acid is present.

Vitamins C and E Although experts continue to debate whether doses beyond the RDA are truly beneficial, vitamins C and E are currently the two most popular vitamins on the market. Since neither one has any significant absorption or interaction problems, the choice (if you choose to take them at all) is whether to buy them in "special" forms—such as natural vitamin E or vitamin C with rose hips or bioflavonids.

"The natural form of vitamin E (which is simply a different configuration of the same chemical compound) is in fact more rapidly absorbed and more avidly maintained in tissue," explains Jeffrey Blumberg, PhD, an antioxidant expert at Tufts University's Human Nutrition Research Center. For that reason, he says, you need more synthetic vitamin E to have the same effect. How much more? Researchers used to think that 1.36 International Units of synthetic vitamin E were equal to one unit of the natural form. But Dr. Blumberg says that recent research indicates the natural form may be nearly twice as strong.

The dose associated with E's potential benefits (protecting against heart disease and boosting immune function), ranges from 100 to 400 units. Depending on how much different preparations cost, it may require doing a bit of math to figure out whether you're better off getting the more expensive natural vitamin E or just taking more of the less costly synthetic form.

Unlike vitamin E, the natural and synthetic forms of vitamin C are equally potent—it doesn't matter whether you get the vitamin from pills, foods, or rose-hip extracts. Paying a premium for esterified vitamin C preparations or "enhancers" like bioflavonoids, which haven't been shown to have any absorption benefits, doesn't appear to be worth the extra money, either.

The best D-fense

Does vitamin D, or the lack of it, have anything to do with breast cancer? With prostate cancer? An interesting new theory says it may. Mortality rates for both cancers are lower in regions where sunlight is most plentiful. Since sunlight is responsible for producing vitamin D in the human body, researchers have wondered if this could be the connection. Some test-tube studies have shown that vitamin D inhibits the growth of cancer cells, including those in the breast and prostate.

Last year a research team at the Northern California Cancer Center analyzed statistics from a survey of a large group of American women and found that women with higher sun exposure and those with a high dietary intake of vitamin D had a lower risk of breast cancer. This was backed up by a study from the University of North Carolina at Chapel Hill.

Any news that might help unravel cancer mysteries is welcome, but this is very preliminary research. Some evidence also points to a link between vitamin D and reduced risk of colon cancer. But all this does not mean you should move south or start sunbathing.

What is this thing called vitamin D?

Unique among the vitamins, vitamin D is a hormone, and like other hormones it is manufactured in the body. It helps the body utilize calcium and phosphorus and builds bones and teeth. Like many other nutrients, it probably has a beneficial effect on the immune system. You don't actually need to consume vitamin D, provided you get a minimal amount of sunlight, which causes your skin cells to manufacture the vitamin.

Some groups of Americans, especially those over 60, tend to be deficient in vitamin D. Thus, last year the Food and Nutrition Board of the National Academy of Sciences revised its vitamin D recommendations upwards for older people: while those under 50 need only 200 IU (international units) daily, those 50 to 70 should get 400 IU, and those over 70 need 600 IU.

If you get even 10 or 15 minutes of sunlight on your arms and face two or three times a week, you will probably manufacture enough vitamin D to meet your needs. And because it is a fat-soluble vitamin, you can store enough to supply you in the days, or even months, when you don't get any sun exposure.

Nevertheless, it's a good idea to drink milk—for many reasons, among them that milk is fortified with vitamin D. Each cup contains 100 IU. Other foods containing vitamin D are fatty fish such as salmon and sardines, egg yolks, and fortified breakfast cereals. (Yogurt is *not*

made from fortified milk.) Too much vitamin D can be toxic, but it's nearly impossible to get too much from food, and it is impossible to get too much from sun exposure.

Is geography a problem? Skin type?

Your ability to make vitamin D from sunlight varies according to your location and the time of year. According to Dr. Michael Holick, an expert in vitamin D at Boston University Medical Center, those who live at a latitude of 42° (a line that runs through Boston, Detroit, Chicago, the middle of Iowa, and southern Oregon) can manufacture sufficient vitamin D from a minimal amount of sun exposure between April through October. That is generally sufficient, because you will store enough vitamin D for the winter. People farther south—in Washington, D.C., for example—can manufacture the vitamin from March through November. The darker Canadian winter may have six months or more when the sun isn't sufficient to manufacture D. But most Canadians (and those living in the northern U.S.) will be all right, particularly if they get some dietary vitamin D.

If you have dark skin, especially if you are African-American, you may need longer exposure to sunlight—perhaps up to twice as much as a light-skinned person—since skin pigmentation screens sunlight and reduces vitamin D production.

Is your age a problem?

As you grow older, your ability to manufacture vitamin D in the sunlight declines, and just increasing your exposure time won't do the trick. By the time you are 70, your vitamin D production is only 30% of what it was when you were 25. That's why you need to increase your dietary intake. Anyone over 60 who doesn't get adequate amounts of vitamin D from foods and also lacks sun exposure will need supplements. Those at highest risk are the homebound or institutionalized, as well as those living in the northern third of this country and in Canada.

Vegans and others who don't drink milk may also need to take a supplement.

Supplements are tricky, however, because even small overdoses of D can be toxic, leading to kidney stones, kidney failure, muscle and bone weakness, and other problems. Danger starts at 2,000 IU a day. *Nearly all documented cases of vitamin D toxicity were caused by supplements.* A daily multivitamin with 400 IU of vitamin D is usually the best solution. But it makes sense to discuss your risk of vitamin D deficiency with a health professional.

Sunscreen note

Sunscreen can reduce or even shut down the synthesis of vitamin D.

This is a problem chiefly for older people, who are often more conscientious about using sunscreen than the young, but who also produce less D. Try to get 15 minutes exposure without sunscreen in the early morning or late afternoon, when the sun is less damaging. Then apply sunscreen if you plan to stay out longer, particularly if you are fair-skinned.

Final word: *You should consider taking 400 IU of vitamin D daily if you fall into one of the following categories:*

■ *Housebound, get little sun.*

■ *Vegan (consume no animal products, and thus no milk, eggs, or fish).*

■ *Over 60, seldom get sun, and drink little or no milk.*

■ *over 70.*

Best source: a multivitamin.

Folate May Offer Protection

In addition to preventing birth defects and heart disease, researchers are discovering that folate may help reduce the risk for cancer. Getting enough of this B vitamin is easy. By eating a diet rich in a variety of vegetables, fruits, beans and whole and enriched grains, you should be getting all you need.

Gᴿᴬᴺᴰᴹᴬ ꜱᴀɪᴅ ɪᴛ ꜰɪʀꜱᴛ. Eating your greens is a good idea. Folate, an essential nutrient found in leafy greens and other plant-based foods, may help protect the body from cancer. Science today is bearing out what this wise woman knew all along.

At the Department of Biochemistry and Molecular Biology at the University of Nebraska Medical Center, Professor Judith Christman, Ph.D., is studying how diets lacking in folate influence the cancer process. With a grant from AICR, Dr. Christman is looking closely at animals to see the genetic abnormalities that can arise when the diet lacks this B vitamin.

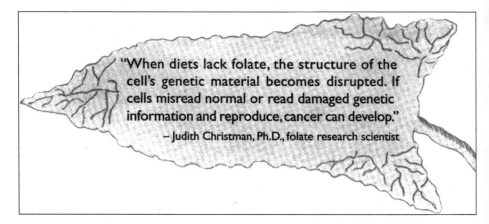

"When diets lack folate, the structure of the cell's genetic material becomes disrupted. If cells misread normal or read damaged genetic information and reproduce, cancer can develop."

– Judith Christman, Ph.D., folate research scientist

Lack of Folate Changes DNA

"When diets lack folate," explains Dr. Christman, "the structure of the cell's genetic material becomes disrupted. If cells misread normal or read damaged genetic information and reproduce, cancer can develop." And the rapidly dividing cells of the body may accumulate more abnormalities. "The more abnormalities in a cell's genetic material, the greater its chances of becoming cancerous," says Dr. Christman.

Links between folate deficiency and lung and uterine cancers are becoming clear. "These are organ sites where cells reproduce quickly," says Dr. Christman. Folate deficiency, along with high alcohol consumption, may also be implicated in cancers of the liver and colon.

Figuring out the exact folate-cancer link is still challenging researchers. "What is clear is that diets lacking in folate have been implicated in a wide variety of chronic diseases," says Dr. Christman.

Folate and Fetal Health, Heart Health

Researchers have found an almost complete absence in spinal cord and brain deformities in babies born to women consuming adequate folate. In other studies, a lack of folate causes homocysteine to accumulate in the blood. High homocysteine levels have been linked to heart attacks, strokes and other vascular diseases.

Get Your Folate

"Fortunately, consuming an adequate amount of folate each day is easier than most people think," says Dr. Christman. In general, diets that feature a variety of vegetables, fruits, whole grains and beans ensure an adequate folate intake. Lentils, soybeans and other beans, peanuts, spinach, kale, asparagus, artichokes, bananas and orange juice are particularly rich sources of this vitamin. In addition, since January 1, 1998, all enriched flour in the U.S. is fortified with folic acid. This means that bread, breakfast cereal and even pasta made with enriched flour are good sources of folate.

How Much Is Enough?

All healthy people are advised to get 400 micrograms (mcg) of folate daily. All pregnant women and women who could become pregnant are advised to get 600 mcg a day and should consider taking a folate supplement.

Supplements are not for everyone, however. In spite of the fact that folate is a water-soluble vitamin with a low risk of toxicity, folate in levels of more than 1000 mcg a day can mask a vitamin B-12 deficiency which could lead to permanent nerve damage if not treated. In addition, studies with cells and animals show that high-level folate supplementation can speed up tumor growth. Although not proven in humans, there may be a danger of promoting an existing cancer with excessive folate supplementation.

Quick Facts . . .

Medications need to be taken at different times relative to meals.

Drugs and medications can interact with nutrients in food.

Consult a physician when health problems persist.

During pregnancy and nursing always consult a physician or pharmacist before taking any medication. Drugs taken by the mother may affect the infant.

Take all medications only with water, unless otherwise advised.

Check with a doctor or pharmacist for the proper way and time to take medication.

Nutrient-Drug Interactions and Food

by J. Anderson and H. Hart[1]

It is a difficult and complex problem to accurately determine the effects of food and nutrients on a particular drug. There are many dramatic results or problems caused by food-drug, drug-drug and alcohol-food-drug interactions. The following table is designed to help the reader become more knowledgeable about drug interactions and their effect on food, a nutrient or another drug that may produce unexpected results or cause additional health problems.

Generic Drugs

Generic drugs often are substituted for brand-name counterparts. They usually are more economical than brand-name drugs. Possible exceptions might be enteric-coated aspirin.

Patients may have concerns about the quality, efficacy, potency or consistency of generic drugs. Generics are therapeutically equivalent to brands approved and rated by the Food and Drug Administration. Many are made by major brand-name companies.

Over-the-Counter (OTC) Drugs

Points to remember:
- OTC drugs usually are meant only to relieve symptoms, not cure a disease or illness.
- Improper use can make symptoms worse or conceal a serious condition that should be brought to a doctor's attention. Never take OTC drugs longer than recommended on the label. If symptoms persist or if new symptoms occur, see a doctor.
- Read the label carefully before taking an OTC product and every time an OTC product is bought. There may be important changes in indications, warnings or directions.
- People with allergies or chronic health problems should be especially careful to read the ingredient, warning and caution statements carefully. If there are any questions, consult a doctor or pharmacist.
- Check expiration dates from time to time. Destroy in the safest way possible any drugs that are outdated or that have deteriorated, such as discolored eyedrops or ointment, or vinegar-smelling aspirin.

Reprinted with permission from Colorado State University Cooperative Extension, Fact Sheet 9.361, December 1998, *Nutrition Quackery,* J. Anderson, L. Patterson, and B. Daly, Dept. of Food Science and Human Nutrition. © 1998 by Colorado State University.

Table 1: Effects of food and nutrients on drugs.

If You Take:	Be Careful With:	Because:
Analgesic and anti-inflammatory agents: Aspirin, Ibuprofen, Indomethacin, Acetaminophen	Co-administration with food.	Absorption rate may be delayed or reduced due to decreased stomach emptying rate.
Antibiotics: Penicillin Erythromycin Tetracycline	Acidic foods: caffeine drinks, tomatoes, fruit juice. Same as penecillin. Foods rich in calcium: milk, cheese, ice cream, yogurt. Don't avoid milk products but take them at a different time.	Increase stomach acid may increase destruction of this drug in the stomach. Empty stomach for better absorption. Calcium, iron preparations and some antacids decrease absorption of the drug or render it ineffective, probably due to chelation and an increase in gastric pH.
Anticoagulants: (Blood Thinners) Dicumarol, Coumadin	Green leafy vegetables, beef liver, broccoli, asparagus, mineral oil, tomato, coffee	These foods contain vitamin K (promotes blood clotting), which interfere with the effect of the blood thinner. Mineral oil decreases the absorption of vitamin K and may increase the effect of the anticoagulant.
Antidepressants: (MAO-monoamine oxidase inhibitors	Tyramine-rich foods: aged cheese, avocados, wine, sour cream, chicken livers, yeast products, pickled herring. Excessive caffeine: chocolate, tea, coffee.	Tyramine may cause potentially lethal increases in blood pressure, fever, terrible headache, vomiting, possibly death.
Antihypertensives: (Drugs for high blood pressure)	Natural licorice. Foods with excessive sodium: cured meats, pickled vegetables, canned soups, processed foods, especially cheese, salted snacks, added salt at table.	Natural licorice contains a substance that causes excessive water retention and thereby increased blood pressure.
Bronchodilators: Theophylline	Charcoal-broiled foods and high carbohydrate diet. Don't eat large amounts of high protein foods: meat, milk, eggs, cheese.	Too much charcoal and carbohydrates decreases absorption of this drug. Protein increases the metabolism of the drug.
Corticosteroids: Prednisone, Solu-medrol, Hydrocortisone	Foods high in sodium: cured meats, pickled vegetables, canned soups, processed foods, especially cheese, salted snacks, added salt at table.	This class of drugs causes increased sodium and water retention leading to edema.
Diuretics: Potassium Wasting: Modiuretic, Naqua, Lasix, Oretic	Natural licorice	See antihypertensives. Diuretics may cause excessive losses of potassium and severe electrolyte disturbances; also loss of vitamin B complex, magnesium, calcium.
Laxatives: Dulcolax	Milk	Laxative becomes ineffective and causes stomach irritation.
Iron supplements:	Taking with bran, or with calcium, zinc or copper supplements.	These minerals and bran make iron unavailable.
Potassium Sparing: Dyrenium, Aldactone	Potassium-rich foods: bananas, figs, wheat germ, orange juice (2 or 3 glasses), salt substitutes, Monosodium glutamate (MSG), sodium-rich foods.	May cause excessive retention of potassium and cardiac problems. Salt substitutes may contain potassium rather than sodium.
Theophylline: Theolair, Somophylline Levodopa (L-Dopa) (for Parkinson's disease)	Co-administration with food. High protein foods: milk, meat, eggs, cheese. Foods rich in vitamin B_6: beef/pork liver, wheat germ, yeast products.	Decreased absorption rate. An increase in protein decreases the absorption of this drug. B_6 antagonizes the drug.

Table 2: Effects of drugs on food or nutrients.

If You Take:	You May Require Extra	Because
Alcohol, particularly excessive use.	Vitamin B_{12}, folate, magnesium.	Turnover of these nutrients increases, and food intake decreases.
Analgesics: Salicylates (aspirin)	Vitamin C, folate, vitamin K.	Aspirin increases loss of vitamin C and competes with folate and vitamin K.
Antacids	Thiamin (Vitamin B_1), taken at a different time., Depending on type of antacid, possibly magnesium, phosphorus, iron, vitamin A, folate.	Inactivates thiamine. These drugs cause decreased absorption of these nutrients.
Antibiotics	Nutrients	Appetite suppression and diarrhea are caused by some of these agents.
Anticancer drugs.	Nutrients	See Antibiotics.
Anticholinergics: Elavil, Thorazine	Fluids	Saliva thickens and loses its ability to prevent tooth decay.
Anticonvulsants	Folate, vitamin D.	These drugs cause decreased absorption of folate, possibly leading to megaloblastic anemia. Increases turnover of vitamin D, especially in children.
Antidepressants: Lithium carbonate, Lithane, Lithobid, Lithonate, Lithotabs, Eskalith	Water (2–3 qts./day) and take with food.	This medication may cause a metallic taste, nausea, vomiting, dry mouth, loss of appetite, weight gain and increased thirst.
Sedatives: Barbiturates	Folate, vitamin D, vitamin B_{12}, thiamin, vitamin C.	Drugs increase the rate these vitamins are used by the body.
Anti-inflammatory agents	Folate	These medications decrease folate absorption.
Cholesterol-lowering medications: Questran	Fat-soluble vitamins: A, D, E, K, folate, iron.	May cause decreased absorption of these vitamins and minerals.
Corticosteroids: Prednisone, Solu-Medrol Hydrocortisone	Protein, potassium, calcium, magnesium, zinc, vitamin C, vitamin B_6.	These drugs cause an increase in excretion.
Diuretics: Potassium wasting; Naqua, Lasix, Oretic	Potassium, calcium, magnesium, zinc.	These drugs cause an increase in excretion of these minerals.
Mineral oil	Fat-soluble vitamins: A, D, E, and K; calcium, phosphorus, potassium.	Mineral oil decreases absorption of these vitamins and minerals.
Oral contraceptives	Vitamin B_6 and folate.	They may cause selective malabsorption or increased metabolism and turnover.
Antacids	Tagamet, Indomethacin, Naprosyn	Antacids inhibit or delay the absorption of these medications.

- Keep all drugs and medications out of the reach of children.
- When pregnant or nursing a baby, check with a health professional before taking any drugs.

Aspirin vs. Acetaminophen vs. Ibuprofen

Aspirin, acetaminophen and ibuprofen all have analgesic (pain control) and antipyretic (fever control) properties. Only aspirin and ibuprofen also contain anti-inflammatory properties. Acetaminophen does not produce the stomach or intestinal irritation or allergic reactions that aspirin can. Gastrointestinal side effects observed with aspirin are greatly reduced with ibuprofen, although patients with aspirin hypersensitivity can have similar reactions.

To reduce stomach upset from ibuprofen, take it with food or an antacid. Avoid alcohol or aspirin with ibuprofen.

Table 3: Effects of drugs on drugs.

If You Take:	Be Careful With	Because:
Anticonvulsant medication: Dilantin	Anticoagulants Digitalis heart medications. Sulfa antibiotics. Antabuse.	Many produce toxic levels of Dilantin and cause hemorrhaging by raising the anticoagulant level. After prolonged anticonvulsant therapy, effectiveness of digatalis medication may decrease. May prevent normal elimination of epilepsy drugs. If taken on top of Dilantin, each drug may independently produce serious side effects. Nervous system toxicity and blood ailments are possibilities.
Antidepressants: Tricyclics: Sinequan Adapin, Elavil Lithium, Norpramin	Alcohol, barbiturates, Tagamet Blood thinners Diuretics Anticonvulsants MAO inhibitors (used for depression or high blood pressure). Minor tranquilizers: Benzodiazepines.	Sedation and drop in body temperature may occur. Decreased absorption. Antidepressant toxicity can occur. Increased anticoagulant effect. Increases effect of Lithium. Antidepressants can increase seizure susceptibility. May cause excitation, delirium, rapid pulse, elevated body temperature and convulsions. Severe sedation may make concentrating difficult and driving dangerous.
Antidiabetic agents (oral and insulin)	Calcium channel blockers: Isoptin, Calan. Oral contraceptives. MAO Inhibitors, Tetracycline.	These medications alter carbohydrate metabolism. Impair glucose tolerance. Hypoglycemia can occur.
Antihistamines	Alcohol	Sedation can occur.
Arthritis medication (potent anti-inflammatory agents)	Blood thinners. Aspirin, aspirin-containing pain relievers. Birth control pills.	Increases susceptibility to internal hemorrhaging. May result in ulcers. Aspirin can diminish the effectiveness of the more powerful drug. Could decrease effectiveness.
Aspirin	Diabetes medicine (oral) Drugs for gout. Vitamin C.	May cause excessive lowering of blood sugar. Aspirin can block the beneficial effects. Never combine them. Large doses of vitamin C can prolong and possibly intensify the action of aspirin. Could produce salicylate side effects (headaches or dizziness) in sensitive people.
Barbiturates	Alcohol.	Increased central nervous system depression.
Benzodiazepine: Valium, Librium, Tranxene, Xanax	Tagamet	Increased sedation can occur.
Blood thinners: Coumadin, Dicumarol	Analgesic pain relievers: aspirin products and arthritis medication. Alcohol Antibiotics. Cholesterol-lowering medications: Atromid-S Thyroid gland supplements. Questran, laxatives, mineral oil.	These enhance blood thinning response, irritate stomach, and may lead to ulcer and hemorrhage. Can increase or decrease blood thinning effects. Decrease vitamin K production increasing chance of hemorrhage. Augments blood thinning response to serious hemorrhage. When combined with anti-coagulant medication, patient is vulnerable to hemorrhage unless dosage is decreased. These drugs decrease absorption.
Calcium channel blockers	Calcium supplements.	Decreased response to blockers.
Corticosteroids: Prednisone, Solu-medrol	Cholesterol-lowering medications.	Inhibits absorption.
Digitalis: Lanoxin	Antacids. Cholesterol-lowering medications. Valium. Diuretics.	Decreased absorption. Decreased length of effect. Increased effect. Digitalis toxicity due to potassium loss.
Oral contraceptives	Valium.	Oral contraceptives enhance effect of Valium.
Tetracycline	Antacids. Zinc, iron supplements.	Cuts down on effectiveness of Tetracycline. Same as antacids.

Naproxen sodium, which has analgesic, antipyretic and anti-inflammatory properties, is indicated for the same conditions as aspirin, ibuprofen and acetaminophen but should not be taken with them. Anyone who generally has three or more alcoholic drinks per day should consult a physician on when and how to take naproxen sodium and other pain relievers.

References

Facts and Comparisons Drug Information. J.B. Lippincott., 1987.

Hansten, P.D., *Drug Interactions.* fifth edition, Lea & Febiger, 1985.

Lewis, K.T., Here's a brief overview of important drug-nutrient interactions. *Pharmacy Times.* May, 1987.

Hecht, Annabel. "OTC Drug Labels: Must Reading," *FDA Consumer,* October 1985, pp. 33–35.

Rados, Bill. "Generic Drugs: Cutting Cost, Not Corners," *FDA Consumer,* October 1985, pp. 27–29.

Handbook: Interactions of Selected Drugs With Nutritional Status, Daphne Roe, American Dietetic Association, 3rd Edition, 1984.

Food and Drug Interaction Guide, L.H. Rottmann, NebGuide (HEG85-206), 1985.

Drug-Nutrient Interactions, Daphne Roe, Hoffman-La Roche, Inc.

Joe Graddon, *The People's Pharmacy 2.* New York: The Hearst Corporation, 1980.

Note

1. J. Anderson, Colorado State University Cooperative Extension foods and nutrition specialist and professor; and H. Hart, associate specialist; food science and human nutrition.

Issued in furtherance of Cooperative Extension work, Acts of May 8 and June 30, 1914, in cooperation with the U.S. Department of Agriculture, Milan A. Rewerts, Director of Cooperative Extension, Colorado State University, Fort Collins, Colorado. Cooperative Extensio programs are available to all without discrimination. No endorsement of products mentioned is intended nor is criticism implied of products not mentioned.

Unit 3

Unit Selections

Key Points to Consider

❖ What are some of the limitations of diet and disease studies?

❖ What are the differences between food allergies and food sensitivities?

❖ What are some of the values added to your diet by eating soy products?

❖ What changes should you make in your lifestyle in order to effectively meet your nutrient needs?

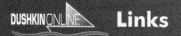 **Links**   **www.dushkin.com/online/**

These sites are annotated on pages 4 and 5.

In Ancient Greece, Hippocrates, the father of medicine, stated in his oath to serve humanity that the physician should use diet as part of his "arsenal" to fight disease. In ancient times, the healing arts included diet, exercise, and the power of the mind to cure disease.

Since those times, research that focuses on the connection between diet and disease has unraveled the role of many nutrients in degenerative disease prevention or reversal, but, frequently, results are controversial and need to be interpreted cautiously before a population-wide health message is mandated. We have also come to better understand the role of genetics in the expression of disease and its importance in how we respond to dietary change. Additionally, research about diet and disease has enabled us to understand the importance and uniqueness of the individual (age, gender, ethnicity, genetics) and his or her particular relation to diet.

With the recent advances in research in the area of phytochemicals such as flavonoids, carotenoids, saponins, indoles, and others in foods, especially fruits and vegetables, and their potential to prevent disease, thereby increasing both quality of life and life expectancy, we are at the zenith of a nutrition revolution. Several articles in this unit describe the role of these compounds in health and disease. The most prevalent degenerative diseases in industrial countries, which are quickly spreading in developing countries, are cancer, cardiovascular disease, diabetes, obesity, and osteoporosis. Phytochemicals have been reported to lower the risk of certain types of cancer and to decrease cholesterol in blood and prevent oxidation of the LDL lipoprotein—risk factors for developing cardiovascular disease. Furthermore, phytochemicals may protect against the development of diabetes and help prevent obesity. A diet rich in fruits and vegetables (not supplements) is the best source of phytochemicals.

But how is the consumer to know what to believe? Even though epidemiological and clinical studies have their pitfalls, the problem is not always the experts but many people who do not understand how science works. This includes much of the media, since information is usually reported out of context, with the goal of creating a sensation. The first article in this unit, entitled "Solving the Diet-and-Disease Puzzle," guides you in what you should look for when evaluating studies and deciding about food purchases.

Heart disease is the number-one killer not only in this country but in most industrial countries. It is well known that consumption of saturated fat increases a person's blood cholesterol, which is one of the primary risk factors for heart disease. The Mediterranean diet, which is enriched in monounsaturated fatty acids and omega-3-fatty acids (found in olive oil and in fish oils) and rich in dietary fiber, antioxidants, and B complex vitamins (found in fruits and vegetables), is cardioprotective. It also prevents heart attacks in people who have suffered them in the past. This diet is well tolerated, tasty, and enjoyable.

High levels of homocysteine, an amino acid that is a metabolic intermediate in methionine metabolism, seem to be a new risk factor related to heart disease. Ensuring that our diet is adequate in folic acid and vitamin B6 by means of eating a balanced diet that is rich in fish, grains, legumes, green leafy vegetables, and fortified cereals will keep our levels of homocysteine normal and will prevent heart disease.

Among the foods leading the phytochemical revolution is soy. Soy is considered to be protective against heart disease, cancer, and osteoporosis and it may ease menopausal symptoms. Again, we must be cautious about potential megadosing through supplements of soy protein isolates.

Another issue that remains controversial is the connection between diet and cancer. Food contains different components that may decrease or increase cancer risk, and since it takes a long time to develop cancer, it is hard to establish a cause-effect relationship between diet and cancer. It has generally been accepted that a diet high in animal products such as red meat increases incidence of cancer and that plant-based diets decrease cancer rates. Is it high-fat diets that raise the risk of cancer? Or are people who eat high-fat diets not physically active, heavier, consumers of more calories, and eat fewer fruits and vegetables? Thus, we cannot pinpoint a clear-cut cause-and-effect relationship. It is prudent to advise that cancer risk decreases if one eats a well-balanced diet, high in whole grains, vegetables, fruits, and beans, and low in fat, saturated fat, and cholesterol. Additionally, maintaining or improving body weight and incorporating physical activity into the daily routine is important.

Even though nearly everyone you talk to thinks that he or she has a true food allergy, the reality is that food allergies affect only 2 to 2.5 percent of the adult population. Food allergies involve the immune system and they can be so severe that they cause death. Food sensitivities do not involve the immune system, but they may produce symptoms that are similar to food allergy. Care needs to be taken when hosting guests with food allergies and sensitivities, according to the third article in this unit.

Since degenerative diseases begin at a young age, establishing healthy eating habits early is crucial for future health and well-being. There has been a significant increase in the prevalence of overweight among children and adolescents in the United States due to the interaction between genetics and the environment. Additionally, calcium intakes do not meet calcium recommendations, a critical dietary factor for developing osteoporosis during adult life. Another nutrient of concern for children is iron. The incidence of iron deficiency is widespread in toddlers and adolescents in the United States. The consequences of iron deficiency anemia for growth development and in long-term health should be taken seriously. Children's diets have been documented to be low in iron, zinc, calcium, and other micronutrients. Intakes are low at home and at day care centers. Since most young children cannot get adequate intakes of these micronutrients without major changes in their diet, nutritionists question whether they should receive routine multivitamin/mineral supplements. Separate food guidelines for children and adolescents promote the development of lifelong eating habits and emphasize the need for parents and childcare providers to serve as positive role models.

Although the elderly seem to have better eating patterns than their grandchildren, their diet still needs improvement. Focus should be placed on the nutrient density of foods since nutrient intake requirements and absorption decrease with age. Diseases, physical limitations, and depression ultimately compromise the nutritional well-being of the elderly population.

The last article in this unit deals with the very important topic of physical activity, which is a critical component to health and well-being and a necessary complement to a healthful diet. Regular, low-impact, moderate-intensity physical activity and a healthful diet reduce the risk of major chronic disease and improve mental health.

Through the Life Span: Diet and Disease

Solving the Diet-and-Disease Puzzle

BY BONNIE LIEBMAN "High-fiber diets don't cut colon cancer," said *USA Today*. ■ In January, the media had itself a juicy "man-bites-dog" story. It wasn't the first time. ■ From beta-carotene (the anti-cancer vitamin that caused cancer) to margarine (the cholesterol-lowering spread that raised cholesterol) to calcium (the mineral that did — oops, didn't—yes, did—prevent osteoporosis), the public has been dragged through a series of flip-flops. ■ Add in the "controversies" over salt, sugar, and eggs that have been created in part by press releases from the food industry and it's no surprise to hear people say that "those experts don't know what they're talking about." ■ The problem isn't always the experts. It's that many people—including much of the media—don't understand how science works.

Remember when the average person never heard about the latest research in *The New England Journal of Medicine*? Back then, a study showing that fiber doesn't prevent colon cancer might not have registered as a flip-flop because only scientists would have read it.

"The press picks up each incremental piece of information as the final answer," says John Baron, a colon cancer expert at Dartmouth College in Hanover, New Hampshire. "Most scientists consider each study a stepping stone to arrive at the truth."

In fact, the fiber story, like many other "surprising new findings," wasn't as much a flip-flop as another piece of a puzzle (see "The Not-Yet-Final Fiber Story").

That's how epidemiologists look at it. They're the people who examine human populations to find links between disease and exposure to foods, medicines, tobacco, exercise, occupational hazards, you name it.

"I think of epidemiology as building a legal argument," says Julie Mares-Perlman of the University of Wisconsin in Madison. "In other

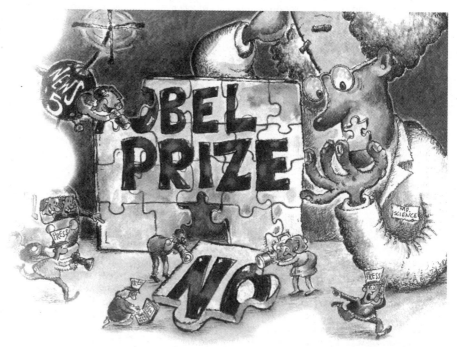

Illustration: Loel Barr.

types of science, you may only need one study, plus another to confirm it. But in epidemiology, two studies can never provide the proof we need."

Diet Difficulties

When you're looking at what people eat, it's even tougher to prove some-

thing. It's a lot easier to remember for how long you've smoked cigarettes, for example, than to remember *how often* you've eaten *what* over the last decade.

"Even the best questionnaires are compromised by changes in the diet, varying portion sizes, and people's inability to tell you what they eat,"

Reprinted from *Nutrition Action Healthletter*, May 1999, pp. 1, 3-8. © 1999 by CSPI, Center for Science in the Public Interest. *Nutrition Action Healthletter*, 1875 Connecticut Ave., NW, Suite 300, Washington, DC 20009-5728 ($24.00 for 10 issues).

says Regina Ziegler, a nutritional epidemiologist at the National Cancer Institute in Bethesda, Maryland. "For example, when people say, 'I eat seven servings of vegetables a week,' do they eat seven full servings or do they count the slice of tomato and lettuce on their sandwich every day?"

And what about the foods people eat at restaurants? Trying to guess how much fat you get when you're served manicotti, chicken curry, beef stroganoff, or even a tuna sandwich is a researcher's nightmare.

What's more, cancer, heart disease, and other illnesses may take a lifetime to develop. Yet most studies don't even attempt to ask people what they've been eating before middle age. "We're gambling that people maintain the same dietary patterns throughout their lives," says Ziegler. That's a big gamble.

Here's a guide to help you interpret the next study that flashes across the evening news. It's not exactly "Epidemiology from A-to-Z." To keep things simple, we've included only three kinds of diet studies and only some of their advantages and limitations.

step: 1
Retrospective Studies

Remember these headlines? "Hot dog consumption tied to leukemia." "Study links coffee use to pancreatic cancer." And just last winter, ketchup ads boasted that "lycopene may help reduce the risk of prostate and cervical cancer."

All of those studies—except for the ones on prostate cancer—were *retrospective,* which means they looked back in time. They're often the first step that researchers take to figure out if Disease X is caused (or prevented) by Food A.

"Sometimes later studies confirm retrospective studies and sometimes they don't," cautions Harvard Medical School researcher Charles Fuchs. In-

deed, later research didn't find a link between coffee and pancreatic cancer. And researchers are still trying to figure out if hot dogs raise the risk of leukemia and if lycopene cuts the risk of cervical (and prostate) cancer.

What researchers usually do:

1. Contact people who were recently diagnosed with Disease X and similar people who were not.

2. Ask both groups what they typically ate during the years before they were diagnosed (and possibly collect blood samples or other information about possible causes of Disease X).

3. See if the people with the disease ate more or less of some foods or nutrients than the people without the disease.

Some advantages

■ **Quick answers.** "Retrospective studies can be done quickly because you don't have to follow a group until they start to develop cancer or other diseases," says Greta Bunin, an epidemiologist at the Children's Hospital of Philadelphia.

■ **Clues to uncommon illnesses.** "Retrospective studies are the only way you can study diseases that are rare, like cancer in children," says Bunin. "It's almost impossible to do a prospective [forward-looking] study on rare cancers because you'd need a lot of people and you'd have to wait a long time."

■ **More details.** "In a retrospective study, you can get a higher level of detail on the disease of interest and the foods and lifestyles that may cause or prevent it," says Ziegler. Instead of asking people questions about everything they eat, you can focus on foods that contain fiber or carotenoids or fat, for example.

Some potential limitations

■ **Inaccuracy.** It's always tough to get a handle on what people eat, but in this case, "you're trying to figure out what they ate ten or 20 years

ago," explains Bunin. "So what they report comes with inaccuracies."

■ **Recall bias.** Let's say that people with colon cancer report eating fewer fruits and vegetables before they got sick than healthy people. "People with cancer might have thought more about what led them to develop cancer, so they may report on their past diets differently than people without disease," says Bunin. If patients have heard news reports that fiber prevents colon cancer, they may think they ate less of it . . . because they have cancer.

■ **Confounding.** Let's say people who eat more fat have a higher risk of colon cancer. Is it the fat—or something else about those people—that matters? "You may think you're looking at high-fat-eaters, but you're actually looking at meat-and-potato-eaters," says Baron. So it could be the meat . . . or the lack of fruits and vegetables . . . or something else about meat-and-potato-eaters that's crucial.

Researchers "adjust" for all the "confounders" they know about, but they can't adjust for the unknown ones or for the ones they can't measure well.

step: 2
Prospective Studies

In 1977, Harvard's Walter Willett transformed the one-year-old Nurses' Health Study into a gold mine of data on diet and health. "Experts were telling the public what to eat, but there was virtually no direct data to support the advice," he explains.

Every two to four years since 1980, 120,000 female nurses have filled out questionnaires about what they eat, how much they weigh, whether they smoke, exercise, take medications, etc. "So far, we have issued more than 300 reports on over a dozen different diseases," says Willett. And as the study goes on—and more

GETTING CLINICAL

"It's an exciting time to be in research," says David Alberts, associate dean for research at the University of Arizona. "About a dozen clinical trials are ongoing and are about to yield results." Many of them study people who have—or have had—a disease, because their chances of getting sick again are much higher than the average person's. A higher risk of disease means that the study can include fewer people.

Name of Study	Diseases Being Studied	Participants	What They're Getting
Randomized Trial of Folate and Colorectal Adenoma (Polyp Prevention Study)	Precancerous colon polyps	750 healthy men & women aged 40 to 75	Folic acid (1,000 mcg/day)
Women's Healthy Eating & Living Study (WHEL)	Breast cancer	3,000 women aged 18 to 70 with breast cancer	Low-fat diet (15-20% of calories) rich in fruits and vegetables (8-10 servings/day) and fiber (30 g/day)
Women's Intervention Nutrition Study (WINS)	Breast cancer	1,750 women treated for localized breast cancer & not already eating a low-fat diet	Low-fat diet (15% of calories)
Carotenoid-Rich Diet Trial to Reverse Cervical Intraepithelial Neoplasm I and II (CAPRE)	Precancerous cervical lesions	326 women with cervical intraepithelial neoplasm (CIN I, II)	Fruits & vegetables rich in carotenoids (8-10 servings/day)
Nutritional Prevention of Cancer	All cancers	1,300 residents of the (low-selenium) Southeastern U.S. who have had non-melanoma skin cancers	Selenium (200-400 mcg/day)
Skin Cancer Prophylaxis by Low-Fat Dietary Intervention	Basal or squamous cell skin cancer	115 people who have had non-melanoma skin cancers	Low-fat diet (20% of calories)
Women's Health Initiative	Breast cancer, colon cancer, heart disease, hip fractures	64,000 postmenopausal women aged 50 to 79	Low-fat diet (20% of calories) and/or calcium (1,000 mg/day) and vitamin D (400 IU/day)
Women's Health Study	Heart attack, stroke, cancers of the breast, lung, and colon, cataracts, macular degeneration	40,000 healthy women aged 45+	Vitamin E (600 IU every other day) and/or aspirin (100 mg every other day)
Women's Antioxidant and Cardiovascular Study (WACS)	Heart attack, stroke, cataracts, macular degeneration	8,000 female health professionals aged 40+ who have heart disease, have had a stroke, or have three or more risk factors for cardiovascular disease	Vitamin C (500 mg/day), vitamin E (600 IU every other day), and/or beta-carotene (50 mg every other day)
Vitamin E Atherosclerosis Prevention Study (VEAPS)	Clogged arteries	353 healthy men & women aged 40 to 85 with high LDL ("bad") cholesterol	Vitamin E (400 IU/day)
Vitamin Intervention for Stroke Prevention (VISP)	Stroke	3,600 people who have had a recent non-disabling stroke and have relatively high blood homocysteine levels	Multivitamin with folic acid (20 mcg or 2,500 mcg/day) and high or low levels of vitamins B-6 and B-12

THE NOT-YET-FINAL FIBER STORY

By Bonnie Liebman

Last January, many people were shocked to hear that fiber might not prevent colon cancer. To the public, it's been conventional wisdom. To many researchers, it's always been a question mark.

"There has been a healthy skepticism about the emphasis on fiber for a long time," says Regina Ziegler, a nutritional epidemiologist at the National Cancer Institute (NCI) in Bethesda, Maryland.

"We know that diets high in fruits, vegetables, whole grains, and legumes are associated with a reduced risk of colon cancer, but whether fiber—or something else in those diets—explains the association has been less clear."

In animals given carcinogens, fiber cuts the number of colon tumors.

"And in retrospective studies, when researchers asked patients with colon cancer about their fiber intake in the past, fiber seemed to be protective," explains Charles Fuchs, one of the Harvard Medical School researchers who last January released data from the Nurses' Health Study showing no link between fiber and cancer.[1]

"But in all of the prospective studies, where we ask a large number of healthy people questions and follow them for a long period, we found nothing," he adds.

Still, Fuchs' results from the Nurses' Health Study aren't the final word on fiber and colon cancer.

Fiber On Trial

Several years ago, faced with the uncertain results of earlier studies, researchers launched two large clinical trials to test a high-fiber diet on the incidence of precancerous colon polyps (adenomas):

■ The Polyp Prevention Trial, sponsored by the National Cancer Institute, involved roughly 2,000 people who had already had at least one colon polyp removed. For three years, each was randomly assigned to eat either an ordinary diet or a low-fat diet that had five to eight servings a day of fruits and vegetables and 18 grams of fiber for every 1,000 calories the person ate.[2] "Most of the people in the high-fiber group were getting more than 35 grams of fiber a day," says the NCI's Elaine Lanza, who co-directs the study.

■ The Wheat Bran Fiber Trial, run by researchers at the University of Arizona Health Sciences Center in Tucson, included more than 1,400 people who had previously had polyps removed. Each was assigned to get either two grams of fiber (the "placebo") or 13 grams of fiber from wheat bran each day for three years.[3] Thirteen grams is what you'd get in a half-cup serving of Kellogg's All-Bran Extra Fiber or General Mills Fiber One cereal.

Both trials are due to release their findings within the next few months. If the fiber-eaters had fewer colon polyps, scientists will have a clear answer that fiber is protective. If they didn't have fewer polyps—which won't be a shock,

given the results of the Nurses' Health Study—it's back to the drawing board.

"Did they use a high enough dose of fiber?" asks John Baron, a colon cancer expert at Dartmouth College in Hanover, New Hampshire. "Did the study start too late in life? What if the participants didn't really eat as much fiber as the researchers told them to?"

"The recurrence of polyps is a ten-year process," says David Alberts, who heads the Wheat Bran Fiber Trial. "The intervention trials lasted three or four years. It could be that only long-term fiber use is associated with a reduction in polyps."

Or maybe fiber simply has nothing to do with colon cancer. "It's a bit surprising compared to what we would have said five or ten years ago," says Harvard University's Walter Willett.

But studies suggest that there is plenty that people can do to cut their risk of the disease.[4-7] "A large majority of the risk for colon cancer can be avoided by staying lean, keeping active, not smoking, avoiding excess red meat, and taking a multivitamin to ensure that you get enough folic acid," says Willett. Calcium may also protect the colon.

Calcium & the Colon

It just goes to show. The cohort study that found no effect of fiber on colon cancer got huge press. Yet just one week before the fiber story broke, the same journal published the results of a clinical trial showing that calcium prevents precancerous colon polyps. It got a yawn.

John Baron and colleagues randomly assigned more than 800 people with a history of polyps to take either a placebo or 1,200 mg a day of calcium (from calcium carbonate).[8] After four years, the calcium-takers averaged 24 percent fewer polyps than the placebo-takers.

"The reduction in risk was relatively modest, so calcium is far from a magic bullet," says Baron. "You can't take a calcium pill and forget about colonoscopies or checking in with your doctor to see if you should do something more aggressive."

And, he cautions, "we studied polyps, not cancer itself. You'd have to do a huge study lasting a long time to look at cancer."

Nevertheless, we now know that the same nutrient that strengthens bones can protect the colon . . . and it's relatively cheap and harmless. "Calcium is generally safe at doses up to 2,000 mg a day," says Baron.

Fiber's Feats

The news was buried in (or left out of) most media reports that fiber doesn't prevent cancer. Earlier research from Walter Willett and colleagues at the Harvard Medical School—the same researchers who found no link between fiber and colon polyps—suggests that people who ate high-fiber diets had a lower risk of not one, but three, major diseases:[9-12]

"These studies found a reduction in the risk of heart disease, diabetes, and high blood pressure," says Harvard's Fuchs. "There are still wonderful benefits from eating fiber."

And it's not just life-threatening diseases that fiber may ward off. "It can reduce the risk of diverticulosis, hemorrhoids, irritable bowel syndrome, and phlebitis in the legs," says Alberts. "It's absolutely essential for normal function, especially of the gastrointestinal tract.

"Even after people finished our trial," he adds, "the majority continued eating the high-fiber cereal because it regulated their bowels. People need fiber to stay healthy. That message hasn't changed."

True, fiber's ability to prevent problems other than constipation has yet to be proven in clinical trials. But that doesn't change the bottom line—that people should eat bran cereals, whole-wheat bread, fruits, vegetables, beans, and other fiber-rich foods. That message got lost amid the "Fiber Benefit Refuted" hoopla. It shouldn't have.

"The press likes controversy," says Fuchs. "It sells papers to say that we thought fiber was good and now it isn't. But that's not my message."

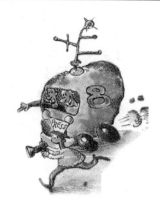

[1] New Eng. J. Med. 340: 169, 223, 1999.
[2] Cancer Epidem. Bio. Prev. 5: 375, 1996.
[3] Cancer Epidem. Bio. Prev. 7: 813, 1998.
[4] Ann. Intern. Med. 129: 517, 1998.
[5] J. Nat. Cancer Inst. 89: 948, 1997.
[6] New Eng. J. Med. 323: 1664, 1990.
[7] J. Nat. Cancer Inst. 86: 183, 192, 1994.
[8] New Eng. J. Med. 340: 101, 1999.
[9] J. Amer. Med. Assoc. 275: 447, 1996.
[10] J. Amer. Med. Assoc. 277: 472, 1997.

of the nurses get sick—it should yield data on less-common illnesses.

That's just one prospective study. Among the others: Harvard's Health Professionals Followup Study (of 40,000 male dentists, veterinarians, and others), the Iowa Women's Health Study (of 29,000 middle-aged Iowans), and the Framingham Heart Study (of 6,000 men and women in Massachusetts).

What researchers usually do:

1. Collect diet, medical, and other information (and sometimes blood samples) on a large group of healthy people (the "cohort").

2. Wait five, ten, or more years to see who gets Disease X, Y, or Z.

3. See if the people who get sick ate less or more of some food or nutrient than the people who stayed healthy.

Some advantages

■ **No recall bias.** "The primary advantage is that we collect dietary data before the disease develops," says Willett, so there's no potential for biased

recall. And the data may be more accurate because researchers ask what the participants are eating now, not what they remember having eaten years before they got sick.

■ **More than one snapshot.** Since the study lasts so long, researchers can ask people what they eat every few years. "With a cohort, you have the opportunity to assess diet at multiple points in time," says Ziegler.

■ **More than one disease.** "Looking at many different diseases is an advantage because sometimes there are trade-offs," notes Willett. "For example, estrogen replacement therapy increases the risk of breast and endometrial cancers but reduces the risk of heart disease. If we recognize the trade-offs, we can give balanced advice."

Some potential limitations

■ **Misclassification.** The Framingham Heart Study never found a higher risk of heart disease in people who ate more saturated fat. Yet laboratory studies show that sat fat raises blood cho-

lesterol. It's hard to estimate how much saturated fat people eat. If some high-sat-fat-eaters were misclassified as low-sat-fat-eaters (or vice versa), that could explain why no link was found.

■ **Diets don't vary enough.** Let's say eating 50 grams of fiber a day prevents colon cancer. A study would find no link at all because very few people eat that much. "You're restricted to what people are typically eating," says Ziegler.

■ **Insensitivity.** Prospective (and retrospective) studies would easily pick up cigarettes as a cause of lung cancer, because smoking accounts for much of the risk. But those studies might miss something that has a minor impact.

For example, some studies find that women who drink alcohol have a higher risk of breast cancer. Other studies don't. One possible explanation: "If you smoked a pack of cigarettes every day for years, your risk of lung cancer would be 1,000-percent higher than a non-smoker's," says Matthew Longnecker of the National Institute of Environmental Health Sciences in North Carolina.

"In comparison, if a woman drank one alcoholic beverage every day for years, on average, her risk of breast cancer would increase by only ten percent."

step: 3
Clinical Trials

Some of the most famous trials are the failures. "Beta-carotene being linked to higher lung cancer risks," announced the headlines in January 1996. It was supposed to do the opposite.[1,2]

Other trials have simply shown no benefit. For example, in 1994 researchers reported no fewer precancerous colon polyps in people given vitamin E, vitamin C, and beta-carotene for four years.[3] Nor did those antioxidants keep arteries from closing up again in people who had undergone angioplasties.[4]

"Controlled clinical trials are the only way to go from questions and hypotheses to definitive answers," explained Richard Klausner, director of the National Cancer Institute, at a 1996 press conference on the unexpected beta-carotene results. "While the results are disappointing," he added, "the research process, I believe, is working." Indeed, many more clinical trials are in progress (see "Getting Clinical").

What researchers usually do:

1. Randomly assign hundreds or thousands of people without Disease X to one of two groups.
2. Give one group the diet (or supplement) that's supposed to prevent Disease X, and give the other an ordinary diet (or a look-alike but inactive placebo supplement).
3. Wait several years to see if one of the two groups has a higher rate of Disease X.

Some advantages,

■ **No misclassification.** In studies other than trials, "there's a lot of measurement error that can obscure an association," says John Baron. If some of the high-vegetable-eaters mistakenly get mixed in with the low-vegetable-eaters, you wouldn't find a link between vegetables and, say, colon cancer, even if vegetables were protective.

In a clinical trial, the researchers decide how much fiber, fat, vitamins, vegetables, or whatever each group gets. That ensures that there is a sizeable difference between the groups.

■ **No confounding.** In prospective studies, "you may not know how diet relates to other lifestyle characteristics," says Baron. But a trial randomly assigns people to one diet or another, so that's the only difference between the groups.

■ **Less-equivocal results.** It's because of trials that we can be fairly certain that folic acid prevents neural tube birth defects, vitamin D prevents hip fractures, and calcium prevents precancerous colon polyps. "Clinical trials are easy to interpret when you find something that lowers the risk of disease," says Mares-Perlman.

Some potential limitations

Clinical trials can be expensive, time-consuming (because you have to wait for a sizeable number of people to get sick), and impractical (for uncommon illnesses). And their results may not apply to everyone. For example, in 1996 researchers found that selenium supplements cut the risk of colon, prostate, and lung cancer in residents of the Southeastern U.S. who had previously had skin cancer.[5] But the results—which researchers are now trying to confirm—may not apply to people who live in other parts of the U.S., where the soil—and the food—has more selenium.

And if trials fail, it's hard to know what happened. Among the possibilities:

■ **Wrong dose?** Maybe a different amount of fiber, vitamin, etc., might have cut the risk of disease.

■ **Wrong people?** Maybe the diet or supplement would have worked in people who were younger, older, healthier, or otherwise different.

■ **Too short or small?** Maybe if the trial had lasted longer . . . or had more people . . . you would have seen a difference in disease rates.

■ **Wrong stuff?** In the lung cancer study, for example, researchers homed in on beta-carotene because people who ate more carotene-rich fruits and vegetables had a lower risk. But maybe something else in those foods prevents cancer.

The Big Picture

With so many pitfalls, it's a wonder that researchers have figured anything out. They've done it by looking at all the evidence, including animal studies, test-tube studies, and short-term clinical studies on people.

Take eggs and cholesterol. Researchers know from hundreds of clinical studies—in which they control every morsel of food the participants eat—that cholesterol in food raises cholesterol in the blood.[6] If a prospective study says otherwise, the study isn't sensitive enough to measure the eggs' impact.

The bottom line is that experts have to look at the big picture. "We need broad and deep knowledge," says Mares-Perlman. "We have to look at the landscape to see if there's a consistent picture in many kinds of studies."

---

[1] *New Eng. J. Med. 330*: 1029, 1994.
[2] *J. Nat. Cancer Inst. 88*: 1550, 1996.
[3] *New Eng. J. Med. 331*: 141, 1994.
[4] *New Eng. J. Med. 337*: 365, 1997.
[5] *J. Amer. Med. Assoc. 277*: 1520, 1996.
[6] *Brit. Med. J. 314*: 112, 1997

PREVENTIVE NUTRITION

FOOD
as disease-fighter

- **Cancer, fruits and vegetables**
- **Phytochemicals and cardiovascular health**
- **Obesity and diabetes**
- **Dietary recommendations**

Eating to stay healthy may not be as easy as it seems. Indeed, a study in the July 16, 1999, issue of Science says that even people living in the United States and other industrialized nations often fail to obtain recommended daily minimums of micronutrients (vitamins and minerals), despite meals containing plenty of calories and a nearly endless variety of food.

Even more alarming, the subsistence diets of many developing countries fail to provide the adequate macronutrients—carbohydrates, fats and proteins—as well as micronutrients needed to meet basic nutritional requirements, the study says.

Besides macronutrients and the 13 vitamins and 17 minerals essential to human health, naturally occurring compounds (called phytochemicals) in plants are receiving increasing attention from researchers looking into the connection between diet and disease.

Phytochemicals (from the Greek word phyto, meaning plant) are unlike vitamins and minerals in that they have no known nutritional value. Some phytochemicals, such as digitalis (extracted from the foxglove) and quinine, have been used for hundreds of years as medicines to treat diseases. Others function as antioxidants, which protect cells from the effects of oxidation and free radicals within the body. They have been recognized only recently as potentially powerful agents that may offer protection from diseases and conditions ranging from some cancers to aging.

"We've known for a long time that the right food choices can improve health and decrease our risks for certain diseases," says Jennifer K. Nelson, a registered dietitian at Mayo Clinic, Rochester, Minn., and associate editor for nutrition at Oasis. "This is especially true for plant foods. What's exciting is that we're realizing these foods are abundant in health-enhancing compounds, and we're discovering how they're used at the cellular level. This brings new meaning to the statement: 'You are what you eat.'"

Phytochemicals

Family	Major Food Sources
Allyl sulfides	Onions, garlic, leeks, chives
Indoles	Cruciferous vegetables (broccoli, cabbage, kale, cauliflower)
Isoflavones	Soybeans (tofu, soy milk)
Phenolic acids	Tomatoes, citrus fruits, carrots, whole grains, nuts
Polyphenols	Green tea, grapes, red wine
Saponins	Beans and legumes
Terpenes	Cherries, citrus fruit peel

Cancer, fruits and vegetables

Since the early 1970s, researchers worldwide have consistently found that people whose diets contained the most fruits and vegetables had the lowest rates of some cancers. Others have found some protective effect from other plant foods such as nuts, grains and seeds. But the strongest evidence suggests that eating plenty of fruits and vegetables can decrease the risk of developing some types of cancer.

For example, researchers have found that perillyl alcohol, found in cherries and lavender, shrinks pancreatic tumors in laboratory animals. And limonene, contained in the peels of citrus fruits, blocks the development of breast tumors and causes existing tumors to shrink in laboratory animals.

Recent links between phytochemicals and lowered cancer risk include:

- A Harvard study that found that a high intake of cruciferous vegetables, such as broccoli and cabbage, may reduce bladder cancer risk in men.
- Another Harvard study found that a diet containing five or more servings of fruits and vegetables daily appears to lower the risk of breast cancer among premenopausal women who have a history of breast cancer or who are moderate drinkers.
- A review published by the National Cancer Institute reported a reduced risk for a variety of cancers among those who often eat tomatoes and tomato-based products.
- Research commissioned by the World Cancer Research Fund and published in the British Medical Journal found that diets high in fruits and vegetables and low in meat are protective against breast, prostate, bowel and other cancers.

"Although we are identifying significant numbers of plant compounds and their roles in fighting disease, there is a growing consensus that a variety of whole foods—not supplements—should be our source for phytochemicals and other compounds important for health," says Nelson.

Phytochemicals and Cardiovascular Health

The phytochemicals in fruits and veggies may help your heart, too. Recent epidemiological studies suggest that a diet rich in fruits and vegetables results in a lowered risk of cardiovascular disease that can't be attributed to major macronutrients or known vitamins and minerals.

According to a review of research by the American Heart Association (AHA), three classes of compounds found in fruits and vegetables—plant sterols, flavonoids, and sulfur-containing compounds—may be important in reducing the risk of atherosclerosis (narrowing of the arteries).

- Sterols are one group of lipids (fat-like substances) found in the body. The most common lipid found in human and animal tissue is cholesterol, an essential part of cell membranes. It's so important, especially to nerve cells, that the body makes its own supply. Cholesterol circulates in the blood in particles called lipoproteins. Researchers have linked certain types of these particles to atherosclerosis, the leading cause of heart attacks and strokes. Atherosclerosis also may contribute to high blood pressure and impotence.

Plant sterols (phytosterols) and cholesterol, from red meat and other dietary sources, compete for absorption during digestion. Large amounts of plant sterols decrease the amount of cholesterol absorbed from food and may have a protective effect.

- Flavonoids have varied chemical structures and are found in fruits, vegetables, nuts and seeds. Some flavonoids have been shown to have an antioxidant effect that prevents damage to cells from free radicals. Others have been shown to make blood cells less "sticky" by limiting the action of platelets. Sources include red wine and soy products (isoflavones).
- Sulfur compounds that occur naturally (the allium family) may lower blood cholesterol and thereby lessen atherosclerosis. Found in onions, garlic and leeks, these compounds have been used as a medicine since ancient times. Garlic oil or cloves have both been shown to lower blood pressure and lipids in humans. Not all of their actions are understood and, according to the AHA, more research needs to be done into the chemistry and pharmacology of sulfur-containing plant compounds.

Obesity and Diabetes

A majority of Americans are now classified as obese, according to the National Institutes of Health (NIH). Obesity is a risk factor for some types of cancer, cardiovascular disease and for type 2 diabetes, commonly called non-insulin-dependent diabetes mellitus (NIDDM) or adult-onset diabetes.

High blood sugar levels from diabetes (hyperglycemia), over time, can cause damage throughout the body. Uncontrolled diabetes can lead to blindness, kidney disease, nerve damage (neuropathy), atherosclerosis, high blood pressure, heart attack and stroke.

Researchers at the Centers for Disease Control and Prevention in Atlanta found that certain carotenoids—plant compounds with antioxidant properties—may protect against the development of type 2 diabetes. Studies also have shown that maintaining a healthful weight by eating a diet that limits calories and includes plenty of fruits and vegetables can reduce the risk of developing diabetes.

Dietary Recommendations

Six national health organizations reviewed dietary guidelines from several agencies, focusing on the scientific evidence supporting them and their effectiveness in preventing coronary heart disease, cancer, obesity and diabetes.

The six groups—the Nutrition Committee of the American Heart Association, the American Cancer Society, the American Dietetic Association, the American Academy of Pediatrics, NIH, and the American Society for Clinical Nutrition—compiled a set of recommendations, drawn from the guidelines.

"For the 2 out of 3 adult Americans who do not smoke and who do not drink excessively, one personal choice seems to influence long-term health prospects more than any other—what we eat," the consensus panel wrote.

The recommendations, published in the July 27, 1999, issue of Circulation: Journal of the American Heart Association, include:

- Balance the food you eat with physical activity. Maintain or improve your weight.
- Choose a diet with plenty of grain products, vegetables and fruits.
- Choose a diet low in fat, saturated fat and cholesterol.
- Choose a diet moderate in sugars.
- Choose a diet moderate in salt and sodium.
- If you drink alcoholic beverages, do so in moderation.

Guess Who's Coming to Dinner?

Just when you think you've thought of everything for your dinner party—food, flowers, music, guests who will enjoy each other—something comes along to remind you that feeding a group of people may present special challenges. In this case, it might be the unexpected food allergy of a guest's date. If only you'd thought to mention that shrimp would be the main course. . . .

Avoiding the above scenario isn't too difficult. It's mostly a matter of communicating with the guests and knowing how to handle certain food allergy issues in the kitchen. This is important because, although an unexpected food allergy situation is inconvenient for the cook, it can be dangerous for the food-allergic guest.

A Food Allergy Primer for the Non-Allergic

Although it may seem that nearly everyone has an allergy to some food or another, in reality true food allergies are quite rare, affecting only 2 to 2.5 percent of the adult population. Food allergies are more common among infants (4 to 6 percent of the population) and children (1 to 2 percent). Many infants outgrow allergies.

There are two types of sensitivities to foods: those that involve the immune system (immunological) and those that don't (non-immunological). All true food allergies are immunological in nature, while non-immunological reactions include a wide variety of adverse food reactions. Here are the basic facts about food al-

lergies, and how they differ from other food sensitivities.

What makes it an allergy?

A true food allergy is a reaction of the body's immune system to something in a food or a food ingredient (virtually always a protein). When a susceptible person is exposed to this protein (called the allergen), the body mistakenly interprets the protein as foreign and produces antibodies to fight it. With repeated exposures to the offending food protein, the body continues to mount its "defense," so that at some point consuming the allergenic food triggers the release of histamine and other powerful chemicals which cause common allergy symptoms (see Chart 1).

The most severe food allergy reaction is called anaphylaxis. This infrequent, yet potentially fatal, response to a food allergen involves several different body systems and results in a number of symptoms instead of the usual one or two seen with a typical food allergy. An anaphylactic reaction can progress quickly from the mild symptom stage—where the individual experiences an itchy tongue or mouth, throat tightening, and wheezing—to the life-threatening stage of cardiac arrest and shock. Immediate medical attention is necessary, and treatment usually includes an injection of epinephrine. "Although they are rare, anaphylactic reactions which are fatal most often occur when the allergic individual is eating away from home and inadvertently consumes the offend-

"Granted, most of the responsibility for avoiding food allergens rests with the person who has the allergy, and one would expect that a life-threatening food allergy would be acknowledged by the individual when he or she is invited to a dinner party."

CHART 1

Food Allergy Symptoms

- <u>Skin symptoms</u>
  Swelling, hives, eczema/atopic dermatitis (skin rash)
- <u>Gastrointestinal symptoms</u>
  Abdominal cramps, nausea, vomiting, diarrhea
- <u>Respiratory symptoms</u>
  Runny nose, asthma/difficulty breathing, tightening of the throat
- <u>Oral symptoms</u>
  Itching, swelling and hives in the mouth, palate and tongue
- <u>Systemic symptoms</u>
  Anaphylactic shock (severe shock involving several body systems)

ing food, fails to recognize the reaction quickly, and there is a delay in epinephrine administration," explains Susan Hefle, Ph.D., co-director of the Food Allergy Research and Resource Program and assistant professor of food science at the University of Nebraska at Lincoln.

Food Sensitivities

Non-immunological food reactions, while not true allergies, can produce symptoms similar to those of a food allergy. This can be confusing to people who suffer from them and is probably one reason why people are quick to say they have a food "allergy" when in fact they may just have a food sensitivity or intolerance of some sort. Food sensitivities are rarely life threatening and the symptoms tend to be more localized.

Lactose intolerance, where the body lacks the enzyme to break down the milk sugar, lactose, is one example of a non-immunological food reaction. Idiosyncratic food reactions, where the cause is unknown, also don't involve the immune system. One example of a food idiosyncrasy is sulfite-induced asthma, which is estimated to affect about 1.7 percent of all asthmatics, according to Hefle.

"Some idiosyncratic reactions, such as a connection between food colors and hyperactivity have been disproved through scientific research, while still others, such as monosodium glutamate (MSG) sensitivity remain unproved," adds Hefle.

Common Causes of Food Allergy

Amazingly, over 160 food allergens have been identified—but only a handful of them account for more than 90 percent of the food allergies in the United States. Most food ingredients (such as aspartame, MSG, food colors, high fructose corn syrup and sugar) are not food allergens.

Food oils, such as peanut oil or soybean oil are generally highly refined, rendering them free of allergenic proteins. In fact, research has shown that people with allergies to the oil's originating food (such as peanut or soybean) do not react to commercially refined and processed oils—the most commonly used oils. Cold-pressed oils, such as various nut oils, can still contain allergenic proteins, which may trigger an allergic reaction in a sensitive individual.

Tips for Hosts: Coping with Food-Allergic Guests

Granted, most of the responsibility for avoiding food allergens rests with the person who has the allergy, and one would expect that a life-threatening food allergy would be acknowl-

edged by the individual when he or she is invited to a dinner party. However, a little planning and preparation can eliminate the need for dealing with a food allergy situation altogether.

Here are some recommendations:

- Ask about food sensitivities when inviting guests and let your guests know what you plan to serve when inviting them. Knowing what you may be dealing with is half the battle. If a guest insists he or she is allergic to a food or ingredient which isn't a known food allergen (and may instead be just a sensitivity) don't get into a debate, simply offer to change the menu.
- Invite guests far enough ahead of time so that the menu can be revised, if necessary.
- Practice safe food handling methods during both the preparation and serving of foods.

Sometimes one can't avoid serving a common food allergen, even when an individual has alerted you to the existence of an allergy. In these cases, it's still possible to have a reaction-free event, but careful cooking and serving is necessary. According to Hefle, measures to take include:

- *Avoiding cross contact by not sharing utensils, food containers, cutting boards and serving dishes. For example, simply wiping off a knife used for a child's peanut* butter sandwich, and then using the same knife to spread mustard on a peanut-allergic child's cheese sandwich is not adequate for preventing a possible allergic reaction. A separate, clean knife, cutting board and plate should be used.

- *Avoiding using the same cooking oil for both allergenic and non-allergenic foods.* Food allergens can survive home cooking temperatures—even when deep-frying. If frying fish and chips, for example, two separate batches of hot oil should be used, as well as separate utensils and serving platters.
- *Avoiding "creative" recipe formulation—"secret ingredients" can*

CHART 2

Common Food Allergies

In Infants: Cow's milk, eggs, peanuts, tree nuts (almond, walnut, hazelnut, Brazil nut, etc.), soybeans, wheat

In Adults: Peanuts, crustacea (shrimp, crab, lobster, crawfish), tree nuts, fish

be dangerous. Many times a food-allergic individual doesn't expect a food allergen to be present in a dish, and will unwittingly consume it only to suffer later. For example, if you know a guest has an allergy to seafood, you should tell him that bottled Asian fish sauce has been used in the salad dressing.

With a few questions and some attention to planning and preparation, both you and your guests can have an enjoyable dinner.

HOMOCYSTEINE: "THE NEW CHOLESTEROL"?

A substance in the blood called homocysteine has made headlines repeatedly over the past few years as a possible new risk factor for cardiac disease. But is it? And if so, what should you do about it? *Heart Advisor* asked Killian Robinson, M.D., a Cleveland Clinic cardiologist who has published widely on the topic of homocysteine, for the facts.

What is homocysteine?

Homocysteine (pronounced HO-mo-SIS-teen) is an amino acid. Several amino acids, including methionine, are essential in human nutrition. Homocysteine is produced when methionine is metabolized. Homocysteine normally stays in the blood only for a short time and is then cleared from the body by the liver.

What makes levels of homocysteine rise? Men have higher levels of homocysteine than women. Medications such as niacin (which is sometimes used for cholesterol lowering) and antifolate drugs (which are used to fight malignant disease) can cause elevated levels. Aging also causes homocysteine to rise.

High levels of homocysteine also occur in a rare inherited disease, homocystinuria, in which a genetic error makes the liver unable to dispose of homocysteine normally. The artery walls of children with this disorder are abnormally thickened and diseased. Patients with homocystinuria may die from blood clots in the brain, heart and kidneys.

Why is homocysteine suspect?

Despite the appearance of the arteries of young victims of homocystinuria, no one suspected that homocysteine played a role in heart disease until a young medical school graduate, Kilmer S. McCully, M.D., published a research paper in 1969. Based on his observations of homocystinuria, Dr. McCully proposed that homocysteine buildup may in fact also be respon-

sible for atherosclerosis. For the most part, the medical community ignored or scoffed at this theory.

Over the past few years, however, the relationship between atherosclerosis and high levels of homocysteine has become a hot "new" topic. In his book *The Homocysteine Revolution,* Dr. McCully surmises that this may be because, over time, physicians have begun to see that traditional risk factors (such as cholesterol and hypertension) cannot account for a large percentage of heart attacks. In fact, people with no recognized risk factors can have coronary disease.

Researchers from Australia and then Europe published the earliest studies revisiting the homocysteine question. The papers strongly suggested a relationship between homocysteine and cardiovascular disease. In this country, a study by The Cleveland Clinic published 1995 in *Circulation* found that high levels of homocysteine increased the risk of heart disease fivefold. That same year, Tufts University researchers found that subjects who had higher levels of homocysteine were also more likely to have blockage of the carotid (neck) artery, a warning sign of the possibility of a stroke or coronary artery disease. They published their findings in *The New England Journal of Medicine.*

In 1997, the *Journal of the American Medical Association (JAMA)* reported that people with the highest levels of homocysteine in the blood had more than twice the risk of clogged arteries in the heart, brain or else-

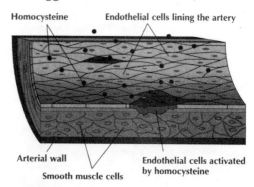

Homocysteine   Endothelial cells lining the artery

Arterial wall

Smooth muscle cells

Endothelial cells activated by homocysteine

 From the *Heart Advisor,* Vol. 2, No. 2, February 1999, pp 4-5. © 1999 by Torstar Publications, Inc. Reprinted by permission.

where. A *New England Journal of Medicine* study, also published in 1997, showed that heart patients with high homocysteine levels had higher mortality rates than patients with low homocysteine levels. And a study that year from the Netherlands, published in *Arteriosclerosis, Thrombosis and Vascular Biology*, determined that every 10 percent increase in homocysteine levels meant about a 10 percent increase in the risk of developing coronary disease.

The evidence was mounting, prompting some researchers to wonder out loud whether homocysteine was "the new cholesterol," an artery-clogging substance previously—and erroneously—considered harmless.

The B vitamin link

Meanwhile, scientists were also looking for a relationship between B vitamins—specifically folate (folic acid), B_6 and B_{12}—and coronary disease. In homocystinuria patients, doses of B vitamin supplements reduced homocysteine levels. Could B vitamin deficiency be linked to cardiac disease?

It seemed so. A 1996 Canadian study in *JAMA* found that participants who did not have diagnosed heart disease at the start of the study but who had the lowest folate levels were much more likely to die of coronary disease than those in the group with the highest levels of folate (who also began the study free of cardiac disease).

The Nurses' Health Study of more than 80,000 nurses found that the women who consumed the lowest amounts of folic acid and B_6 were more likely to develop heart disease, despite the fact that they had no known heart problems at the start of the study. The women who got the most folic acid and B_6 over the years cut their risk of heart disease in half.

A case-control study by Dr. Robinson and members of the European Concerted Action group, published in the Feb. 10, 1998, issue of *Circulation,* determined that lower levels of folate and B_6 conferred an increased risk of atherosclerosis. The study examined 1,550 patients under age 60 in 19 countries.

Results of a double-blinded, placebo-controlled study reported at the 1998 International Joint Conference on Stroke and Cerebral Circulation showed that a combination of folic acid, B_6 and B_{12} could lower homocysteine levels in patients who had had a stroke.

At the August 1998 Congress of the European Society of Cardiology in Vienna, it was reported that heart disease patients who are folate deficient are 1.7 times more likely to have a heart attack than those who have normal levels.

But findings from other, "prospective" studies (in which the research question is posed before the data are collected) have been less consistent. Some have shown a definite relationship between coronary artery

What's a normal homocysteine level?

Before the dangers of cholesterol were understood, levels as high as 300 milligrams per deciliter (mg/dL) were considered safe. Today, normal is defined as under 200 in otherwise healthy people, and levels over 240 mg/dL call for medical treatment.

In a similar vein, the definition of normal levels of homocysteine is the subject of some debate. Different physicians believe "normal" is anywhere from five to 12 micromoles per liter.

"Studies show that the risk of cardiovascular disease rises as homocysteine levels go above 10 to 12," Dr. Robinson says. People who are vitamin deficient, taking certain drugs or in renal failure can have levels as high as 100 to 200.

Homocysteine levels are measured by a blood test, best done after fasting. Your physician won't necessarily test you for homocysteine, however, unless you are routinely seen at a teaching hospital where there is an academic interest in the question.

If you have been diagnosed with heart disease, or are at risk, you can request a homocysteine test, which may be covered by health insurance.

disease and elevated homocysteine levels as well as an inverse correlation with B vitamins. Yet other large, well-designed studies—for example, The Atherosclerosis Risk in Communities (ARIC)—have not. In the July 21, 1998, issue of *Circulation,* ARIC authors stated that they could find no consistent relationship between homocysteine and the risk of disease.

The differences could be because of design problems or methodological limitations of the different studies, or even differences in tests used to measure homocysteine and sample size.

"It is perturbing that the prospective studies do not always bear out the findings of earlier case-control studies," Dr. Robinson says. "We need to determine whether there is a true cause-and-effect connection between heart disease and homocysteine.

"Of course, an association does not always prove causality. It's possible that what we are seeing when homocysteine levels are high is an 'epiphenomenon,' or a fellow traveler of vascular disease rather than a cause of it.

"The true question at this point in time," Dr. Robinson continues, "is if you treat the problem—high homocysteine—does the risk of cardiac disease disappear? This is what current trials are designed to find out."

What you can do

In general, doctors are loath to recommend any kind of treatment when a theory is still unproven. However, the intervention needed to keep homocysteine levels low—increasing your B vitamin intake—is so benign that many doctors are recommending it as a safe course of action until the study results become available in the next four to five years.

Dr. Robinson recommends starting with a heart-healthy diet that includes good sources of B vitamins. It's fairly easy to get enough B_6 and B_{12}—good sources include fish, poultry, lean meat, bananas, prunes, dried beans and whole grains.

It's a bit harder to reach the recommended dietary allowance (RDA) for folic acid, which was recently raised to 400 micrograms (mcg). Green leafy vegetables such as spinach and brussels sprouts, dried peas, beans, lentils and nuts are your best bets, in addition to some fortified cereals.

The government recently began fortifying breads and grains with folic acid, primarily to prevent birth defects that have been associated with folate deficiency. Check the nutrition label on foods you buy made with grain—there may be added folic acid.

Many doctors are advising their cardiac patients to take a multivitamin tablet daily to ensure adequate folic acid. "There's probably very little risk to taking a multivitamin supplement," Dr. Robinson says.

Warning

If you choose to supplement your diet with folic acid, it may be wise to also take 500 mcg of vitamin B_{12}. "Too much folic acid can mask a deficiency of B_{12} that is more common as we age," Dr. Robinson explains. "The deficiency may lead to nerve damage that could persist or worsen if undiscovered."

Alternatively, you could have your levels of B_{12} checked by your physician every six months. If they're normal, you would not need to add B_{12}.

Note: Even multivitamin pills should be taken under medical supervision if you have had a heart attack.

Soy: CAUSE FOR JOY?

By Jack Raso and Dr. Ruth Kava

The soybean, a legume that has for millennia been a staple in tropical and warm temperate regions of East Asia, has in the West recently been described as a superfood "leading the phytochemical revolution." Phytochemicals are diverse compounds whose common denominator is that plants produce them. The word usually refers to plant compounds termed "bioactive non-nutrients," and the vitamins that plants make are not conventionally referred to as phytochemicals. Ingesting phytochemicals, unlike ingesting vitamins and certain minerals, is not considered essential for maintaining human lives. But scientific findings tentatively suggest that habitual ample intakes of such compounds may contribute to disease prevention.

For example, such findings associate phenolic phytochemicals called "isoflavones" with the prevention of cancer, coronary heart disease (CHD), and osteoporosis. Isoflavones are a class of phytoestrogens, or "plant estrogens"—i.e., phytochemicals that have low estrogenic activity—and have been termed "dietary estrogens," "estrogeno-mimetics," and "estrogen mimics." Because of the isoflavone concentration in soy—which is greater than that in any of the other known edible-plant sources of these chemicals (chickpeas, for instance)—soybeans are exceptionally high in phytoestrogens. (Phytoestrogens also include certain "lignins"—noncarbohydrate dietary fibers.)

More than 2,500 varieties of soy are being cultivated. Soybeans are used to make many foods, including miso (a fermented paste), *natto* (soybeans that have been steamed, fermented, and mashed), soymilk, tempeh (fermented soy; also spelled "tempe"), tofu (bean curd), and certain meat substitutes and noodles. Miso, regular soymilk, roasted soy nuts, soy flour, tempeh, tofu, and textured vegetable protein (TVP) are rich in isoflavones. But soy oil, soy sauce, and some other soy products lack them.

> *Cholesterol reduction can result from ingesting as few as 25 grams of soy protein daily. . . .*

The most abundant isoflavone in soy is genistein, which has been the focus of most isoflavone research. Genistein and daidzein, another of the major isoflavones in soy, are structurally similar to the sex hormone estradiol—the main form of estrogen that the ovaries produce (and the form that occurs naturally in plants). Soybeans are the only significant dietary source of genistein and daidzein. Researchers attribute the healthful effects of consuming soybeans and soyfoods largely to the hormonal and other actions of these isoflavones and to the ability of soy protein to reduce cholesterol and low-density lipoprotein (LDL, or "bad") cholesterol in the blood.

But soybeans contain other compounds that might be preventive or have therapeutic utility in humans—for example, the Bowman-Birk inhibitor (BBI) and other protease* inhibitors; inositol hexaphosphate (IP6); and soaplike sugar derivatives called "saponins." The BBI may have utility in preventing and suppressing carcinogenesis. IP6—which is also a constituent of other legumes, rice, wheat bran, and virtually all mammalian cells—apparently can normalize various cancerous cells in mice. Saponins (many of which have a steroid portion) may have utility in preventing colon cancer and in reducing blood cholesterol. Moreover, soybeans are high in fiber (e.g., possibly anticarcinegenic lignins); folic acid; the trace element boron; and the essential minerals calcium, iron, magnesium, and zinc.

Heart Disease

About 34 million Americans have excessive cholesterol in their blood. That elevated plasma cholesterol is a major risk factor for CHD has been established. A decrease in plasma cholesterol of 1 percent decreases the risk of CHD by 2 percent.

---

* Proteases are enzymes that speed protein decomposition.

Reprinted with permission from *Priorities*, Vol. 11, No. 1, 1999, pp. 15-17, 24. © 1999 by the American Council on Science and Health, Inc., 1995 Broadway, New York, NY 10023-5860.

Cardiovascular disease (CVD)—which includes heart disease,* hypertension, and strokes—is the leading cause of death in the United States. But in Japan, for example, the incidence of CVD is low, and the difference in CVD incidence between the U.S. and Japan has been linked to dietary factors, such as soy-product consumption and daily calorie intake (which is lower in Japan than in the U.S.). The inhabitants of the Far East and Southeast Asia typically derive about 10 percent of their daily protein intakes from soybeans, whereas in the U.S. soybeans contribute minimally to such intake.

> **. . . [T]he daily calorie intake in countries characterized by high soyfood consumption is much less than that in the U.S.**

In a study published in *The New England Journal of Medicine* in 1995, researchers compared data from 38 clinical trials performed over 25 years that had focused on the effects of soy protein consumption on blood lipid levels. They concluded that soy protein consumption can reduce plasma cholesterol by 9.3 percent. If this is so—and if a 1 percent reduction of plasma cholesterol reduces the risk of CHD by 2 percent—appropriate intakes of soy protein might reduce CHD risk by nearly 19 percent.

The cholesterol-lowering effect of soy protein seems independent of fat intake and is most pronounced in persons whose plasma cholesterol is elevated. Cholesterol reduction can result from ingesting as few as 25 grams of soy protein daily (as from one cup of soybeans, though 40 grams may be optimal for some persons), and this effect increases according to one's in-

take. The mechanism by which soy protein lowers blood cholesterol has not been elucidated but is an object of continuing scientific investigation. In any case, because soybeans have no cholesterol and are low in saturated fat and high in fiber (that soy fiber can reduce blood cholesterol has also been demonstrated), they are an appropriate food for most persons with heart disease.

In November 1998 the U.S. Food and Drug Administration proposed, pending public comments, to allow the labeling of foods that contain at least 6.25 grams of soy protein per serving as able—in the context of a diet low in saturated fat and cholesterol—to lower CHD risk.

Cancer

Cancer is the second leading cause of death in the U.S. In China, Japan, and other countries where soyfood intake is ample, the prevalence of breast, colon, and prostate cancers is much lower than that in the U.S. Scientific findings suggest that soy and soyfood consumption may be partly responsible for this low prevalence. But it is notable that the daily calorie intake in countries characterized by high soyfood consumption is much less than that in the U.S.

> **The soy isoflavones diadzein and genistein are similar to ipriflavone, a synthetic drug used widely in Asia and Europe that tends to prevent decreases in bone mass.**

Estrogen can promote tumors, and high estrogen levels increase one's risk of developing breast cancer. Because isoflavones bind to receptors to which estrogen would otherwise have

bound, they can, theoretically, prevent or lessen interactions between estrogen and tumors.

Isolated isoflavones have appeared beneficial against cancer in *in vitro* tests and, at very high levels, in animal experiments. Thus, the hypothesis that soybeans and soyfoods are protective against cancer in humans deserves testing. But whether ingesting soybeans, soyfoods, or isolated isoflavones in adulthood lowers one's risk of developing cancer is far from settled. For example, some reports of laboratory studies indicate that genistein stops the growth of human breast-cancer cells, while others indicate it contributes to such growth. Factors, dietary (e.g., a relatively low daily calorie intake) and nondietary (e.g., relatively high activity), that tend to accompany the consumption of soybeans and soyfoods may well explain differences in cancer incidence. Lifestyles and overall diets in Japan, for example, differ considerably from those in Western countries.

Osteoporosis

Osteoporosis is a disease marked by a loss of bone mass that increases the risk of fractures. One of every five American women over age 65 has had at least one bone fracture. Diet and exercise affect bone mass and the risk of osteoporosis. The mineral chiefly responsible for maintaining bone mass is calcium. High protein intakes—because they retard the deposition of calcium in bone and promote the release of calcium therefrom and its removal from the body—can eventually cause a decrease in bone mass.

Soy protein is anabolically equivalent to animal protein (i.e., equivalent in its ability to maintain bodily tissues) in all humans except premature infants. But—like other vegetable proteins—soy protein does not induce as much urinary removal of calcium from the body as does animal protein. Moreover, whole soybeans and many soyfoods—for example, fortified soymilk, tempeh, tofu made with a

---

* "Heart disease" refers to any heart or coronary-artery condition that adversely affects circulation.

> *The proportion of soy isoflavones, or of various soy constituents, may be crucial to the heathfulness of consuming soy.*

calcium-containing reagent (such as calcium sulfate), and TVP—are rich in calcium, and the human body absorbs soy calcium well.

The soy isoflavones daidzein and genistein are similar to ipriflavone, a synthetic drug used widely in Asia and Europe that tends to prevent decreases in bone mass. Animal-research findings suggest that genistein may also do so—at quantities attainable with conventional foods. Genistein binds almost as well as estrogen does to *ER beta*, the type of estrogen receptor that predominates in bone (and in the cardiovascular system). Evidence from research on the relationship between soy and osteoporosis suggests that daily ingestion of both soy protein and isoflavones at quantities comfortably attainable with conventional foods can favorably affect bone. But such evidence is insufficient for offering definitive nutritional advice.

Menopausal Problems

Menopause is the period during which ovarian production of estrogen diminishes and a woman naturally and permanently ceases menstruating. Menopausal estrogen reduction has both physical and psychological effects.

Hot flashes and "night sweats," for instance, are commonly reported. But reports worldwide of how severe and how frequent such effects are, are inconsistent. For example, the likelihood of a menopausal Japanese being thus affected is apparently one third that of a menopausal American. The hypothesis that soy isoflavone consumption is partly responsible for this apparent difference deserves testing. The estrogenic activity of soy isoflavones might moderate the effects of the reduction in ovarian estrogen. But the scientific data concerning whether soy isoflavones can ease menopausal complaints are inconsistent, and the healthful menopausal effects found in isoflavone research have been moderate.

Caution Is Advisable

In the context of a healthful diet and lifestyle, consuming soybeans and traditional soyfoods can lower the risk of coronary heart disease, might contribute to preventing cancer and osteoporosis, and might ease menopausal complaints. Furthermore, evidence is lacking that ingesting isoflavones at quantities attainable with traditional soy products has adverse effects.

Nevertheless, caution is in order:

- Some soy products are high in fat and/or sodium and are therefore inappropriate as central dietary items for some persons with cardiovascular disease.
- Genistein can have toxic side effects at high intakes.
- Theoretically, isoflavones, because of their estrogenic activity, may have adverse side effects similar to those of ovarian estrogen.
- The human health repercussions of long-term consumption of isolated soy isoflavones (as pill ingredients, for instance), and that of soy protein isolates (which often contain isoflavones and other water-soluble soy constituents), are unknown. The proportion of soy isoflavones, or of various soy constituents, may be crucial to the healthfulness of consuming soy.

In 1996, at the Second International Symposium on the Role of Soy in Preventing and Treating Chronic Disease, noted soy researcher Kenneth D. Setchell, Ph.D., who identified phytoestyrogens in human blood and urine some 20 years ago, said in conclusion that "negative effects" are likely from high supplemental intakes of isoflavones and that "the potential for self-induced mega-dosing with [over-the-counter soy isoflavone preparations] should be a serious concern for the future."

Findings from research on the health effects of eating soy have enabled only very tentative conclusions. Pending further clinical-research data, we can prudently use soy as a preventive by consuming soybeans and soyfoods in the context of a diet distinguished by high intakes of varied plant foods.

JACK RASO, M.S., R.D., IS ACSH'S DIRECTOR OF PUBLICATIONS. RUTH KAVA, PH.D., R.D., IS ACSH'S DIRECTOR OF NUTRITION.

Questions and Answers about Cancer, Diet and Fats

Research is evolving about the relationship of diet to cancer. Cancer is a very complex disease, having few definitive answers regarding its cause. Factors to be considered include:

- There are well over 100 different types of cancers, with many differing causes.
- The average diet contains a tremendous amount of different components, some of which may lower the risk of cancer, while others may raise it.
- Unlike heart disease in which blood cholesterol levels serve as an indicator of risk, there are no similar types of markers to indicate a cancer may be developing.
- Cancer takes a long time to develop, which makes it difficult to establish a cause and effect relationship.
- Because of the many questions about diet and cancer that remain unanswered, dietary recommendations should be based on the body of scientific evidence, not just one study. Research published in peer-reviewed journals is the most reliable source of emerging information about diet and cancer.

What can be done to help reduce my risk for developing cancer?

More than 100 types of cancers exist with as many different causes which are not yet completely understood. For that reason, there is no sure way to prevent cancer. But health experts agree there is one general approach to take to help reduce your risk for developing cancer: Adopt a healthy lifestyle that includes getting regular physical activity, eating a balanced diet and not smoking. A healthy lifestyle plays a major role in determining cancer risk.

How does diet affect cancer risk?

Several dietary factors appear to affect the risk of cancer. The type of food is one factor. Diets rich in plant foods such as whole grains, vegetables, fruits and beans may reduce risk for some types of cancer such as colorectal, oral and esophageal. In addition, some studies have linked a diet high in animal products such as red meat with an increase in cancer of the colon and prostate. Recent research, however, indicates the potential link between red meat and colon and prostate cancer can be explained by many other diet and lifestyle factors and needs to be investigated more thoroughly.

Obesity is another risk factor for cancer that is affected by diet. Consuming more calories than you need can lead to obesity. Physical activity has a doubled impact here—it not only helps reduce risk for obesity, it also independently helps reduce the risk of developing certain cancers.

What is the most important dietary step to help reduce risk of cancer?

The strongest evidence points to a well-balanced diet high in whole grains, vegetables, fruits and beans. These foods contain fiber, which is believed to reduce the risk of getting cancers of the rectum and colon. They are also rich in other substances including antioxidant vitamins and minerals and other phytochemicals that may play an important role in reducing cancer risk. For example, lycopene, a carotenoid found abundantly in tomato-based foods, has been found to have potent antioxidant properties that appear to be particularly effective against prostate cancer.

What role does dietary fat play in cancer risk?

The role of dietary fat in the development of cancer, if any, is still unclear. Epidemiological research, which can only propose but not prove associations, suggests high-fat diets may increase risk for some cancers in some people. But other influences, such as that people who eat high-fat diets tend to be heavier and eat more calories and fewer fruits and vegetables, may play a greater role in the development of cancer.

From *International Food Information Council*, May 27, 1999, pp. 1-3. Reprinted with permission from the International Food Information Council Foundation.

According to the 1996 Dietary Guidelines of the American Cancer Society, high-fat diets have been associated with the development of colon, rectal and prostate cancers. However, increasing consumption of whole grains, vegetables, fruits, beans and other fiber-containing foods seems to be more important than decreasing fat intake to reduce the risk of cancers that have been associated with a high-fat diet. More research is needed to determine clearly whether fat plays a direct role in the development of these cancers.

Diets high in fat have not been shown to be a factor in cancers of the stomach, kidney, esophagus, and larynx.

Does fat intake affect risk of breast cancer?

Scientists are still trying to determine if dietary fat plays a role in breast cancer. Breast cancer is associated with circulating hormone levels throughout life, which are influenced by several factors including obesity and physical activity. A recent study of 90,000 women in the United States and Europe found only no significant association between diets high in dietary fat and breast cancer.

To lower risk of breast cancer, the American Cancer Society advises women to eat a diet rich in fruits and vegetables, be physically active, avoid obesity, and limit intake of alcoholic beverages.

Do the individual types of fats affect cancer risk?

The relationship of types of fat to cancer risk is being actively investigated, but it is not yet clear how saturated, monounsaturated or polyunsaturated fatty acids may affect cancer risk. Although several animal studies suggest polyunsaturated fats may increase tumor growth, no relationship has been found between polyunsaturated fats and cancer in humans. Likewise, studies in animals have found that omega-3 fatty acids suppress cancer formation, but there is no direct evidence for protective effects in humans at this time. The most recent review of the literature on trans fats and cancer concluded that there is no evidence that the intake of trans fats affects risk for cancer.

What advice do health experts give for cancer prevention?

Health experts advise a total approach to cancer prevention that includes getting enough physical activity, eating a healthful diet and not smoking.

The recommendations to help prevent chronic disease, including cancer, are embodied in the *Dietary Guide-lines for Americans,* which are tenets for an overall healthful lifestyle for all:

- *Eat a variety of foods.* To make sure you get all of the nutrients and other substances needed for health, choose the recommended number of daily servings from each of the five major food groups displayed in the Food Guide Pyramid.
- *Balance the food you eat with physical activity— maintain or improve your weight.* If you are sedentary, try to become more active. If you are already very active, try to continue the same level of activity as you age. If your weight is not in the healthy range, try to reduce health risks through better eating and exercise habits.
- *Choose a diet with plenty of grain products, vegetables and fruits.* Eat more grain and whole-grain products (breads, cereals, pasta, rice), vegetables, fruits, beans, lentils and peas.
- *Choose a diet low in fat, saturated fat, and cholesterol.* Some dietary fat is needed for good health. But to keep fat intake in a healthful range, use fats and oils in moderation, and frequently choose lean and lower-fat foods. The Nutrition Facts label helps you choose foods lower in fat, saturated fat, and cholesterol.
- *Choose a diet moderate in sugars.* Use sugars in moderation—sparingly if your calorie needs are low. Read the Nutrition Facts label on foods you buy.
- *Choose a diet moderate in salt and sodium.* Read the Nutrition Facts label to compare and help identify foods lower in sodium within each group. Use herbs and spices to flavor food. Try to choose forms of foods that you frequently consume that are lower in sodium and salt.
- *If you drink alcoholic beverages, do so in moderation.* If you drink alcoholic beverages, do so in moderation, with meals, and when consumption does not put you or others at risk.

References

Giovannucci, E., Ascherio, A., Rimm, E.B., et al. *Intake of carotenoids and retinol in relation to risk of prostate cancer.* J Natl Cancer Inst, Dec 1995, 87(23): 1767–1776.

Guidelines on Diet, Nutrition, and Cancer Prevention: Reducing the Risk of Cancer with Healthy Food Choices and Physical Activity. Atlanta, GA: The American Cancer Society, 1996.

Ip, C. and Marshall, J. *Trans Fatty Acids and Cancer.* Nutrition Reviews, May 1996, 54: 5: 138–145.

U.S. Department of Agriculture and U.S. Department of Health and Human Services. *Nutrition and Your Health: Dietary Guidelines for Americans,* 4th ed. Home and Garden Bulletin 232. Washington, DC: Government Printing Office, 1995.

Willett, W.C., Hunter, D.J., Stampfer, M.J., et al. *Dietary fat and fiber in relation to risk of breast cancer.* An 8-year follow-up. J Amer Med Assoc, Oct. 21, 1992, 268(15): 2037–2044.

For more information contact: International Food Information Council 100 Connecticut Avenue, NW Ste. 430 Washington, DC 20036

Micronutrient Shortfalls in Young Children's Diets: Common, and owing to inadequate intakes both at home and at child care centers

Numerous studies documented low intakes of iron, zinc, calcium, and other micronutrients in young children. A recent report suggests that intakes are low in both home food and food provided at day care centers. Most of the young children in that study could not have obtained adequate intakes of key micronutrients without major dietary changes. Is it time to recommend routine multivitamin/mineral supplementation for all young children?

Recommended Dietary Allowances (RDA),[1] I and the more recent Dietary Reference Intakes (DRI),[2] provide the best current estimates of the nutrition needs of different population groups. It is therefore disturbing to read yet another survey documenting that young children have extremely low intakes of iron, zinc, and other key micronutrients relative to RDAs and DRIs.[3] Other surveys recently identified the same problem,[4,5] with iron, zinc, calcium, vitamin A, and vitamin B_6 being the nutrients most frequently consumed in inadequate amounts. There is also some evidence that the nutrition adequacy of young children's diets has decreased, with calcium intake in particular being considerably lower in recent surveys than in previous ones. [5,6]

Dietary data alone do not provide conclusive evidence of widespread nutrition deficiencies. This is partly because the accuracy of dietary reporting can be poor.[7] In addition, the RDAs for all nutrients except energy are set higher than the true need of most individuals to allow for variability in individual requirements).[1] National and regional surveys involving collection of blood samples, however, also observed a significant percentage of young children with low levels of nutrients measurable in blood (e.g., iron),[8] providing further evidence that many children consume nutritionally inadequate diets.

As reviewed elsewhere, several studies suggested that micronutrient shortages in early childhood have serious adverse consequences that may be only partly reversible.[9–12] Iron deficiency is of particular concern because it is extremely common (affecting an estimated 15 million children worldwide),[13] and is linked to long-term impairments in brain maturation, attention span, intelligence scores, and school performance, as well as an increased risk of mental retardation.[14–16] It should be noted that these studies are not individually conclusive because they are observational in nature rather than randomized clinical trials. Many studies reported the same result, however, and intervention studies to reverse anemia in infants

diagnosed with iron deficiency suggested that the potential for reversal of developmental impairments associated with iron deficiency is, at best, limited.[17–20] This latter finding is consistent with animal studies suggesting irreversible effects of iron deficiency on brain iron content and hence on development.[21] Although the reasons why iron deficiency has long-term developmental effects are not well defined, the well-known need of iron for myelination of developing neurons within the central nervous system and the fact that iron is an essential component of several neurotransmitters may be part of the explanation.[11]

Briley et al.[3] reported that only 6% of young children in their study consumed the RDA for zinc and that 45% of the subjects consumed less than two-thirds of the RDA. Zinc is a component of at least 200 enzymes in the human body, forms part of biomembranes, and is thought to be necessary for RNA, DNA, and ribosome stabilization.[22] It is therefore not surprising that permanent growth retardation is one of the

From *Nutrition Reviews*, Vol. 58, No. 1, pp. 27-29, 2000. © 2000 by Susan B. Roberts and Melvin B. Heyman. Reprinted by permission.

early signs of zinc deficiency.[22–25] Recent work also suggested depressed immunity and reduced muscle accretion as features of moderate zinc deficiency in childhood, even when linear growth is not compromised.[26]

Low calcium intakes during childhood are also predicted to have long-term consequences. In particular, calcium is required for accretion of bone mass, and hence bone strength, which occurs almost exclusively during childhood and adolescence. Thus inadequate calcium intake in early life is expected to reduce peak bone mass and increase the risk of osteoporosis later in life.[27,28] There is even recent data suggesting that calcium intakes much higher than the RDAs[1] (which are themselves higher than the new DRIs for children younger than 3 years)[2] may further increase bone mass accretion and hence reduce the risk of future fractures.[29] When combined with work on iron and zinc, these studies emphasize the importance of preventing micronutrient deficiencies in all young children while ongoing research further quantifies the deleterious effects of micronutrient deficiencies and their mechanisms of action.

The issue of why micronutrients are so limiting in the diet of today's children relates in part to children's need for high levels of micronutrients relative to energy. It is also relevant that recent studies of total energy expenditure indicated that the true energy requirements of young children are 15–20% lower than the estimates given in the most recent RDAs.[30] With true energy requirements being low, it can be challenging for young children with normal appetites to physically consume enough food to meet the RDAs for many micronutrients. This is especially true if their diet contains a relatively high proportion of added sugar, fat, and other low-micronutrient items, which is currently the case in the typical diet of most American children.[5] In addition, it is likely that micronutrient intakes were considerably higher during the

evolution of Homo sapiens. Eaton et al.[31] estimated that paleolithic man consumed 5.8 times as much iron, 2.7 times as much zinc, 1.67 times as much calcium, and 1.7–8.40 times as much of other micronutrients as do modern humans, owing to the predominance of micronutrient-rich foods such as meat, legumes, roots, nuts, and fruits in the diet. Thus, during the time when natural selection of human lineages was active, humans did not eat the low micronutrient intakes present in the diet of modern children, a fact that may help to explain the apparent lack of effective mechanisms to prevent the harmful long-term consequences of low micronutrient intakes.

An additional finding in the study by Briley et al.[3] was that home food and food from child care centers provided comparable intakes of dairy products, meat, beans, eggs, fruit, and vegetables relative to the amount of time the children spent in each place. However, cereal, bread, and pasta intakes were much lower at the child care center, and sugar and fat intakes were much higher at home. Although increasing cereal intake in child care centers was suggested as a potential solution to low daily iron and zinc intakes, a focus on home food may be more effective. This is because replacement of high sugar and fat intakes at home with more nutritionally balanced items could have potential nutrition benefits without the loss of the more micronutrient-dense items consumed at the child care center.

Another issue related to making recommendations of dietary improvement for young children is whether it is even reasonable to expect food to be effective in filling all nutrient gaps. Calcium needs are theoretically easy to meet with food because dairy products are such rich sources. There are, however, few very rich food sources for micronutrients such as iron and zinc. For the 45% of children in the study by Briley et al.[3] who consumed less than two-thirds the requirement for zinc, an additional approximately 1

½ cups per day of fortified cereal served with ¾ cup of milk would have had to be consumed for nutrition adequacy (assuming the use of cereal fortified with zinc and containing 15–30% of the Daily Value[32] per 1 cup serving). This amount of cereal represents approximately 20% of the total energy requirement of a 3-year-old child and is therefore an unfeasible and undesirable goal unless balanced by a substantial decrease in other foods. Moreover, even if it were possible to induce young children to eat regular large portions of cereal, the loss of those other foods could decrease micronutrient intakes and have an unpredictable effect on the overall nutrition balance, depending on which foods were replaced.

A practical solution to ensure the nutrition adequacy of young children is routine use of a multivitamin/mineral supplement containing key limiting nutrients that cannot easily be obtained from food. Although nutrition supplements are not currently considered necessary for general use,[33] it may be time to recognize that multivitamin/mineral supplements are a realistic solution to the problem of widespread inadequacies of critical nutrients. This proposed solution,[34] which is both relatively inexpensive and feasible, could be highly effective against the current nutrient shortfalls and could also help safeguard children against further undesirable decreases in iron and zinc intakes. With respect to the latter possibility, it should be noted that decreases in iron and zinc intake could occur in association with any general reduction in dietary quality but are also a possible consequence of greater adherence to the Dietary Guidelines for Americans.[35] This is because red meat and eggs are two of the richest sources of iron and zinc but contain high levels of both saturated fat and cholesterol, which should be limited in people older than 2 years of age, according to the current Dietary Guidelines for Americans.[35]

In summary, multiple dietary surveys documented low micronutrient intakes by young children. Routine recommendation of multivitamin/mineral supplements for young children, combined with practical advice to parents and child care providers regarding ways to improve overall childhood nutrition, may help prevent the adverse effects of early-life nutrition deficiencies suggested in multiple recent studies.

Notes

1. National Research Council. Recommended dietary allowances, 10th edition. Washington, DC: National Academy Press, 1989

2. Yates AA, Schlicker SA, Suitor CW. Dietary reference intakes: the new basis for recommendations for calcium and related nutrients, B vitamins, and choline. J Am Diet Assoc 1998;98:699–706

3. Briley ME, Jastrow S, Vickers J, Roberts-Gray C. Dietary intake at child-care centers and away: are parents and care providers working as partners or at cross-purposes? J Am Diet Assoc 1999;99:950-4

4. Stanek K, Abbott D, Cramer S. Diet quality and the eating environment of preschool children. J Am Diet Assoc 1990;90:1582–4

5. Kennedy E, Goldberg J. What are American children eating? Implications for public policy. Nutr Rev 1995;53:111–26

6. Albertson AM, Tobelmann RC, Engstrom A, Asp EH. Nutrient intakes of 2- to 10-year-old American children: 10-year trends. J Am Diet Assoc 1992;92:1492–6

7. Schoeller DA. How accurate is self-reported dietary energy intake? Nutr Rev 1990;48:373–9

8. Looker AC, Dallman PR, Carroll MID, et al. Prevalence of iron deficiency in the United States. JAMA 1997;277:973–6

9. Pollitt E. Iron deficiency and cognitive function. Annu Rev Nutr 1993;13:521–37

10. Beard J. One person's view of iron deficiency, development, and cognitive function. Am J Clin Nutr 1995;62:709–10

11. Lubin BH, Golden C, Kelley P, Oski FA. Nutritional anemias. In: Walker WA, Watkins JB, eds. Nutrition in pediatrics, 2nd edition. Hamilton, ON, Canada: B.C. Decker Inc, 1996;660–77

12. Kretchmer N, Beard JL, Carlson S. The role of nutrition in the development of normal cognition. Am J Clin Nutr 1996;63(suppl):997S–1001S

13. DeMaeyer F, Adiels-Tegman M. The prevalence of anemia in the world. World Health Stat Q 1985;38:302–16

14. Lozoff B, Jimenez E, Wolf AW. Long-term developmental outcome of infants with iron deficiency. New Engl J Med 1991;325:687–94

15. Roncagliolo M, Garrido M, Walter T, et al. Evidence of altered central nervous system development in infants with iron deficiency anemia at 6 mo: delayed maturation of auditory brainstem responses. Am J Clin Nutr 1998;68:683–90

16. Hurtado EK, Claussen AH, Scott KG. Early childhood anemia and mild or moderate mental retardation. Am J Clin Nutr 1999;69:115–9

17. Lozoff B, Brittenham GM, Viteri FE, et al. The effects of short-term oral iron therapy on developmental deficits in iron-deficient anemic infants. J Pediatr 1982;100:351–7

18. Pollitt E, Leibel RL, Greenfield IDB. Iron-deficiency and cognitive test performance in preschool children. Nutr Behav 1983;1:137–46

19. Aukett MA, Parks YA, Scott PH, Wharton BA. Treatment with iron increases weight gain and psychomotor development. Arch Dis Child 1986;61:849-57

20. Walter T. Infancy: mental and motor development. Am J Clin Nutr 1989;50:655–66

21. Dallman PR, Siimes MN, Manies EC. Brain iron: persistent deficiency following short-term iron deprivation in the young rat. Br J Haematol 1975;31:209–15

22. King JC, Keen CL. Zinc. In: Shils ME, Olson JA, Shike M, eds. Modern nutrition in health and disease, volume 1. Philadelphia: Lea & Febiger, 1994;214–30

23. Walravens PA, Hambidge KM. Growth of infants fed a zinc supplemented formula. Am J Clin Nutr 1976;29:1114–21

24. Walravens PA, Krebs NF, Hambidge KM. Linear growth of low-income preschool children receiving a zinc supplement. Am J Clin Nutr 1983;38:195-201

25. Walravens PA, Hambidge KM, Koepfer DM. Zinc supplementation of infants with a nutritional pattern of failure to thrive: a double-blind, controlled trial. Pediatrics 1989;83:532–8

26. Kikafunda JK, Walker AF, Allan EF, Tumwine JK. Effect of zinc supplementation on growth and body composition of Ugandan preschool children: a randomized, controlled intervention trial. Am J Clin Nutr 1998;68:1261–6

27. Allen LH, Wood RJ. Calcium and phosphorous. In: Shils ME, Olson JA, Shike M, eds. Modern nutrition in health and disease, 8th edition. Philadelphia: Lea & Febiger, 1994;144–63

28. Prentice A. Calcium requirements of children. Nutr Rev 1995;53:37–45

29. Johnson CCJ, Miller JZ, Slemenda CW, et al. Calcium supplementation and increases in bone mineral density in children. N Engl J Med 1992;327:82-7

30. Prentice AM, Lucas A, Vasquez–Velasquez L, et al. Are current dietary guidelines for young children a prescription for overfeeding? Lancet 1988;2:1066-8

31. Eaton SIB, Eaton III SIB, Konner MJ. Paleolithic nutrition revisited: a twelve-year retrospective on its nature and implications. Eur J Clin Nutr 1997;51:207–16

32. Mahan LK, Escott-Stump S. Krause's food, nutrition, & diet therapy, 9th edition. Philadelphia: W.B. Saunders Co, 1996;331

33. Committee on Nutrition, American Academy of Pediatrics. Pediatric nutrition handbook, 4th edition. Kleinman RE, ed. Elk Grove Village, IL: American Academy of Pediatrics, 1998

34. Roberts SB, Heyman MB, Tracy L. Feeding your child for lifelong health. New York: Bantam, 1999

35. U.S. Department of Agriculture. Dietary guidelines for Americans, 4th edition, Home and Garden bulletin 232. Washington, DC: U.S. Department of Agriculture, 1995

This review was prepared by Susan B. Roberts, Ph.D., and Melvin B. Heyman, M.D., M.RH. Dr. Roberts is Professor of Nutrition and Psychiatry at Tufts University and Chief of the Energy Metabolism Laboratory at the Jean Mayer USDA Human Nutrition Research Center on Aging at Tufts University, Boston, MA 02111, USA. Dr. Heyman is Professor of Pediatrics and Chief of the Division of Pediatric Gastroenterology and Nutrition at the University of California, San Francisco, CA 94143, USA.

A Focus on Nutrition for the Elderly:
It's Time to Take a Closer Look

Longevity trends, combined with the swelling wave of aging "baby boomers," are contributing to an explosive growth in the U.S. elderly population, aged 65 and over, which has grown 11-fold during the 20th century[1]. By 2050 about 19 million Americans (24 percent of elderly Americans) will be aged 85 and over[1]. Older people may not know that their nutrient requirements can change from their younger years. The process of aging can introduce other factors—chronic disease, physical disabilities, poor economic status, social isolation, prescription medications, and altered mental status that may cause poor eating habits that do not meet an older person's current nutrient needs. The elderly face the challenge of choosing a nutrient dense diet, one that provides an adequate intake of nutrients at a time when their activity levels and energy needs decline. Assessing the diet quality of the elderly is critical to addressing issues relevant to their health and nutritional status.

This *Nutritional Insight* summarizes the overall diet quality of three age groups of independent, free-living elderly Americans—the young-old, 65–74 years; the old, 75–84 years; and the oldest-old, 85 + years— using the Healthy Eating Index (HEI)[2]. Data from USDA's Continuing Survey of Food Intakes by Individuals (CSFII) 1994–96, a nationally representative survey containing information on people's consumption of foods and nutrients, were used in the analysis. Scores for the elderly groups are compared with the overall IIEI for "pre-elderly" adults aged 45–64.

About the Healthy Eating Index

The HEI is a summary measure of people's overall diet quality. It is an excellent tool both for assessing the quality of Americans' diets and for understanding better the influence of food choices on Americans' health. The HEI is expressed as one score on a scale of 1–100 but is comprised of the sum of 10 components. Each component score can range between 0 and 10. Components 1–5 measure the degree to which a person's diet conforms to the serving recommendations from the USDA Food Guide Pyramid's five major food groups: Grains, vegetables, fruits, milk, and meat. A high score for these components is reached by maximizing consumption of recommended amounts. Components 6–9 measure compliance of to-

tal fat and saturated fat intake according to the *Dietary Guidelines for Americans* and of cholesterol and sodium from the *Daily Values* listed on the Nutrition Facts Label. A high score is reached by consuming at or below recommended amounts. The last component evaluates variety in the diet. A person consuming 8 or more different foods each day will score 10 points. A summary HEI score above 80 implies a "good" diet; a score between 51–80 implies a diet that "needs improvement"; and a score less than 51 implies a "poor" diet.

Overall HEI Snapshot

The CSFII 1994–96 data show the average HEI score for elderly persons 65 + years old is 67.2 out of a possible score of 100. The average HEI score for the pre-elderly group aged 45–64 is 63.4. Both fall midway in the "needs improvement" range.

Among the three elderly groups, as age increases, those with an overall diet quality of "good" remain consistent at around 20–21 percent (fig. 1). Most movement in diet quality occurs between the "needs improvement" and "poor" ratings. The data indicate that with an increase in age there is a slight, but gradual, increase in the percentage of elderly with a "poor" diet (12 to 15 percent). In comparison, fewer individuals in the pre-elderly group (aged 45–64) achieve a "good" diet, and more of them have a diet rated as "needs improvement" or "poor." However, the elderly people's mean HEI scores decrease as income levels decrease, indicating a greater risk for a poor diet quality among lower socio-economic groups.

Figure 1. Overall diet quality, older age groups

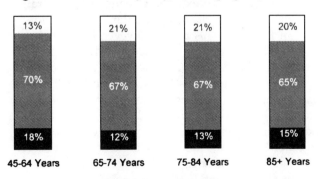

■Poor (HEI < 51) ▨Needs Improvement (HEI 51-80) ☐Good (HEI > 80)

From *Nutrition Insights,* July 1999, pp. 1-2. Reprinted by permission of the USDA Center for Nutrition Policy and Promotion.

Looking Closer at the Components

A closer look at the HEI component scores reveals more pronounced differences between age groups (fig. 2). Among the three elderly age groups, the median scores for each of five components—total fat, saturated fat, cholesterol, sodium, and variety—are 8.0 or better. Despite good scores, the pre-elderly group's component scores were not as high as the elderly groups' scores in three of those same five components. A high score for total fat, saturated fat, cholesterol, and sodium is reached by consuming at or below recommended amounts: thus interpretation of these high scores may be deceiving. A review of CSFII food energy intake data showed that an elderly person's caloric intake declines by as much as 500 calories between ages 65 and 85. Therefore, although the score is high, without further study, it is not possible to know whether reduced food intake is keeping the intake of these components low, or whether the elderly are receiving well-balanced nutrition assistance.

The fruits and milk components had the lowest HEI scores for all age groups. Median fruit scores for the three elderly age groups ranged from 4.6 to 4.9. A slight decrease is noted with advancing age. Median fruit scores for the pre-elderly age group hovered around 3.1, much lower than even the lowest fruit score of the three elderly age groups. Milk component median scores "see-sawed" tightly with advancing age.

In terms of age group, the HEI component scores of the younger, pre-elderly group lagged behind those of the elderly age groups in 3 of the 10 food components (fruit, total fat, and sodium), but they either met or exceeded the elders' scores in 6 other components (grains, vegetables, milk, meat, saturated fat, and variety). All ages studied have a median score of 10.0 for cholesterol.

As Aging Advances

A noticeable, but not extreme, decline in the overall diet quality of Americans aged 65 and over is indicated in Figure 1. This trend, however, is more clearly observed by looking at their median HEI component scores in Figure 2. Only milk, total fat, and sodium scores deviated from this trend. Milk and total fat component scores vacillated from 4.3 to 5.0 and from 7.4 to 8.4, respectively, among all age groups studied. Sodium component scores showed a reverse trend— the older the group, the higher the component score. Until age 85, the groups' median variety score remained at a constant 10.0. After age 85, the group's score dropped dramatically to 8.0.

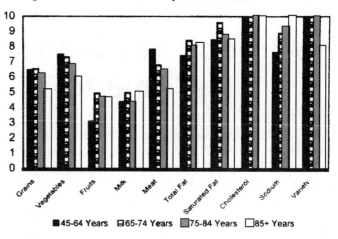

Figure 2. Median HEI component scores

■ 45-64 Years ▥ 65-74 Years ▨ 75-84 Years □ 85+ Years

Conclusions

The overall diet quality of the elderly seems to be better than for their pre-elderly counterparts, but it still falls into the "needs improvement" category. The data indicate the elderly are consuming enough different foods (i.e., variety). However, research efforts and nutrition education strategies should target the quantity and nutrient density of foods the elderly consume, because both quantity and nutrient density are integral to meeting the recommended intake levels of the five major food groups. Inadequate intake of the milk and fruits components, in particular, needs addressing. In addition to eating patterns and income status, poor HEI scores also may be affected by other influential risk factors, such as physical limitations, depression, and non-participation in nutrition programs. Such factors should be considered when conducting research and developing nutrition communications that lead to successful aging.

The United Nations International Year of the Older Person is being celebrated during 1999. Its theme "Healthy Aging, Healthy Living—Start Now!" is indicative that it is time to focus more of our nutrition research, nutrition policy development, and nutrition promotion efforts on the elderly now and into the next millennium.

Contributors: Nancy W. Gaston, M.A., R.D., Anne Mardis, M.D., M.P.H., Shirley Gerrior, Ph.D., R.D., Nadine Sahyoun, Ph.D., R.D., and Rajen S. Anand, Ph.D.

References

1. U.S. Department of Commerce. Economics and Statistics Administration (visited 1998, December 9). U.S. Census Bureau the Official Statistics Statistical Brief, "Sixty-five plus in the United States," May 1995 [WWW document]. URL http://www.census.gov/socdemo /www/agebrief.html.

2. Bowman, S.A., Lino, M., Gerrior, S.A., and Basiotis, P.P. 1998. The Healthy Eating Index: 1994–96. U.S. Department of Agriculture, Center for Nutrition Policy and Promotion. CNPP-5. Available at http://www.usda.gov/cnpp

PHYSICAL ACTIVITY AND NUTRITION: A WINNING COMBINATION FOR HEALTH

INTRODUCTION

Health professionals and the federal government recognize the importance of regular physical activity and a healthful diet to reduce the risk of major chronic diseases and improve well-being (1–9). In recent years, scientific evidence of the health benefits of being physically active, from early childhood throughout later adult years, has led to specific recommendations and/or practical suggestions to increase physical activity (2, 4–8).

Regardless of age, everyone benefits from a physically active lifestyle. Compared to their sedentary peers, physically active children tend to be at lower risk of overweight (10) and are more likely to become physically active adults (11). For adults, regular physical activity, along with a healthful diet, helps to reduce the risk of major chronic diseases such as cardiovascular disease, hypertension, obesity, adult-onset diabetes mellitus, osteoporosis, and some cancers (1–3, 5–9).

Improved mental health or psychological well-being is another benefit of physical activity (6). For older adults, regular physical activity improves muscle strength, functional mobility/independence, and quality of life (12, 13). A physically active lifestyle also delays all-cause mortality (6, 14–16).

Despite a growing consensus and awareness of the substantial health benefits of regular physical activity, many Americans lead relatively sedentary lifestyles (2, 6, 10, 17–20). According to the Surgeon General's Report on Physical Activity and Health (6), only 22% of adults in the U.S. engage in physical activity sufficient to derive health benefits; 53% are somewhat active but not active enough to derive health benefits; and 25% are completely sedentary. Children also lead relatively sedentary lifestyles (6, 10). Only 22% of children participate in 30 minutes of vigorous activity a day and one in four children receives no physical education in school, according to a recent survey of 1,504 families with children in grades 4–12 (10).

The current levels of physical activity among both young and old make it unlikely that many of the federal government's *Healthy People 2000* objectives for physical activity will be achieved (18, 19). Americans give several reasons for their relatively sedentary lifestyles. These include lack of time, injury or other physical difficulties, inclement weather, a dislike for exercise, fear of crime in their neighborhoods, and our "information age" which fosters time spent in front of the computer, television, and video screen (2).

This *Digest* reviews recent research findings supporting the beneficial role of regular physical activity and a healthful diet throughout life, from early childhood through later adult years. Also presented are current recommendations for physical activity offered by various health organizations.

CHILDHOOD AND ADOLESCENCE

Regular physical activity benefits children and adolescents by improving their strength and endurance, helping to control body weight, building healthy bones, and reducing anxiety and stress (21). A growing proportion of children and adolescents in the U.S. are overweight (22–25). Approximately 14% of children aged 6 to 11 years and 12% of adolescents aged 12 to 17 years are overweight (22). Not only is overweight highly preva-

Physical inactivity is a major public health concern in the U.S. In general, females are less physically active than males and physical activity declines with age.

lent among young people, but this condition has continued to rise over the years (22) and affect younger and younger children (24, 25). This situation, coupled with recognition that overweight in children and adolescents may increase the likelihood of adult morbidity and mortality (26), has drawn attention to contributing factors (23, 27).

Physical inactivity is regarded as a major contributing factor to overweight among children and adolescents (6, 10, 23). Because childhood and adolescence can set the stage for lifelong physical activities (11), parents, care providers, teachers, athletic coaches, and others are urged to encourage children to become more physically active (5, 6, 10, 21). Care should be taken to ensure that efforts to prevent overweight in children do not compromise children's growth and development (5).

Physical activity and nutrition, especially adequate calcium intake, play an important role in the development of genetically-determined bone mass (6, 28–31). Maximizing peak bone mass, which occurs between ages 19 and 30 years depending on specific bones, and reducing bone loss in later years lower the risk of osteoporosis. Physical activity during childhood can strengthen bones and contribute to increased peak bone mass in adulthood (6, 28–31). In a prospective study of 470 healthy children ages 8 to 16 years, weight-bearing physical activity and a high calcium intake increased forearm trabecular bone mineral density (30). A study of over 200 women ages 18 to 31 years found that those who were more physically active during their high school years exhibited higher hip bone density, total body and spine bone mineral content, and total body bone mineral density than their less physically active counterparts (31).

Physical activity during childhood and adolescence may favorably influence blood lipid profiles (6, 32). The Cardiovascular Risk in Young Finns Study involving more than 2,300 children and young adults links higher levels of physical activity with increased blood levels of high density lipoprotein (HDL) cholesterol in males and lower triglyceride levels in females (32).

Regular physical activity also reduces anxiety and stress, increases self-esteem (21), and allows an increase in caloric intake without weight gain which enables an individual to increase food choices and improve nutrient intake. A recent cross-sectional study of nearly 500 low-income children 9 to 12 years of age in Montreal found that children who were more physically active consumed more calories, calcium, iron, zinc, and fiber, but did not gain more weight than their inactive peers (33).

ADULTHOOD

Cardiovascular Disease. Numerous studies have established that physical activity reduces the risk of cardiovascular disease, particularly among previously inactive individuals (1, 6, 8, 34, 35).

Regular physical activity and a healthful diet throughout life reduce the risk of major chronic diseases and improve overall health and well-being.

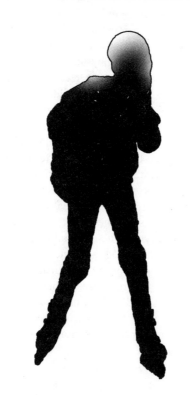

Physical activity exerts its beneficial effect on cardiovascular health through a variety of direct and indirect mechanisms. Physical activity favorably influences the blood lipid profile, specifically raising HDL cholesterol and lowering elevated blood levels of total and low density lipoprotein (LDL) cholesterol and triglyceride levels (6–8, 35–37). In addition, physical activity increases lipoprotein lipase, an enzyme that

removes cholesterol and free fatty acids from the blood, decreases plasma viscosity thereby influencing blood flow, and favorably affects blood clotting and fibrinolytic mechanisms (1, 6, 7, 38). Physical activity may also reduce risk of cardiovascular disease by its beneficial effects on other cardiovascular disease risk factors such as high blood pressure, obesity, and adult-onset diabetes mellitus (6, 7, 35). The cardiovascular benefits of regular physical activity have been demonstrated in both males and females (36, 38–41), as well as in patients with cardiovascular disease or individuals at high risk of developing this disease (42).

To reduce the risk of heart disease, the NIH Consensus Panel on Physical Activity and Cardiovascular Health (7) recommends that children and adults participate in moderate intensity physical activity for at least 30 minutes on most, and preferably all, days of the week. The American Heart Association recommends that adults should also participate in resistance exercise (e.g., lifting weights) for a minimum of two days a week (8).

Hypertension. Physical inactivity contributes to high blood pressure, an established risk factor for cardiovascular disease (6, 8, 39, 43). Sedentary normotensive individuals exhibit a 20% to 50% higher risk of developing hypertension than do their more physically active counterparts (43). Moderately intense physical activity such as brisk walking for 30 to 45 minutes on most days of the week can lower blood pressure (43).

Overweight. Paralleling the trend observed among children, the prevalence of overweight among U.S. adults has markedly increased, specifically from about 25% between 1960 and 1980 to 33% in 1988–91 (18, 44). Physical inactivity is an important contributor to the rise in overweight among U.S. adults (6, 45).

Studies report lower body weight, body mass index, or skinfold measures among physically active adults than among their sedentary counterparts (3, 5–7, 39). Regular physical activity contributes to weight maintenance and/or reduction by increasing caloric expenditure (1, 6, 46). Research indicates that physical activity does not necessarily produce a compensatory increase in appetite or energy intake (6, 47).

As a component of a weight reduction program, physical activity favors the loss of body fat and helps to preserve lean body tissue (6, 46, 48). Minimizing lean tissue loss helps to protect against a decrease in metabolic rate which can increase the propensity to regain weight (48). Physical activity in conjunction with moderate energy restriction may also enhance dietary compliance (49), help to maintain weight loss (6, 7, 50, 51), and improve maximal oxygen consumption or functional capacity (52).

The 1995 *Dietary Guidelines for Americans* (5) recognizes the importance of physical activity, along with a healthful diet, to maintain a healthy body weight. These guidelines call for 30 minutes or more of moderate physical activity on most, and preferably all, days of the week. Health professional organization such as The American Dietetic Association support this position (3).

Diabetes Mellitus. The goals of managing adult-onset or non-insulin dependent diabetes mellitus (NIDDM) include achieving and maintaining normal blood glucose, lipid, and blood pressure levels (1, 53). Although there are few data regarding the effects of combined dietary modification and physical activity on NIDDM, regular physical activity is recommended to help achieve and maintain normal blood glucose levels and a reasonable body weight (1, 6, 53). Epidemiological data indicate a protective effect of physical activity against developing NIDDM (6, 54, 55). The benefits of physical activity appear to be most pronounced for individuals at high risk for developing NIDDM (1, 55).

Cancer. Epidemiological studies provide fairly consistent support for a protective effect of regular physical activity against colon cancer, the third most common cancer among adults (6, 9). Physical activity may reduce colon cancer risk by stimulating colon peristalsis, thereby speeding up the movement of dietary factors, bile acids, and carcinogens through the gastrointestinal tract. Physical activity may also favorably affect the immune system (9, 56), alter prostaglandin synthesis (6), and, in association with a lower body mass, create a metabolic environment less conducive to the growth of cancer (9).

"Successful weight management for adults requires a life-long commitment to healthful behaviors emphasizing eating practices and daily physical activity that are sustainable and enjoyable," states the American Dietetic Association (3).

Although less consistent than for colon cancer, epidemiological findings indicate that regular physical activity may reduce the risk of breast cancer, especially in premenopausal or younger women (6, 9, 57, 58). Evidence is too limited or inconsistent to support conclusions regarding the effect of physical activity on other cancers (6, 9).

Osteoporosis. Throughout life, regular weight-bearing physical activity helps to maintain the normal structure and functional strength of bone (1, 6). Increasing peak bone mass reached by age 30 and protecting against bone loss in later years reduces the risk of osteoporosis, a debilitating bone-thinning disease affecting 20 million women and 7 to 12 million men in the U.S. (59).

Numerous studies indicate that regular weight-bearing physical activity, especially throughout life, helps to protect against osteoporosis (6, 60–65). However, physical activity alone is insufficient to protect against this disease (66). In addition to physical activity, diet (especially adequate calcium and vitamin D intake), and hormonal status (estrogen) contribute to skeletal health (66).

Increased physical activity and calcium intake have been demonstrated to increase bone density and decrease bone loss at various skeletal sites (61, 67–70). A review of 17 trials found that physical activity exerted beneficial effects on bone mineral density at the lumbar spine at high calcium intakes (i.e., > 1,000 mg/day), but not at calcium intakes less than 1,000 mg/day (67). Other studies indicate independent effects of physical activity and dietary calcium on bone health (61, 69, 70). In a recent investigation involving 422 women ages 25 to 65 years in Finland, both high physical activity and high calcium intake (i.e., 1,475 mg/day versus 638 mg/day) were associated with higher total bone mineral content than in participants who were less physically active and consumed lower amounts of calcium (70).

Weight-bearing aerobic activities such as walking, tennis, and low impact aerobics, as well as high-intensity strength training, improve bone density (6, 68). When 39 postmenopausal, sedentary women participated in either high-intensity strength training exercises two days a week for one year or remained sedentary, bone density in the exercise group increased by an average of 1.5%, whereas it declined by about 2% in the sedentary women (68). The high-intensity strength training not only helped to preserve bone density, but it also increased muscle strength and balance, all of which can reduce the risk of future osteoporotic fractures (68).

Clearly, regular weight-bearing exercise benefits bone health at all ages. Because the benefits of weight-bearing exercise are site specific, it is best to participate in a variety of physical activities.

LATER ADULT YEARS

Physical activity is especially important for older adults because of their often low functional status and high incidence of major chronic diseases (6, 12, 71, 72). A recent cross-sectional study involving over 2,000 adults 65 years of age and older associated high intensity physical activity with lower blood insulin, triglyceride, and fibrinogen levels, reduced obesity, higher HDL cholesterol levels, and reduced risk of heart attacks and heart injury (72). Similarly, physical activity in later adult years positively affects multiple risk factors for osteoporotic fractures (i.e., skeletal fragility, muscle weakness, and deteriorating balance) (6, 8, 68).

Physical activity in later adult years may help improve muscle strength, aerobic endurance, functional capacity, gait, joint flexibility, balance, reaction time, and overall quality of life (6, 8, 12, 13, 68). Reduced muscle strength is a major cause of disability among older adults (12). Resistance or strength training has been demonstrated to be beneficial for even frail, institutionalized elderly adults aged 72 to 98 years (13). Also, the increased energy needs resulting from a more physically active lifestyle may allow older adults to improve their overall nutritional intake when energy needs are met by nutrient-dense foods.

RECOMMENDATIONS FOR A PHYSICALLY ACTIVE LIFESTYLE

There is a general consensus among medical and physical activity experts that all Americans, children and adults, should participate in about 30 minutes of moderate intensity physical activity on most, and preferably all, days of the week (2, 5–8). It is now widely recognized that moderate intensity activity equivalent to brisk walking at 3 to 4 mph, and not necessarily a structured, vigorous exercise program, confers health benefits. Resistance or strength exercise at a moderate intensity for two to three days a week is also recommended, especially for older adults (8, 13, 61, 68, 73).

Motivating sedentary individuals to become more physically active is a major challenge (35, 74). The key to

encouraging individuals to lead more physically active lifestyles is to help them identify activities that they enjoy, feel competent and safe doing, and fit into their schedules and budgets (8, 35).

Physical activity alone is not the answer to health. Rather, physical activity should be combined with a healthful diet made up of a variety of foods in moderation from the major

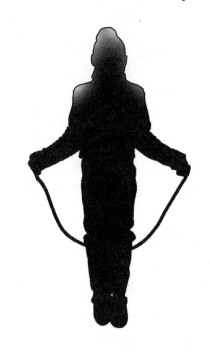

All Americans, children and adults, are encouraged to participate in about 30 minutes of moderate intensity physical activity on most, and preferably all, days of the week.

food groups (3, 5). To help the public put food, nutrition, and physical activity messages into action, the Dietary Guidelines Alliance (4) has implemented a campaign called "It's All About You." This campaign provides action tips for the following five supporting messages: "Be Realistic," "Be Adventurous," "Be Flexible," "Be Sen-

sible," and "Be Active" (4). The "Be Active" message encourages the public to think fun and remember that small amounts of physical activity add up over time (4).

REFERENCES

1. Blair, S.N., E. Horton, A. S. Leon, et. al. Med. Sci. Sports Exerc. *28 (3)*: 335, 1996.
2. Pate, R. R., M. Pratt, S. N. Blair, et. al. JAMA *273:* 402, 1995.
3. The American Dietetic Association. J. Am. Diet. Assoc. *97:* 71, 1997.
4. The Dietary Guidelines Alliance. *Reaching Consumers With Meaningful Health Messages. A Handbook for Nutrition and Health Communicators.* A project of the Dietary Guidelines Alliance, 1996.
5. U.S. Department of Agriculture and U.S. Department of Health and Human Services. *Nutrition and Your Health: Dietary Guidelines for Americans.* 4th edition. Home & Garden Bulletin No. 232. Washington, DC: U.S. Government Printing Office, 1995.
6. U.S. Department of Health and Human Services. *Physical Activity and Health: A Report of the Surgeon General.* Atlanta, GA: U.S. Department of Health and Human Services, Centers for Disease Control and Prevention, National Center for Chronic Disease Prevention and Health Promotion, 1996.
7. NIH Consensus Development Panel on Physical Activity and Cardiovascular Health, JAMA *276:* 241, 1996.
8. Fletcher, G. F., G. Balady, S. N. Blair, et. al. Circulation *94:* 857, 1996.
9. World Cancer Research Fund in association with American Institute for Cancer Research. *Food, Nutrition and the Prevention of Cancer: a Global Perspective.* Washington, DC: American Institute for Cancer Research, 1997.
10. International Life Sciences Institute. *Improving Children's Health Through Physical Activity: A New Opportunity.* A Survey of Parents and Children About Physical Activity Patterns. July 1997.
11. Telama, R., L. Laakso, X. Yang, et. al. Am. J. Prev. Med. *13:* 317, 1997.
12. Evans, W. J., and D. Cyr-Campbell. J. Am. Diet. Assoc. *97:* 632, 1997.
13. Fiatarone, M. A., E. F. O'Neill, N. D. Ryan, et. al. N. Engl. J. Med. *330:* 1769, 1994.
14. Paffenbarger, R.S., Jr., J. B. Kampert, I. -M. Lee, et. al. Med. Sci. Sports Exerc. *26 (7):* 857, 1994.
15. Kushi, L. H., R. M. Fee, A. R. Folsom, et. al. JAMA *277:* 1287, 1997.
16. Kujala, U. M., J. Kaprio, S. Sarna, et. al. JAMA *279:* 440, 1998.
17. The American Dietetic Association. *Nutrition Trends Survey 1997.* September 1997.
18. Federation of American Societies for Experimental Biology, Life Sciences Research Office. Prepared for the Interagency Board for Nutrition Monitoring and Related Research. *Third Report on Nutrition Monitoring in the United States: Executive Summary.* Washington, DC: U.S. Government Printing Office, December 1995.

19. National Center for Health Statistics. *Healthy People 2000 Review, 1995–96.* Hyattsville, MD: Public Health Service, 1996.

20. U.S. Department of Agriculture, Agricultural Research Service. Data tables: results from USDA's 1996 Continuing Survey of Food Intakes by Individuals and 1996 Diet and Health Knowledge Survey, [Online]. ARS Food Surveys Research Group. December, 1997. Available (under "Releases"): http://www.barc.usda.gov/bhnrc/foodsurvey/home.htm[February 25, 1988].

21. Centers for Disease Control and Prevention, U.S. Department of Health and Human Services, National Center for Chronic Disease Prevention and Health Promotion. *CDC's Guidelines for School and Community Programs to Promote Lifelong Physical Activity Among Young People.* March 1997.

22. Division of Health Examination Statistics, National Center for Health Statistics, Division of Nutrition and Physical Activity, National Center for Chronic Disease Prevention and Health Promotion, DCD. *MMWR 46 (9) (March 7):* 199, 1997.

23. Bar-Or, O., J. Foreyt, C. Bouchard, et. al. Med. Sci. Sports Exerc. *30:* 2, 1998.

24. Ogden, C. L., R. P. Troiano, R. R. Briefel, et. al. Pediatrics 99 (4): e[1], 1997.

25. Mei, Z., K. S. Scanlon, L. M. Grummer-Strawn, et. al. Pediatrics *101 (1):* e12, 1997.

26. Dietz, W. H. J. Nutr. *128:* 411s, 1998.

27. Christoffel, K. K., and A. Ariza. Pediatrics *101:* 103, 1998.

28. Vuori, I. Nutr. Rev. *54 (4):* 11s, 1996.

29. Dyson, K., C. J. R. Blimkie, K. S. Davison, et. al. Med. Sci. Sports Exerc. 29 (4): 443, 1997.

30. Gunnes, M., and E. H. Lehmann. Acta Paediatr. *85:* 19, 1996.

31. Teegarden, D., W. R. Proulx, M. Kern, et. al. Med. Sci. Sports Exerc. *28:* 105, 1996.

32. Raitakari, O. T., S. Taimela, K. V. K. Porkka, et. al. Med. Sci Sports Exerc. 29 (8): 1055, 1997.

33. Johnson-Down, L., J. O'Loughlin, K. G. Koski, et. al. J. Nutr. *127:* 2310, 1997.

34. Blair, S. N., J. B. Kampert, H. W. Kohl, III, et. al. JAMA 276: 205, 1996.

35. Clark, K. L., In: *Cardiovascular Nutrition. Strategies and Tools for Disease Management and Prevention.* P. Kris-Etherton and J. H. Burns (Eds). Chicago, IL: The American Dietetic Association, 1998, p. 27.

36. Marragat, J., R. Elosua, M. -I. Covas, et. al. Am. J. Epidemiol. *143:* 562, 1996.

37. Leaf, D. A., D. L. Parker, and D. Schaad. Med. Sci. Sports Exerc. 29 (9): 1152, 1997.

38. Koenig, W., M. Sund, A. Doring, et. al. Circulation 95: 335, 1997.

39. Pols, M. A., P. H. M. Peeters, J. W. R. Twisk, et. al. Am. J. Epidemiol. *146:* 322, 1997.

40. Folsom, A. R., D. K. Arnett, R. G. Hutchinson, et. al. Med. Sci. Sports Exerc. 29 (7): 901, 1997.

41. Mensink, G. B. M., D. W. Heerstrass, S. E. Neppelenbroek, et. al. Med. Sci. Sports Exerc. 29 (9): 1192, 1997.

42. Niebauer, J., R. Hambrecht, T. Velich, et. al. Circulation 96: 2534, 1997.

43. The Sixth Report of the Joint National Committee on Prevention, Detection, Evaluation, and Treatment of High Blood Pressure. Arch. Intern. Med. *157:* 2413, 1997.

44. Kuczmarski, R., K. M. Flegal, S. M. Campbell, et. al. JAMA 272: 205, 1994.

45. National Institute of Diabetes and Digestive and Kidney Diseases, National Institutes of Health. *Physical Activity and Weight Control.* NIH Publ. No. 96-4031, April 1996.

46. Hill, J. O., and R. Commerford. Int. J. Sports Nutr. 6: 80, 1996.

47. King, N. A., A. Tremblay, and J. E. Blundell. Med. Sci. Sports Exerc. *29:* 1076, 1997.

48. Pritchard, J. E., C. A. Nowson, and J. D. Wark. J. Am Diet. Assoc. 97: 37, 1997.

49. Racette, S. B., D. A. Schoeller, R. F. Kushner, et. al. Am. J. Clin. Nutr. 62: 345, 1995.

50. Grodstein, F., R. Levine, L. Troy, et. al. Arch. Intern. Med. *156:* 1302, 1996.

51. Schoeller, D.A., K. Shay, and R. F. Kushner. Am. J. Clin. Nutr. 66: 551, 1997.

52. Kraemer, W. J., J. S. Volek, K. L. Clark, et. al. J. Appl. Physiol. 83(1): 270, 1997.

53. American Diabetes Association. Diabetes Care 21 (suppl. 1): 32, 1998.

54. Burchfiel, C. M., D. S. Sharp, J. D. Curb, et. al. Am. J. Epidemiol. *141:* 360, 1995.

55. Lynch, J., S. P. Helmrich, T. A. Lakka, et. al. Arch. Intern. Med. *156:* 1307, 1996.

56. Hoffman-Goetz, L. Nutr. Rev. *56(s):* 126, 1998.

57. Thune, I., T. Brenn, E. Lund, et. al. N. Engl. J. Med. *336 (18):* 1269, 1997.

58. Gammon, M. D., E. M. John, and J. A. Britton. J. Natl. Cancer Inst. 90: 100, 1998.

59. Looker, A. C., E. S. Orwoll, C. C. Johnston, Jr., et. al. J. Bone Miner. Res. 12 (11): 1761, 1997.

60. American College of Sports Medicine. Med. Sci. Sports Exerc. 27 (4): i, 1995.

61. Nelson, M. E., E. C. Fisher, F. A. Dilmanian, et. al. Am. J. Clin. Nutr. *53:* 1304, 1991.

62. Etherington, J., P. A. Harris, D. Nandra, et. al. J. Bone Miner. Res. 11 (9): 1333, 1996.

63. Alekel, L., J. L. Clasey, P. C. Fehling, et. al. Med. Sci. Sports Exerc. 27 (11): 1477, 1996.

64. Taffe, D. R., T. L. Robinson, C. M. Snow, et. al. J. Bone Miner. Res. 12 (2): 255, 1997.

65. Dook, J. E., C. James, N. K. Henderson, et. al. Med. Sci. Sports Exerc. 29 (3): 291, 1997.

66. Heaney, R. P. Nutr. Rev. 54 (4): 3s, 1996.

67. Specker, B. L. J. Bone Miner. Res. 11 (10): 1539, 1996.

68. Nelson, M. E., M. A. Fiatarone, C. M. Morganti, et. al. JAMA 272: 1909, 1994.

69. Suleiman, S., M. Nelson, F. Li, et. al. Am. J. Clin. Nutr. 66: 937, 1997.

70. Uusi-rasi, K., H. Sievanen, I. Vuori, et, al. J. Bone Miner. Res. 13 (1): 133, 1998.

71. Evans, W. J. Nutr. Rev. 54 (1): 35s, 1996.

72. Siscovick, D. S., L. Fried, M. Mittelmark, et. al. Am. J. Epidemiol. 145 (11): 977, 1997.

73. Nelson, M. E., and S. Wernick. *Strong Women Stay Young.* New York: Bantam Books, 1997.

74. Andersen, R. E., S. N. Blair, L. J. Cheskin, et. al. Ann. Intern. Med. *127:* 395, 1997.

ACKNOWLEDGMENTS

National Dairy Council® assumes the responsibility for this publication. However, we would like to acknowledge the help and suggestions of the following reviewers in its preparation:

■ Kristine L. Clark, Ph.D., R. D.
Director, Sports Nutrition Program
Assistant Professor of Nutrition
Center for Sports Medicine Pennsylvania State University University Park, PA

■ Miriam E. Nelson, Ph.D.
Associate Chief, Human Physiology Laboratory at the Jean Mayer USDA
Human Nutrition Research Center on Aging
Tufts University Boston, MA

The *Dairy Council Digest*® is written and edited by Lois D. McBean, M. S., R. D.

Unit 4

Unit Selections

Key Points to Consider

❖ As the incidence of obesity increases, how can it best be prevented?

❖ What sort of health risks can be affected by some of the more popular weight-loss methods?

❖ What are some of the causes behind a person's becoming obese?

❖ What sort of predictors would indicate dangerous eating disorders?

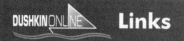 **Links**   **www.dushkin.com/online/**

These sites are annotated on pages 4 and 5.

Overweight and obesity have become epidemic in the United States during the last century and are rising at a dangerous rate worldwide. Approximately 5 million adults are overweight or obese according to the new standards set by the U.S. government using a body mass index (BMI) of 30 to 39.9. Reports suggest that by the year 2050, half of the U.S. population would be considered obese. This problem is prevalent in both genders and all ages, races, and ethnic groups. Twenty-five percent of U.S. children and adolescents are overweight or at risk, which emphasizes the need for prevention, as obese children become obese adults. The catastrophic health consequences of obesity are heart disease, diabetes, gallbladder disease, osteoarthritis, and some cancers. The cost for treating this degenerative disease in the United States is approximately $100 billion per year.

Even though professionals have tried hard to prevent and combat obesity with behavior modification, a healthy diet, and exercise, it seems that these traditional ways have not proven effective. In a society where fast-food eateries are the mainstay of meals, where "big," including food servings, is better, where there is a universal reliance on automobiles, and where the food industry is more interested in profit than in the health of the population, we should not be surprised that obesity has become an epidemic.

Thus, there is a great need for a multifaceted public health approach that would include health officials, researchers, educators, legislators, transportation experts, urban planners, and businesses, which would cooperate in formulating ways to combat obesity. Some of the articles in this unit question the NIH's (National Institute of Health) definition of obesity and argue that the NIH focuses on weight loss rather than on improved health. They offer arguments against the dictum that weight loss makes one healthier and give evidence that the NIH guidelines serve the weight-loss industry better than the consumer. A sound public health policy would require that weight-loss therapies have long-term maintenance and relapse-prevention measures built into them. One of the many factors that predispose a person to weight gain is genetics. Professionals are considering how genes interact with a person's environment. At least 130 genes that cause obesity have been discovered. Some determine how quickly the stomach informs the brain that it is full; others decide how efficiently the body converts extra calories to body fat. This discovery also explains the genetic variability among individuals and emphasizes the importance of individualized treatment rather than one-size-fits-all remedies. It also alerts us to the fact that each person's weight and body shape is a mark of his or her individuality.

There is a plethora of weight loss programs, "quick and easy" diets, and fad diet books that promise quick weight loss and perpetuate the obsession of the population with losing weight. Most people want a quick fix for the present and are

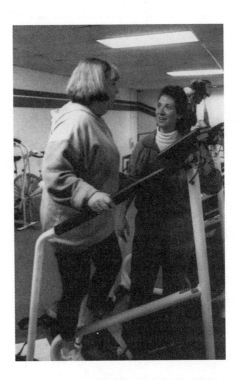

deceiving themselves into thinking that weight will not be regained when they get off the fad diets. Ways to get around the quick-fix mentality are described in some of the articles and the strengths and weaknesses of the most popular weight-loss diets and books are included in this unit.

It seems that the message of professionals to reduce fat calories has been misinterpreted by Americans. Most Americans think that eating certain types of food while avoiding others is more critical to weight management than reducing their portion sizes and, thus, caloric intake. Again the theme of "quick-fix" remedies reemerges. Portion sizes are getting larger in restaurants or other food establishments. Plates have increased from 10 inch to 12 inch sizes and most Americans are unaware of this change. The total daily intake for Americans has increase by 184 calories per day over the last 20 years.

In a country where obesity has become an epidemic it becomes an oxymoron that eating disorders, especially *anorexia nervosa,* are reaching epidemic proportions. Approximately 5 million Americans, especially young women, battle eating disorders and the deleterious effects on health that these disorders bring. Many symptoms that we surmised to be unique to anorexia and *bulimia nervosa* have been found to be the result of starvation. The focus on slimness and dieting all over the world, the use of "skinny" fashion models by the fashion industry, and the preoccupation of a culture with outward appearance, other sociocultural influences, and family dynamics are some of the causes of the above syndromes. Emphasizing "healthy" bodies and fitness, commitment to lifelong healthy eating, preparing children for the changes of puberty, and praising them for goals that they accomplish should be the focus of our society rather than thinness.

Halting the Obesity Epidemic: A Public Health Policy Approach

Marion Nestle, PhD MPH
Michael F. Jacobson, PhD

IN 1974, AN EDITORIAL IN The Lancet identified obesity as "the most important nutritional disease in the affluent countries of the world,"[1] yet a quarter century later, its prevalence has increased sharply among American adults, adolescents, and children.[2-4] The deleterious effects of obesity on chronic disease risk, morbidity, and mortality;[5,6] its high medical, psychological, and social costs;[7,8] its multiplicity of causes;[9] its persistence from childhood into adulthood[10]; the paucity of successful treatment options;[11] the hazards of pharmacologic treatments;[12] and the complexities of treatment guidelines[13] all argue for increased attention to the *prevention* of excessive weight gain starting as early in life as possible. Prevention, however, requires changes in individual behavioral patterns as well as eliminating environmental barriers to healthy food choices and active lifestyles—both exceedingly difficult to achieve.

Because obesity results from chronic consumption of energy (calories) in excess of that used by the body, prevention requires people to balance the energy they consume from food and drinks with the energy expended through metabolic and muscular activity. Although the precise relationship between the diet and activity components of this "equation" is still under investigation,[14,15] it is intuitively obvious that successful prevention strategies—individual and societal—must address both elements.[16]

SYNOPSIS

Traditional ways of preventing and treating overweight and obesity have almost invariably focused on changing the behavior of individuals, an approach that has proven woefully inadequate, as indicated by the rising rates of both conditions. Considering the many aspects of American culture that promote obesity, from the proliferation of fast-food outlets to almost universal reliance on automobiles, reversing current trends will require a multifaceted public health policy approach as well as considerable funding. National leadership is needed to ensure the participation of health officials and researchers, educators and legislators, transportation experts and urban planners, and businesses and nonprofit groups in formulating a public health campaign with a better chance of success. The authors outline a broad range of policy recommendations and suggest that an obesity prevention campaign might be funded, in part, with revenues from small taxes on selected products that provide "empty" calories—such as soft drinks—or that reduce physical activity—such as automobiles.

GUIDELINES FOCUS ON INDIVIDUALS

Concern about obesity is not new. By 1952, the American Heart Association had already identified obesity as a cardiac risk factor modifiable through diet and exercise.[17] Subsequently, a number of federal agencies and private organizations devoted to general health promotion or to prevention of chronic conditions for which obesity is a risk factor—coronary heart disease, cancer, stroke, and diabetes-issued guidelines advising Americans to reduce energy intake, raise energy expenditure, or do both to maintain healthy weight (Figure 1). Typically, these guidelines focused on individuals and tended to state the obvious. For example, the otherwise landmark 1977 Senate report on diet and chronic disease prevention, *Dietary Goals for the United States,* omitted any mention of obesity. (The second edition was amended to advise:

From *Public Health Reports,* January/February 2000, pp. 12-16. © 2000 by Oxford University Press. Reprinted by permission.

Figure 1. Examples of policy guidelines published by US government agencies and health organizations for prevention of obesity through diet, exercise, or both

1952 American Heart Association: *Food for Your Heart*[17]
1965 American Heart Association: *Diet and Heart Disease*
1968 American Heart Association: *Diet and Heart Disease*
1970 White House Conference on Food, Nutrition, and Health[19]
1971 American Diabetes Association: *Principles of Nutrition and Dietary Recommendations*
1974 National Institutes of Health: *Obesity in Perspective*
1974 American Heart Association: *Diet and Coronary Heart Disease*
1977 National Institutes of Health: *Obesity in America*[20,,22]
1977 US Senate Select Committee on Nutrition and Human Needs: *Dietary Goals for the United States, 2nd Edition*[18]
1978 American Heart Association: *Diet and Coronary Heart Disease*
1979 US Department of Health, Education, and Welfare: *Healthy People: The Surgeon General's Report on Health Promotion and Disease Prevention*
1979 National Cancer Institute: *Statement on Diet, Nutrition, and Cancer*
1979 American Diabetes Association: *Principles of Nutrition and Dietary Recommendations*
1980 US Department of Agriculture and US Department of Health and Human Services: *Dietary Guidelines for Americans*[24]
1984 National Institutes of Health: *Lowering Blood Cholesterol to Prevent Heart Disease*
1984 American Cancer Society: *Nutrition and Cancer: Cause and Prevention*
1985 National Institutes of Health: *Consensus Development Conference Statement*
1985 US Department of Agriculture and US Department of Health and Human Services: *Dietary Guidelines for Americans, 2nd Edition*
1986 American Heart Association: *Dietary Guidelines for Healthy American Adults*

1986 American Diabetes Association: *Nutritional Recommendations and Principles*
1988 US Department of Health and Human Services: *The Surgeon General's Report on Nutrition and Health*
1988 American Heart Association: *Dietary Guidelines for Healthy American Adults*
1988 National Cancer Institute: *NCI Dietary Guidelines*
1988 National Heart, Lung, and Blood Institute: *National Cholesterol Education Program*
1989 National Research Council: *Diet and Health: Implications for Reducing Chronic Disease Risk*
1990 US Department of Agriculture and US Department of Health and Human Services: *Dietary Guidelines for Americans, 3rd Edition*
1991 American Cancer Society: *Guidelines on Diet, Nutrition, and Cancer*
1993 National Heart, Lung, and Blood Institute: *National Cholesterol Education Program*
1994 American Diabetes Association: *Nutrition Principles for the Management of Diabetes and Related Complications*
1995 US Department of Agriculture and US Department of Health and Human Services: *Dietary Guidelines for Americans, 4th Edition*
1996 American Heart Association: *Dietary Guidelines for Healthy American Adults*
1996 American Cancer Society: *Guidelines on Diet, Nutrition, and Cancer Prevention*
1996 American Diabetes Association: *Nutrition Recommendations and Principles*
1997 American Heart Association: *Guide to Primary Prevention of Cardiovascular Disease*
1997 World Cancer Research Fund and American Institute for Cancer Research: *Food, Nutrition and the Prevention of Cancer: A Global Perspective*
1999 American Heart Association: *Preventive Nutrition: Pediatrics to Geriatrics*

NOTE: References not indicated are available from the authors on request.

"To avoid overweight, consume only as much energy [calories] as is expended; if overweight, decrease energy intake and increase energy expenditure."[18]) Overall, the nearly half-century history of such banal recommendations is notable for addressing both physical activity and dietary patterns, but also for lack of creativity, a focus on individual behavior change, and ineffectiveness.

Only rarely did such guidelines deal with factors in society and the environment that might contribute to obesity. Participants in the 1969 White House Conference on Food, Nutrition, and Health recommended a major national effort to reverse the trend toward inactivity in the population through a

mass-media campaign focused on milder forms of exercise such as walking or stair-climbing; school physical education programs; and federal funding for community recreation facilities.[19] The 1977 *Dietary Goals* report described certain societal influences on dietary intake, such as television advertising, but made no recommendations for government action beyond education, research, and food labeling.[18]

The most notable exception was the report of a 1977 conference organized by the National Institutes of Health (NIH) to review research and develop recommendations for obesity prevention and management. In one paper, A. J. Stunkard thoroughly reviewed social and environmental influences on obe-

sity.[20] As a result, the conference report included an extraordinarily broad list of proposals for federal, community, and private actions to foster dietary improvements and more active lifestyles. These ranged from coordinated health education and model school programs to changes in regulations for grades of meat, advertising, taxes, and insurance premiums.[21] Some of the proposals cut right to the core of the matter: "Propose that any national health insurance program ... recognize obesity as a disease and include within its benefits coverage for the treatment of it." "Make nutrition counseling reimbursable under Medicare." and "Fund demonstration projects at the worksite."[22] Perhaps because the recommendations

Figure 2. Principal US Public Health Service objectives for reducing the prevalence of obesity through improved nutrition and physical fitness

Promoting Health/Preventing Disease (1980)[23]

By 1990:

- Reduce the prevalence of significant overweight (>120% ideal weight) among adult men to 10% and among adult women to 17% without nutritional impairment.
- 50% of the overweight population should have adopted weight loss regimens, combining an appropriate balance of diet and physical activity.
- 90% of adults should understand that to lose weight people must either consume foods that contain fewer calories or increase physical activity, or both.

Healthy People 2000 (1990)[26]

By 2000:

- Reduce the prevalence of overweight to no more than 20% of adults and 15% of adolescents.
- Increase to 50% the proportion of overweight people ages 12 and older who have adopted sound dietary practices combined with regular physical activity to attain an appropriate body weight.

Healthy People 2010 (2000)[30]

By 2010:

- Increase to at least 60% the prevalence of healthy weight (body mass index [BMI] 19–25) among adults.
- Reduce to 15% the proportion of adults with BMI ≥30.
- Reduce to 5% or less the prevalence of obesity in children and adolescents.
- Increase the proportion of schools that teach essential nutrition topics such as balancing food intake and physical activity in at least three grades.
- Increase to at least 85% the proportion of worksites that offer nutrition education and/or weight management programs for employees.
- Increase to at least 75% the proportion of primary care providers who provide or order weight reduction services for patients with cardiovascular disease and diabetes mellitus diagnoses.

The *Healthy People 2010* objectives also address obesity indirectly through specific objectives for increasing moderate and physical activity among children and adults; for encouraging consumption of more healthful diets; for increasing the use of nutrition labels; for reducing sources of unnecessary calories in food products and in restaurant and school meals; for increasing nutrition and physical education in schools; and for improving access to community recreational facilities.[30]

took 23 pages to list, conveyed no sense of priority, would be expensive to implement, but specified no means of funding, they were largely ignored and soon forgotten. Subsequent reports on obesity prevention continued to emphasize individual approaches to decreasing energy intake and increasing energy expenditure without much consideration of the factors in society that act as barriers to such approaches.

NATIONAL OBJECTIVES

Prevention of obesity by individuals and population groups has been an explicit goal of national public health policy since 1980 (see Figure 2). In developing its successive 10-year plans to reduce behavioral risks for disease through specific and measurable health objectives, the US Public Health Service (PHS) said that the government should "lead, catalyze, and provide strategic support" for implementation through collaboration with professional and industry groups.[23] In developing the specific *Promoting Health/Preventing Disease* objectives for obesity prevention and the methods to implement them, PHS suggested that government agencies do such things as work with public and private agencies to distribute copies of the *Dietary Guidelines for Americans*[24] and other educational materials; encourage development of nutrition education and fitness programs through grants to states; and support research on methods to prevent and control obesity among adults and children. Although these obesity objectives were assigned to the Department of Health and Human Services (DHHS), the implementation activities were distributed among multiple agencies within the Department, with no one agency taking lead responsibility. Thus, the Centers for Disease Control and Prevention (CDC) were to encourage adoption of model school curricula, the Food and Drug Administration (FDA) was to develop a mass-media campaign to educate the public about food labels, and NIH was to sponsor workshops and research on obesity. Implementation steps to achieve the physical activity objectives were distributed among at least nine federal agencies.[25] The words used to describe the implementation steps reflected—and continue to reflect—political and funding realities. Government agencies can encourage, publicize, and cooperate with—but usually cannot implement—programs to achieve national obesity objectives.

Nevertheless, evidence of rising rates of obesity in the late 1980s and 1990s[2,13] has focused increasing attention on the need for prevention strategies. In PHS's second 10-year plan, *Healthy People 2000,* the section on physical activity and fitness appears first among the 22 priority areas for behavior change, and the nutrition objectives appear second, emphasizing PHS's view of obesity as a priority public health problem. Among the objectives in these areas, reducing rates of overweight among adults and adolescents appeared second in order only to prevention of cardiovascular disease.

Healthy People 2000 listed specific objectives for promotion of nutrition and physical education in schools, work sites, and communities—public health approaches that would surely create a more favorable environment for prevention of obesity (see Figure 2).[26]

Despite these efforts, the activity levels of Americans appear to have changed little, if at all, from the 1970s to the 1990s.[5,27] Discerning such trends is exceedingly difficult due to the lack of reliable methods for measuring energy expenditure in the population. Moreover, the average caloric intake reported by Americans rose from 1826 kilocalories per day (kcal/d) in 1977–1978 and 1774 kcal/d in 1989–1991[28] to 2002 kcal/d in 1994–1996.[29] No matter how imprecise the data, these trends suggest why average body weights are increasing so significantly. According to data from the 1976–80 and 1988–1994 National Health and Nutrition Examination Surveys, the prevalence of overweight (defined as at or above the 85th percentile of body mass index [BMI] in 1976–1980) rose from 25.4% to 34.9% among American adults, from 24.1% to 33.3% among men and from 26.5% to 36.4% among women; nearly doubled among children ages 6–11 years from 7.6% to 13.7%; and rose from 5.7% to 11.5% among adolescents.[2,4] (The BMI is defined as body weight in kilograms divided by height in meters squared [kg/m^2].) According to the results of telephone surveys conducted by the CDC, the prevalence of obesity (defined as a BMI ≥ 30), increased from 12% to nearly 18% in just the few years from 1991 to 1998.[2] Trends in prevention and treatment of obesity are also moving in precisely the wrong direction. The proportions of schools offering physical education, overweight people who report dieting and exercising to lose weight, and primary-care physicians who counsel patients about behavioral risk factors for obesity and other conditions have all declined.[7]

In response to these alarming developments, the third PHS 10-year plan, *Healthy People 2010,* continues to emphasize goals related to regular exercise, noting that people with risk factors for coronary heart disease, such as obesity and hypertension, may particularly benefit from physical activity.[30] The first *three* objectives in the nutrition section now focus on increasing the prevalence of healthy weight (BMI 19–25), reducing the prevalence of obesity, and reducing overweight among children and adolescents (Figure 2). But the plan offers little guidance as to how the objectives are expected to be achieved beyond calling for "a concerted public effort" in that direction.[30]

BARRIERS TO OBESITY PREVENTION

Although the impact of obesity on health has been recognized for nearly a half century and its increasing prevalence among adults and children shows no sign of reversal, national action plans consist mostly of wishful thinking and admonitions to individuals rather than public health strategies that could promote more healthful lifestyles (such as those presented by Stunkard in 1977 and later).[20,21] Public health officials need to recognize that when it comes to obesity, our society's environment is "toxic."[31] Unintended consequences of our post-industrial society are deeply rooted cultural, social, and economic factors that actively encourage overeating and sedentary behavior and discourage alterations in these patterns, a situation that calls for more active and comprehensive intervention strategies.

Energy intake. The data indicate that Americans are consuming more calories but are not compensating for them with increased physical activity. If recommendations to consume fewer calories have so little effect, it may be in part because such advice runs counter to the economic imperatives of our food system.[32] While not the sole reason for high caloric intake, massive efforts by food manufacturers and restaurant chains to encourage people to buy their brands must undoubtedly play a role. Promotions, pricing, packaging, and availability all encourage Americans to eat more food, not less.

The food industry spends about $11 billion annually on advertising and another $22 billion or so on trade shows, supermarket "slotting fees," incentives, and other consumer promotions.[33] In 1998, promotion costs for popular candy bars were $10 million to $50 million, for soft drinks up to $115.5 million, and for the McDonald's restaurant chain just over a billion dollars.[34] Such figures dwarf the National Cancer Institute's $1 million annual investment in the educational component of its 5-A-Day campaign to increase consumption of fruit and vegetables[35] or the $1.5 million budget of the National Heart, Lung, and Blood Institute's National Cholesterol Education Campaign.[36] American children are bombarded daily with dozens of television commercials promoting fast foods, snack foods, and soft drinks.[37] Advertisements for such products are even commonplace in schools, thanks to Channel One, a private venture that provides free video equipment and a daily television "news" program in exchange for mandatory viewing of commercials by students,[38] and school district contracts for exclusive marketing of one or another soft drink in vending machines and sports facilities.[39] Advertising directly affects the food choices of children,[40] who now have far more disposable income than they had several decades ago and far greater influence on their parents' buying habits.[41]

Americans spend about half of their food budget and consume about one-third their daily energy[42] on meals and drinks consumed outside the home, where it is exceedingly difficult to estimate the energy content of the food. About 170,000 fast-food restaurants[43] and three million soft drink vending machines[44] help ensure that Americans are not more than a few steps from immediate sources of relatively non-nutritious foods. As a Coca-Cola Company executive proclaimed, "[T]o build pervasiveness of our products, we're putting ice-cold Coca-Cola classic and our other brands within reach, wherever you look: at the supermarket, the video store, the soccer field, the gas station—everywhere."[45]

Food eaten outside the home, on average, is higher in fat and lower in micronutrients than food prepared at home.[42] Many popular table-service restaurant meals—lunch or dinner—provide 1000 to 2000 kcal each,[46] amounts equivalent to 35% to 100% of a full day's energy requirement for most adults.[47] Restaurants and movie theaters charge just a few cents more for larger-size orders of soft drinks, popcorn, and French fries, and the standard serving sizes of these and other foods have increased greatly in the past decade.[48] For example, in the 1950s, Coca-Cola was packaged only in 6.5-oz bottles; single-serving containers expanded first to 12-oz cans and, more recently, to 20-oz bottles. A 12-oz soft drink provides about 150 kcal, all from sugars, but contains no other nutrients of significance.[49]

Taken together, such changes in the food environment help explain why it requires more and more will power for Americans to maintain an appropriate intake of energy.

Energy expenditure, Influencing Americans to increase energy expenditure is as daunting a task as encouraging reductions in energy intake. Twentieth-century labor-saving devices, from automobiles to e-mail, are ubiquitous and have reduced energy needs, as has the shift of a large proportion of the workforce from manual

Figure 3. Reducing the prevalence of obesity: policy recommendations

Education

- Provide federal funding to state public health departments for mass media health promotion campaigns that emphasize healthful eating and physical activity patterns.
- Require instruction in nutrition and weight management as part of the school curriculum for future health-education teachers.
- Make a plant-based diet the focus of dietary guidance.
- Ban required watching of commercials for foods high in calories, fat, or sugar on school television programs (for example, Channel One).
- Declare and organize an annual National "No-TV" Week.
- Require and fund daily physical education and sports programs in primary and secondary schools, extending the school day if necessary.
- Develop culturally relevant obesity prevention campaigns for high-risk and low-income Americans.
- Promote healthy eating in government cafeterias, Veterans Administration medical centers, military installations, prisons, and other venues.
- Institute campaigns to promote healthy eating and activity patterns among federal and state employees in all departments.

Food labeling and advertising

- Require chain restaurants to provide information about calorie content on menus or menu boards and nutrition labeling on wrappers.
- Require that containers for soft drinks and snacks sold in movie theaters, convenience stores, and other venues bear information about calorie, fat, or sugar content.
- Require nutrition labeling on fresh meat and poultry products.
- Restrict advertising of high-calorie, low-nutrient foods on television shows commonly watched by children or require broadcasters to provide equal time for messages promoting healthy eating and physical activity.
- Require print advertisements to disclose the caloric content of the foods being marketed.

Food assistance programs

- Protect school food programs by eliminating the sale of soft drinks, candy bars, and foods high in calories, fat, or sugar in school buildings.
- Require that any foods that compete with school meals be consistent with federal recommendations for fat, saturated fat, cholesterol, sugar, and sodium content.
- Develop an incentive system to encourage Food Stamp recipients to purchase fruits, vegetables, whole grains, and other healthful foods, such as by earmarking increases in Food Stamp benefits for the purchase of those foods.

Health care and training

- Require medical, nursing, and other health professions curricula to teach the principles and benefits of healthful diet and exercise patterns.
- Require health care providers to learn about behavioral risks for obesity and how to counsel patients about health-promoting behavior change.
- Develop and fund a research agenda focused on behavioral as well as metabolic determinants of weight gain and maintenance, and on the most cost-effective methods for promoting healthful diet and activity patterns.
- Revise Medicaid and Medicare regulations to provide incentives to health care providers for nutrition and obesity counseling and other interventions that meet specified standards of cost and effectiveness.

Transportation and urban development

- Provide funding and other incentives for bicycle paths, recreation centers, swimming pools, parks, and sidewalks.
- Develop and provide guides for cities, zoning authorities, and urban planners on ways to modify zoning requirements, designate downtown areas as pedestrian malls and automobile-free zones, and modify residential neighborhoods, workplaces, and shopping centers to promote physical activity.

Taxes

- Levy city, state, or federal taxes on soft drinks and other foods high in calories, fat, or sugar to fund campaigns to promote good nutrition and physical activity.
- Subsidize the costs of low-calorie nutritious foods, perhaps by raising the costs of selected high-calorie, low-nutrient foods.
- Remove sales taxes on, or provide other incentives for, purchase of exercise equipment.
- Provide tax incentives to encourage employers to provide weight management programs.

Policy development

- Use the National Nutrition Summit to develop a national campaign to prevent obesity.
- Produce a Surgeon General's Report on Obesity Prevention.
- Expand the scope of the President's Council on Physical Fitness and Sports to include nutrition and to emphasize obesity prevention.
- Develop a coordinated federal implementation plan for the Healthy People 2010 nutrition and physical activity objectives.

labor to white-collar jobs that require nothing more active than pressing keys on a computer.[50] Wonders of modern civilization such as central heating lessen the energy cost of maintaining body temperature, and air conditioning makes it much more comfortable on hot summer days to stay inside and watch television or play computer games than to engage in outdoor activities. Dangerous neighborhoods—or the perception of danger—discourage people from walking dogs, pushing strollers, playing ball, jogging, or permitting children to play outdoors.[51] Many suburban neighborhoods are structured for the convenience of automobile drivers; they may not have sidewalks and may lack stores, entertainment, or other destinations within walking distance. Meanwhile, the decline in tax support for many public school systems and the need to fulfill competing academic priorities have forced them to relegate physical education to the category of "frill." Many school districts have had to eliminate physical education classes entirely, and fewer and fewer schools offer any opportunity for students to be physically active during the school day.[6] Such barriers make it clear why an attempt to "detoxify" the present environment and create one that fosters healthful activity patterns deserves far more attention than it has received since the 1977 recommendations in *Obesity in America*.[20,22]

PUBLIC HEALTH APPROACHES

In an environment so antagonistic to healthful lifestyles, no quick and easy solution to the problem of obesity should be expected. Meaningful efforts must include the development of government policies and programs that address both the "energy in" and "energy out" components of weight maintenance. Although privately funded campaigns to educate the public and mobilize physicians to combat obesity, such as Shape Up America,[52] are useful adjuncts, they cannot be expected to achieve significant population-wide behavior change. What is needed is substantial involvement of and investment by government at all levels. Governmental policies and programs affect many of the environmental determinants of poor diets and sedentary lifestyles. Communities, workplaces, schools, medical centers, and many other venues are subject to federal and other governmental regulations that could be modified to make the environment more conducive to healthful diet and

activity patterns. Just as the environmental crisis spurred the public to make a huge financial investment in seeking solutions, so should the obesity epidemic.

In Figure 3, we provide recommendations for a variety of such modifications along with suggestions for new policies targeted to obesity prevention. These recommendations, reflecting the disparate influences on diet and activity, address education, food regulation and advertising, food assistance, health care and the training of health professionals, transportation and urban development, taxation, and the development of federal policy. We offer the suggestions, some of which have been proposed by others,[20,22,53,54] to stimulate discussion of a much wider range of approaches than is typically considered. In doing so, we suggest changes in existing policies and practices that affect health behaviors. We believe these proposals are politically and economically feasible and, collectively, capable of producing a significant effect in helping people to maintain healthy weight. Each of the suggestions could benefit from further discussion and analysis. Here, we comment on just a few of them.

Using media campaigns. Media advertising should be a vital part of any campaign to reduce obesity through promotion of positive changes in behavior, such as eating more fruits, vegetables, and whole grains; switching to lower-fat meat or dairy products; eating fewer hamburgers and steaks; and drinking water instead of soda. Campaigns of this kind can be remarkably effective. For example, the Center for Science in the Public Interest's "1% Or Less" program doubled the market share of low-fat and fat-free milk in several communities through intensive, seven-week paid advertising and public relations campaigns that cost as little as 22 cents per person.[56–58] Those efforts illustrate that advertising can be an affordable, effective method for promoting dietary change—even in the context of media advertising for less nutritious foods. Similar mass-media motivational campaigns could be developed to encourage people to walk, jog, bicycle, and engage in other enjoyable activities that expend energy.

Discouraging TV watching and junk-food advertising. Anti-obesity measures need to address television watching, a major sedentary activity as well as one that exposes viewers to countless commercials for high-calorie foods. The average American child between the ages of 8 and 18 spends more than three hours daily watching television and another three or four

hours with other media.[59] Television is an increasingly well-established risk factor for obesity and its health consequences in both adults and children.[60,61] At least one study now shows that reducing the number of hours spent watching television or playing video games is a promising approach to preventing obesity in children.[62] Government and private organizations could sponsor an annual "No TV Week" to remind people that life is possible, even better, with little or no television and that watching television could well be replaced by physical and social activities that expend more energy. The Department of Education and DHHS could sponsor a national campaign, building on previous work by the nonprofit TV-Free America.[63]

Advertisements for candy, snacks, fast foods, and soft drinks should not be allowed on television shows commonly watched by children younger than age 10. Researchers have shown that younger children do not understand the concept of advertising—that it differs from program content and is designed to sell, not inform—and that children of all ages are highly influenced by television commercials to buy or demand the products that they see advertised.[64] It makes no sense for a society to allow private interests to misshape the eating habits of the next generation, and it is time for Congress to repeal the law that blocks the Federal Trade Commission from promulgating industry-wide rules to control advertising during children's television programs.[65]

Promoting physical activity. Federal and state government agencies could do more to make physical activity more attractive and convenient. They could provide incentives to communities to develop safe bicycle paths and jogging trails; to build more public swimming pools, tennis courts, and ball fields; to pass zoning rules favoring sidewalks in residential and commercial areas, traffic-free areas, and traffic patterns that encourage people to walk to school, work, and shopping; and safety protection for streets, parks, and playgrounds. Government could also provide incentives to use mass transit, and disincentives to drive private cars, thereby encouraging people to walk to bus stops and train stations.

Reaching children through the schools. State boards of education and local school boards have an obligation to promote healthful lifestyles. Physical education should again be required, preferably on a daily basis, to encourage students to expend energy and to help them develop lifelong enjoyment of jogging, ball games, swimming, and other low-cost activities. School boards should be encouraged to resist efforts of marketers to sell soda and high-calorie, low-nutrient snack foods in hallways and cafeterias. Congress could support more healthful school meals by insisting that the US Department of Agriculture (USDA) set stricter limits on sales of foods high in energy (calories), fat, and sugar that compete with the sale of balanced breakfasts and lunches.

Adjusting food prices. Price is a factor in food purchases. Lowering by half the prices of fruits and vegetables in vending machines and school cafeterias can result in doubling their sales.[66] The government could adopt policies to decrease the prices of more healthful foods and increase the prices of foods high in energy.[67] Local governments and the media might offer free publicity, awards, or other incentives to restaurants to offer free salads with meals, to charge more for less nutritious foods, and to reduce the prices of more nutritious foods.

FINANCING OBESITY PREVENTION

The principal barrier to meaningful health-promotion programs is almost always lack of funds, and the educational campaigns and certain other measures we propose would not be inexpensive. But to put such costs in perspective, it is important to understand that the annual costs of direct health care and lost productivity resulting from obesity and its consequences have been estimated at 5.7% of total US health care expenditures, or $52 billion in 1995 dollars.[68] More conservative estimates still suggest that obesity accounts for 1% to 4% of total health care costs.[7] Notwithstanding these enormous costs, Congress and state legislatures provide virtually no funding specifically targeted to anti-obesity measures other than basic research. The $5 million recently granted to the CDC for nutrition and obesity programs represents a small but important step in the right direction.

To compensate for state and federal legislatures' failure to apply general revenues to anti-obesity measures, other commentators have suggested that revenues from taxes on "junk foods" be used to subsidize the costs of more healthful foods.[31] While onerous taxes on commonly purchased products would be highly unpopular and politically unrealistic, small taxes are feasible. Such taxes would likely have little effect on overall sales but could

generate sufficient revenues to fund some of the measures that we are suggesting. Legislatures have long levied taxes on products deemed to be unhealthful. Thus, the federal government and states impose taxes on alcoholic beverages and cigarettes; these taxes are supported by large public majorities, especially when the revenues are earmarked for health purposes.[69] Several states currently tax soft drinks and snack foods. In California, for example, soft drinks are the only foods subject to the 7.25% sales tax; we calculate on the basis of population[43] and consumption[70] statistics that this tax alone raises about $200 million per year. A two-cent-per-can tax on soft drinks in Arkansas raises $40 million per year (Personal communication, Tamra Huff, Arkansas Department of Finance and Administration, September 1998). In these and several other states, the tax revenues go into the general treasury. West Virginia, however, uses the revenues from its soft drink tax to support its state medical, dental, and nursing schools, and Tennessee earmarks 21% of the revenues from its tax for cleaning up highway litter.

To fund the television advertisements, physical education teachers, bicycle paths, swimming pools, and other measures that we propose, we suggest that small taxes be levied on several widely used products that are likely to contribute to obesity. We estimate that each of the following hypothetical taxes would generate revenues of about $1 billion per year:

- A 2/3-cent tax per 12 oz on soft drinks.[70]
- A 5% tax on new televisions and video equipment.[43]
- A $65 tax on each new motor vehicle (about 0.3% on a $20,000 car), or an extra penny tax per gallon of gasoline.[43]

A national survey found that 45% of adults would support a one-cent tax on a can of soft drink, pound of potato chips, or pound of butter it the revenues funded a national health education program.[71] Such taxes are too small to raise serious concerns about their regressive nature.

TOWARD NATIONAL ACTION

The USDA and DHHS have announced plans for a National Nutrition Summit, scheduled for May 30–31, 2000. This Summit could catalyze an unprecedented effort to reverse the

obesity epidemic. Its focus will be on behavioral factors—especially those that could help prevent overweight and obesity.[72] The Summit provides an ideal opportunity for public and private institutions to initiate the kinds of policies and programs that we are advocating. We believe that the Summit should emphasize ways to improve both government policies and corporate practices that affect individual behavior change.

Government officials could use the Summit to announce actions, including proposed legislation, that their departments will seek to implement (see Figure 3). For example, USDA could announce incentives to encourage Food Stamp recipients to buy more produce, whole grains, and reduced-fat animal products. The Surgeon General could announce a campaign to reduce television watching. Justice Department officials could announce initiatives for reducing inner-city crime to make playing outside safer for children, while the Department of Housing and Urban Development could announce grants for inner-city recreational facilities. The Department of Transportation could announce increased funding to enable states to expand mass transit and provide more bicycle paths. Finally, the futility of current efforts demonstrates the urgent need for research on which to base more effective public health policies. Ending the obesity epidemic will require much greater knowledge of effective diet and activity strategies than is currently available. The research focus must extend beyond genetic, metabolic, and drug development studies to encompass—and emphasize—population-based behavioral interventions, policy development, and program evaluation.

Thus, we propose that the measures outlined in Figure 3 be implemented on a trial basis and evaluated for their effectiveness. We do not pretend that these suggestions alone will eliminate obesity from American society, but they will be valuable if they help to produce even small reductions in the rate of obesity, as even modest weight loss confers substantial health and economic benefits.[73] Without such a national commitment and effective new approaches to making the environment more favorable to maintaining healthy weight, we doubt that the current trends can be reversed.

REFERENCES

1. Infant and adult obesity [editorial]. Lancet 1974;i:17–18.

2. Mokdad AH, Serdula MK, Dietz WH, Bowman BA, Marks JS, Koplan JP. The spread of the obesity epidemic in the United States, 1991–1998. JAMA 1999;282:1519–22.

3. Troiano RP, Flegal KM, Kuczmarski RJ, Campbell SM, Johnson CL. Overweight prevalence and trends for children and adolescents. Arch Pediatr Adolesc Med 1995;149:1085–91.

4. Update: prevalence of overweight among children, adolescents, and adults—United States, 1988–1994. MMWR Morb Mortal Wkly Rep 1997;46:199–202.

5. Must A, Spadano J, Coakley EH, Field AE, Colditz G, Dietz WH. The disease burden associated with overweight and obesity. JAMA 1999;282:1523–9.

6. Allison DB, Fontaine KR, Manson JE, Stevens J, Vanltallie TB. Annual deaths attributable to obesity in the United States. JAMA 1999;282:1530–8.

7. Allison DB, Zannolli R, Narayan KMV. The direct health care costs of obesity in the United States. Am J Public Health 1999;89:1194–9.

8. Rippe JM, Aronne LJ, Gilligan VF, Kumanyika S, Miller S, Owens GM, et al. Public policy statement on obesity and health from the Interdisciplinary Council on Lifestyle and Obesity Management. Nutr Clin Care 1998;1:34–7.

9. Grundy SM. Multifactorial causation of obesity: implications for prevention. Am J Clin Nutr 1998;67(3 Suppl):5365–725.

10. Whitaker RC, Wright JA, Pepe MS, Seidel KD, Dietz WH. Predicting obesity in young adulthood from childhood and parental obesity. N Engl J Med 1997;337:869–73.

11. Methods for voluntary weight loss and control: Technology Assessment Conference statement. Bethesda (MD): National Institutes of Health (US); 1992.

12. Williamson DF. Pharmacotherapy for obesity. JAMA 1999;281:278–80.

13. Expert Panel on the Identification, Evaluation, and Treatment of Overweight in Adults. Clinical guidelines on the identification, evaluation, and treatment of overweight in adults. Bethesda (MD): National Institutes of Health (US); 1998.

14. US Preventive Services Task Force. Guide to clinical preventive services. 2nd ed. Alexandria (VA): International Medical Publishing; 1996.

15. Dalton S. Overweight and weight management. Gaithersburg (MD): Aspen; 1997.

16. Koplan JP, Dietz WH. Caloric imbalance and public health policy. JAMA 1999;282:1579–80.

17. Harvard School of Public Health, Department of Nutrition. Food for your heart: a manual for patient and physician. New York: American Heart Association; 1952.

18. Senate Select Committee on Nutrition and Human Needs (US). Dietary goals for the United States. 2nd ed. Washington: Government Printing Office; 1977.

19. White House Conference on Food, Nutrition, and Health: final report. Washington: Government Printing Office; 1970.

20. Stunkard AJ. Obesity and the social environment: current status, future prospects. In: Bray GA, editor. Obesity in America. Washington: Department of Health, Education, and Welfare (US); 1979. NIH Pub. No.: 79–359.

21. Stunkard A. The social environment and the control of obesity. In: Stunkard AJ, editor. Obesity. Philadelphia: WB Saunders; 1980. p. 438–62.

22. Fullarton JE. Matrix for action: nutrition and dietary practices [appendix]. In: Bray GA, editor. Obesity in America. Washington: Department of Health, Education, and Welfare (US); 1979. p. 241–64. NIH Pub. No.: 7–359.

23. Department of Health and Human Services (US). Promoting health/preventing disease: objectives for the nation. Washington: Government Printing Office; 1980.

24. Department of Agriculture (US) and Department and Health and Human Services (US). Nutrition and your health: dietary guidelines for Americans. Washington: Government Printing Office; 1980,

25. Department of Health and Human Services (US). Promoting health/preventing disease: Public Health Service implementation plans for attaining the objectives for the nation. Public Health Rep 1983;Sept-Oct Suppl.

26. Department of Health and Human Services (US). Healthy People: national health promotion and disease prevention objectives. Washington: Government Printing Office; 1990.

27. Department of Health and Human Services (US). The 1990 Health Objectives for the Nation: a midcourse review. Washington: Office of Disease Prevention and Health Promotion (US); 1986.

28. Life Sciences Research Office, Federation of American Societies for Experimental Biology. Third report on nutrition monitoring in the United States. Vol 2. Prepared for Interagency Board for Nutrition Monitoring and Related Research, US Department of Health and Human Services, US Department of Agriculture. Washington: Government Printing Office; 1995.

29. Department of Agriculture (US). Data Tables: Results from USDA's 1994–96 Continuing Survey of Food Intakes by Individuals and 1994–96 Diet and Health Knowledge Survey, December 1997 [cited 1999 Feb 23]. Available from: URL: http://www.barc.usda.gov/bhnrc/foodsurvey/home.htm

30. Department of Health and Human Services (US). Healthy People 2010: understanding and improving health. Conference edition. Washington: Government Printing Office; 2000.

31. Battle EK, Brownell KD. Confronting a rising tide of eating disorders and obesity: treatment vs. prevention and policy. Addict Behav 1996;21:755–65.

32. Department of Agriculture, Economic Research Service (US). U.S. Food Expenditures [cited 1999 Dec II]. Available from: URL: http://www.econ.ag.gov/

33. Gallo AE. The food marketing system in 1996. Agricultural Information Bulletin No. 743. Washington: Department of Agriculture (US); 1998.

34. 44th annual: 100 leading national advertisers. Advertising Age 1999 Sept 27;S1–S46.

35. Gov't & industry launch fruit and vegetable push; but NCI takes back seat. Nutr Week 1992;22(26):1–2.

36. Cleeman JI, Lenfant C. The National Cholesterol Education Program: progress and prospects. JAMA 1998;280:2099–104.

37. Kotz K, Story M. Food advertisements during children's Saturday morning television programming: are they consistent with dietary recommendations? J Am Diet Assoc 1994;94:1296–1300.

38. Hays CL. Channel One's mixed grades in schools. New York Times 1999 Dec 5;Sect. C:1,14–15.

39. Hays CL. Be true to your cola, rah! rah!: battle for soft-drink loyalties moves to public schools. New York Times 1998 Mar &Sect. D:1,4.

40. Sylvester GP, Achterberg C, Williams J. Children's television and nutrition: friends or foes. Nutr Today 1995;30(1):6–15.

41. McNeal JU. The kids market: myths and realities. Ithaca (NY): Paramount Market Publishing; 1999.

42. Lin B-H, Frazao E, Guthrie J. Away-from-home foods increasingly important to quality of American diet. Agricultural Information Bulletin No. 749. Washington: Department of Agriculture (US); 1999.

43. Bureau of the Census (US). Statistical abstract of the United States: the national data book: 1997. 117th ed. Washington: Government Printing Office; 1997.

44. Vended bottled drinks. Vending Times 1998;38(9):15,21–2.

45. Annual Report. Atlanta: Coca-Cola Co.; 1997. Available from Coca-Cola Co., One Coca-Cola Plaza, Atlanta GA 30313.

46. Burros M. Losing count of calories as plates fill up. New York Times 1997 Apr 2;Sect. C:1,4.

47. National Research Council. Recommended dietary allowances. 9th rev. ed. Washington: National Academy Press; 1989.

48. Young LR, Nestle M. Portion sizes in dietary assessment: issues and policy implications. Nutr Rev 1995;53:149–58.

49. Jacobson MF. Liquid candy: how soft drinks are harming Americans' health. Washington: Center for Science in the Public Interest; 1998.

50. President's Council on Physical Fitness and Sports (US). Physical activity and health: a report of the Surgeon General. Washington: Department of Health and Human Services (US); 1996.

51. Neighborhood safety and the prevalence of physical inactivity—selected states, 1996. MMWR Morb Mortal Wkly Rep 1999;48:143–6.

52. Welcome to Shape Up America! [cited 1999 Dec 4]. Available from: URL: http://www.shapeup.org/

53. Jeffery RW. Public health approaches to the management of obesity. In: Brownell KD, Fairburn CG, editors. Eating disorders and obesity: a comprehensive handbook. New York: Guilford Press; 1995. p. 558–63.

54. Hirsch J. Obesity prevention initiative. Obes Res 1994;2:569–84.

55. Zepezauer M, Naiman A. Take the rich off welfare. Tucson (AZ): Odonlan Press; 1996.

56. Reger B, Wootan MG, Booth-Butterfield S. Using mass media to promote healthy eating: a community-based demonstration project. Prev Med 1999;29:414–21.

57. Reger B, Wootan MG, Booth-Butterfield S, Smith H. 1% or less: a community-based nutrition campaign. Public Health Rep 1998;113:410–19.

58. Nestle M. Toward more healthful dietary patterns—a matter of policy. Public Health Rep 1998;113;420–3.

59. McClain DL. Where is today's child? probably watching TV. New York Times 1999 Dec 6;Sect. C:18.

60. Anderson RE, Crespo CJ, Bartlett SJ, Cheskin LJ, Pratt M. Relationship of physical activity and television watching with body weight and level of fatness among children: results from the Third National Health and Nutrition Examination Survey. JAMA 1998;279:938–42.

61. Jeffery RW, French SA. Epidemic obesity in the United States: are fast foods and television viewing contributing? Am J Public Health 1998;88:277–80.

62. Robinson TN. Reducing children's television viewing to prevent obesity: a randomized controlled trial. JAMA 1999;282:1561–7.

63. Ryan M. Are you ready for TV-Turnoff Week? Parade 1998 Apr 12;18–19.

64. Fox RF. Harvesting minds: how TV commercials control kids. Westport (CN): Praeger; 1996.

65. Federal Trade Commission Improvements Act of 1980, Pub. L No. 96–252, 94 Stat. 374 (1980).

66. French SA, Story M, Jeffery RW, Snyder P, Eisenberg M, Sidebottom A, Murray D. Pricing strategy to promote fruit and vegetable purchase in high school cafeterias. J Am Diet Assoc 1997;97:1008–10.

67. French SA, Jeffery RW, Story M, Harman P, Snyder M. A pricing strategy to promote low-fat snack choices through vending machines. Am J Public Health 1997;87:849–51.

68. Wolf AM, Colditz GA. Current estimates of the economic cost of obesity in the United States. Obes Res 1998;6:97–106.

69. Conference Research Center. Special consumer survey report: to tax or not to tax. New York: Conference Board; 1993 Jun.

70. Putnam JJ, Allshouse JE. Food consumption, prices, and expenditures, 1970–97. Statistical Bulletin No. 965. Washington: Department of Agriculture (US); 1999.

71. Bruskin-Goldring Research. Potato chip labels/health programs, January 30–31, 1999. Edison (NJ): Center for Science in the Public Interest; 1999.

72. Department of Agriculture (US) and Department of Health and Human Services (US). National Nutrition Summit: notice of a public meeting to solicit input in the planning of a National Nutrition Summit. Fed Reg 1999; 64(Nov 26):66451.

73. Oster G, Thompson D, Edelsberg J, Bird AP, Colditz GA. Lifetime health and economic benefits of weight loss among obese persons. Am J Public Health 1999;89:1536–42.

This analysis was supported in part by research challenge grants from New York University (NYU) and the NYU School of Education. The authors thank Margo Wootan, DSc, of the Center for Science in the Public Interest (CSPI), for her contributions to the policy suggestions, and Suzanne Rostler of NYU, Stacey Freis of NYU, and Geoffrey Barron of CSPI for research assistance.

Dr. Nestle is Professor and Chair, Department of Nutrition and Food Studies, New York University. Dr. Jacobson is the Executive Director, Center for Science in the Public Interest, Washington, DC.

Address correspondence to: Dr. Nestle, Dept. of Nutrition and Food Studies, NYU, New York NY 10012; tel. 212-998-5595; fax 212-995-4194; e-mail arion.nestle@nyu.edu.

NIH Guidelines: An Evaluation

by Frances M. Berg, MS

The first National institutes of Health guidelines on the treatment of obesity were released on June 17, 1998, to a storm of controversy. The *Clinical Guidelines on the Identification, Evaluation, and Treatment of Overweight and Obesity in Adults,* developed by a 24-member panel of specialists convened by the National Heart, Lung, and Blood Institute in cooperation with the National Institute of Diabetes and Digestive and Kidney Diseases, bring together much valuable information, but at the same time raise numerous questions.[1]

Their purpose is to furnish health professionals with the best available information about who is at risk and what treatment is most appropriate. However, the guidelines are based on two assumptions which seem invalid to many experts in the field. These are, first, that a body mass index (BMI) of 25 constitutes a health risk and, second, that safe and effective weight loss therapy exists. The guidelines lower the level at which a person is defined as overweight and at health risk and includes 55 percent of American adults. (This lowers the previous level of a BMI of 27.3 for women and 27.8 for men set by the National Center for Health Statistics.) They also provide six weight loss methods said to be effective.

They focus on weight loss rather than improved health. They do not warn of potential harm from the recommendations given, or evaluate research on the risks of dieting and weight loss, dysfunctional eating, eating disorders, weight cycling, fraudulent weight loss promotions, or the difficulty in long-term weight loss maintenance. They barely mention obesity prevention, and then, oddly, mainly in connection with preventing weight regain after weight loss.

Validity of claim for risks at a body mass index of 25

"All overweight and obese adults with a BMI of 25 or more are considered at risk," the guidelines state.

What is the evidence that these people are at risk?

Slight increases in risk factors may occur at lower weights for some conditions, the report suggests, but it clearly regards most differences at this level, if any, as minimal. Nearly all research discussed by the guidelines on the risks of related conditions focus on risks at a BMI of 30 or more. Exceptions are its numerous references to the Nurses' Health Study, which finds higher risks above a BMI of 22 for several disease conditions. However, the NIH guidelines profess to be based on research from 236 randomized controlled trials, so it lessens credibility to extensively reference a self-reported, nonrandomized, noncontrolled study such as the Nurses' Study. It also raises the question: if stronger references were available, would they not have been cited instead?

The guidelines report that a BMI of close to 25 (24.8 for white men and 24.3 for white women) is the level of lowest morality. For ethnic and racial minorities they find this to be higher, about 27 for African-Americans, and much higher or no relationship at all for Pima Indian men and women. For older adults, age 55 to 74, the report says the lowest mortality occurs in the BMI range of 25 to 30, even after adjusting for smoking status and pre-existing illness.

This leaves two weak reasons for the cut-off level of a BMI of 25. In defense, its most vocal proponent, George Bray, MD, of the Pennington Biomedical Research Center, Baton Rouge, Louisiana, says that increments of 5 are a good way to divide categories, simple and easy to use; cutoff points of 20, 25, 30, 35, and 40 provide "simplicity and reasonableness."[2] Second, he says that using a BMI of 25 brings the NIH recommendations in line with what other groups advise. He fails to mention that others have adopted this standard through the efforts of like-minded people with whom he has networked for the past 20 years. Obesity experts worldwide are a small group who network extensively. Bray is listed as a background author for the 1998 World Health Organization report *Obesity: Preventing and Managing the Global Epidemic* which adopts the same standard.[3] Even in this latest defense by Bray, published in *Obesity Research,* he acknowledges that for men a BMI of 24 is associated with the lowest mortality, and for women it differs (rises) with age.

Thus, there appears to be no reasonable justification for setting a BMI of 25 as the level at which a person is defined as overweight and at health risk. The research cited in the report refutes the claim that this was an evidence-based decision.

Validity of efficacy claim

The guidelines claim, "A variety of effective options exist for the management of overweight and obese patients, including dietary therapy approaches such as low-calorie diets and lower-fat diets; altering physical activity patterns; behavior therapy techniques; pharmacotherapy; surgery; and combinations of these techniques." In support of this statement, the panel evaluated a great many short-term studies of 4 months or more and defined 1-year studies as being long term.

However, it is well known that both levels are far too short a time to be relevant.

Long-term weight loss is not 1 year, but keeping off lost weight for 2 years or more after the end of any maintenance program, according to the Federal Trade Commission. The American Heart Association guidelines call for 5 years: "If there are no data to demonstrate that program participants maintain their weight losses for 5 years or more, there is no scientific evidence of long-term results of the program."[4]

The NIH guidelines recommend losing 10 percent of baseline weight, or about 1 to 2 pounds per week for 6 months, with "subsequent strategy based on the amount of weight lost." They recommend that a weight maintenance program begin at 6 months, but are vague about its nature or how successful it might be.

Most studies suggest such a maintenance program has little likelihood of success.

"No plan has demonstrated significant success in weight maintenance beyond 6 to 12 months," writes Ann Coulston, MS, RD, senior research dietitian with the General Clinical Research Center at Stanford University Medical Center, in the lead article of the recent obesity supplement to the *Journal of the American Dietetic Association.*[5]

Thus, the standards for evaluating weight loss therapy in the NIH guidelines lack credibility, despite the many studies cited. No credible case has been made for the effectiveness of the six methods recommended.

Other evidence suggests that current methods are neither safe nor effective in the long term. Questioning the value of all methods of current obesity treatment in their January 1, 1998, editorial, Jerome P. Kassirer, MD, and Marcia Angell, MD, editors of the *New England Journal of Medicine,* made these four points:

- *Since many people cannot lose much weight no matter how hard they try, and promptly regain whatever they do lose, the vast amounts of money spent on diet clubs, special foods, and over-the-counter remedies, estimated to be on the order of $30 to $50 billion yearly, is wasted.*
- *The latest magical cures are neither magical nor harmless.... Until we have better data about the risks of being overweight and the benefits and risks of trying to lose weight, we should remember that the cure for obesity may be worse than the condition.*
- *The data linking overweight and death are limited, fragmentary, and often ambiguous.*
- *Even granting an association between increasing body weight and higher mortality, at least for younger people, it does not follow that losing weight will reduce the risk. We simply do not know.*[6,7]

The NIH guidelines reveal strong evidence that physical activity alone, without weight loss, reduces the risk for cardiovascular disease and other disease factors. Yet physical activity is emphasized primarily as a component of weight loss therapy. It is not advanced on its own as a safe and proven method of reducing risk factors associated with obesity.

In one about-face, the panel members do not recommend the very low calorie diet of 800 calories or less, even though it has been long endorsed by obesity specialists and National Institute of Diabetes and Digestive and Kidney Diseases official policy, and could be justified as readily as the six other methods on the basis of 4-month trials.

Why are these experts now willing to acknowledge that the very low calorie diet has been unsuccessful in achieving long-term weight loss, that it risks nutritional inadequacies, causes increased risk of gallstones, means more weight is usually regained, and does not allow for gradual eating behavior change? How will they admit this for other methods?

The panel members considered patient motivation a key factor, despite acknowledging that they could find no evidence that motivation makes any difference in successful weight loss. Yet they urge physicians to heighten patients' motivation, and recommend two strategies. First, the doctor is to explain the dangers of obesity and, second, how "the new treatment plan will be different."

This is astonishing advice that seems to encourage physicians to manipulate their patients with scare tactics and false promises. How the new plan will be different is not explained, since the six weight loss methods described have been in use for many decades and often have failed both patient and doctor. It seems inconceivable that many experienced physicians will follow this advice.

Whose needs do the guidelines serve?

Again, the professed purpose of the NIH guidelines is to advise health professionals in the best ways to treat their large patients by determining who is at risk and what treatment is most appropriate. But an objective evaluation can only conclude that they accomplish neither of these objectives.

Is there, then, perhaps a hidden agenda? And if so, could it be to get more people on weight loss programs, regardless of the consequences? Such question lead inevitably to another: Are the NIH guidelines aimed in part at serving the needs of the weight loss industry?

If true, this would explain one paradox contained in the guidelines. The NIH guidelines seem to advocate separating maintenance from weight loss, defining them as two separate therapies, as in this advice: "After 6 months, efforts to maintain weight loss should be put in place."

A sounder public health policy than is in place today would require weight loss therapy to prove long-term maintenance before any weight is lost, thus avoiding the risks of weight cycling

---

Weight loss maintenance then becomes a part of obesity prevention, as in this definition: "Prevention includes primary prevention of overweight or obesity itself, *secondary prevention or avoidance of weight regain following weight loss,* and prevention of further weight increases in obese individuals unable to lose weight."

This makes no apparent sense and confuses both issues. However, it can serve the needs of the weight loss industry. If this concept is accepted, the industry can continue to document success for short-term weight loss and avoid the need to show long-term maintenance.

However, logic suggests that weight loss and maintenance belong together, placing the responsibility for long-term results with the weight loss program itself. A sounder public health policy than is in place today would require weight loss therapy to prove long-term maintenance before any weight is lost, thus avoiding the risks of weight cycling. It would no longer be acceptable to urge people to lose weight, by any method, and then in 6 months—as advocated here—begin some vague kind of maintenance program that has no track record of success.

Similarly, a clearer definition of prevention would include as the primary goal preventing overweight, and as secondary goals preventing further weight increases and associated risks. This is a definition that can be implemented now and begin to move prevention efforts forward.

Vested interests may play a role

As timely as ever is the protest of Thaddeus Prout, MD, former chair of the Food and Drug Administration Committee on Anorectic Drugs, and of the Committee on Drugs for the American Board of Internal Medicine,

when he testified before the 1990 Congressional hearings investigating the weight loss industry: "The same faces, the same people who have been doing industry-paid research for two decades are before us. . . . In July of 1983 we discussed this same question . . . We listened to their data, looked at their paltry studies. We are hearing all the exaggerated claims of success again. . . . The medical profession has learned that they need not waste the time or postage [with] an entrenched and persuasive pharmaceutical industry. What can we do? Shall we wait another decade and have a new generation of concerned physicians wringing their hands and bumping their heads against the stone wall of industry?"[8]

The issue of vested interests is complex, yet cannot be ignored. How many of the 24 NIH panel members have vested interests in the diet industry, or feel pressures to comply with its demands? These are respected scientists making health decisions in the national interest according to their highest ethics. Yet one may argue that many academics make accommodations almost daily to the issues of research funding, financial affiliations, consultancies, and the politics of power. Disclosure of financial affiliations was not requested from members of the panel, chaired by F. Xavier Pi-Sunyer, director of the federally-funded Obesity Research Center, St. Luke's/ Roosevelt Hospital Center in New York City.

It appears the NIH guidelines serve the weight loss industry better than health professionals or consumers

---

However, when disclosure was required of a related group for the *Journal of the American Medical Association,* it was revealed that eight of the nine members of the National Task Force on the Prevention and Treatment of Obesity were receiving funding from at least two and as many as eight commercial weight-loss companies.[9] At that time, Pi-Sunyer's financial affiliations included being on the advisory boards of Wyeth-Ayerst and Knoll pharmacueticals, and being a consultant to Lilly Pharmaceuticals, Genentech, Hoffman-LaRoche, Knoll, Weight Watchers, and Neutrogen. Others on both the NIH panel and the Task Force are William H. Dietz, James O. Hill, and G. Terence Wilson, each listed as having at least two financial affiliations with these same companies.

It also may be suggested that the new guidelines appear designed to replace the industry-financed "Guidance for Treatment of Adult Obesity" distributed to physicians by Shape Up America and the American Obesity Association in 1996, and made obsolete when the drugs it advocated were withdrawn from the market.

In recent months, drug companies involved in producing diet drugs have distributed versions of the NIH guidelines to health professionals at medical conferences and financed special editions on obesity for subscribers of medical, health, and nutrition journals.

Conclusion

In summary, it appears the NIH guidelines serve the weight loss industry better than they serve health professionals or consumers. They overestimate the risks of obesity and the number of people at risk, assume that people can easily lose 10 percent of their weight and keep it off, promote weight loss treatments that have little chance of long-term success, encourage physicians to manipulate their patients with scare tactics and false promises, and appear likely to spread a sense of alarm, while doing nothing to further prevention efforts. Thus, the new NIH guidelines are unlikely to benefit the public, or to help health care providers deal in effective ways with the problems of obesity.

References

1. Clinical guidelines on the identification, evaluation, and treatment of overweight and obesity in adults: the evidence report. Bethesda, MD: National Institutes of Health, National Heart, Lung, and Blood Institute. Preprint June 1998.
2. Bray G. In defense of a body mass index of 25 as the cut-off point for defining overweight. Obes Res 1998; 6:461–462.
3. Obesity: Preventing and managing the global epidemic: report of a WHO consultation on obesity. WHO/NUT/NCD/98.1. Geneva, Switzerland: World Health Organization, 1998.
4. American Heart Association Guidelines. HWJ 1997; 11:108–110.
5. Coulston AM. Obesity as an epidemic: facing the challenge. J Am Diet Assoc 1998; 98:10(Suppl. 2):16–22.
6. Kassirer JP, Angell M. Losing weight—an ill-fated New Year's resolution. N Engl J Med 1998; 338:52–54.
7. Berg F. Medical journal questions obesity treatment. HWJ 1998; 12:36.
8. Berg F. Witnesses charge diet drug is hazardous. Obes Health 1991; 5:9–12. (Sept 24, 1990, Congressional hearings, U.S. House of Representatives Small Business Subcommittee on Regulation, Business Opportunities and Energy).
9. National Task Force on the Prevention and Treatment of Obesity. Drug therapy. JAMA. 1996; 276:1907–1915. (Berg F. Task Force advises against diet drugs. HWJ 1997; 11:27).

WHY WE GET FAT

The good news is recent research indicates fat might not be your fault. The bad news is you might not be able to do much about it

By Shawna Vogel

John Rossi was a model employee at Kragen Auto Parts in Berkeley, California. In his ten years there, first as a clerk and then as a manager, he had missed only three days of work and had regularly put in 50- to 60-hour weeks. So it was something of a surprise when Rossi's manager told him one day in 1991 not to come to work anymore.

A spokesman for the store later said that Rossi was fired for poor job performance. But the only reason Rossi could see for his dismissal was his weight. A high school

> ## Genes predispose some toward toe tapping, hair twirling, and other calorie-burning fidgeting

football star, Rossi had struggled with obesity throughout his adult life. By the age of 21, when he started working at Kragen, he weighed 275 pounds. Over the next decade he tried everything from fasting to hypnosis, and at one point had his jaws wired shut. On the day he was fired, Rossi weighed about 400 pounds.

Still, laudatory letters from customers and the company's own evaluations were clear: weight had never affected Rossi's job performance. So he decided to sue. In 1995, jurors awarded him $1,035,652 for lost compensation and emotional distress. They concluded that Rossi couldn't legally be dismissed for a condition beyond his control. What convinced them, says Rossi's lawyer, Barbara Lawless, was testimony from a medical witness that each person's weight is controlled primarily by genet-

ics—the witness attributed 80 percent to genes and only 20 percent to environment.

The jury's decision reflects a profound shift in the way our culture views people who are excessively overweight. No longer can we equate significant weight with lack of willpower. With every passing month, scientists announce the discovery of new genes and gene neighborhoods that can be associated with obesity. The count is up to 130 and climbing. In each of us, these genes combine to produce different results. Richard Atkinson, an obesity researcher at the University of Wisconsin in Madison, says, "If you think about all the combinations and permutations of those 130 genes, there are going to be dozens, hundreds, thousands of different kinds of obesity." But knowledge is power, too. An understanding of the genetics of weight control is helping researchers develop a new generation of drugs for weight control.

What does it mean for a gene to be associated with obesity? Although all human beings share the same basic genetic blueprint, genes that make up that blueprint, or genome, vary from individual to individual. For example, imagine two people, each dressed in the same garments: underwear, pants, socks, shoes, shirt, and so on. If one wears a cashmere sweater and the other a cotton sweater, the one in cashmere will probably be warmer. But not necessarily. What if the cashmere-clad person is caught in an Arctic snowstorm while the cotton wearer visits a Florida beach? In that case, the one in cashmere will feel considerably chillier despite the warm sweater because of the different environment. Similarly, someone who inherits the version of a particular gene that's associated with obesity will be more likely to wind up fat than someone who inherits a normal version, but that tendency can be affected by environmental factors such as how much fattening food is available. So once re-

WHEN IT'S NOT YOUR FAULT

With John Wayne bluntness, David West, a geneticist and obesity physician at Parke-Davis in Alameda, California, says, "Some people have the good genes, some people don't. Some patients, especially the very morbidly obese, are pretty much a biological problem. They have a real nasty set of genes. As long as they have enough calories to eat, they're going to be fat no matter what environment they're in and despite their best efforts."

Nevertheless, West says most people don't get fat unless they follow a certain style of life. To gain weight they have to work at it: sit behind a desk all day, wolf down a big lunch, collapse at home with a few beers, then wake up the next day and repeat the process. Genes may make them susceptible to weight gain, but a fattening environment makes the gain happen.

In a way, most of us are a lot like a group of mice West has been studying for the past six years. The mice get fat only when they are fed a delectable brand of rat chow that resembles cookie dough—sugar, condensed milk, minerals, and powdered rodent food. As in a typical North American diet, 40 percent of the calories come from fat. And one group of rats in related experiments become obese only when they are offered many different, tasty items at once. Researchers call that a "supermarket" or "cafeteria" diet, and its similarity to the food available to most Americans needs no elaboration.

When West's mice become fat, they show all the associated biological changes that people do. Their blood sugar goes up, they get more gallbladder and cardiovascular diseases, and they develop problems with insulin similar to human type II diabetes. Geneticists have shown that this reaction to a rich environment stems from not just one gene but a multitude of genes that contribute to the animals' susceptibility, and they believe people have a similar genetic profile.

But just as genes can make us susceptible to obesity, they can also make us resistant. Intriguingly, some strains of mice never become obese despite efforts to fatten them up. Studying these animals may help us understand why some people can eat more than others and never gain weight. The same idea of genetic resistance and susceptibility applies not only to obesity but also to obesity-related illnesses. West says that "there are a fair number of people walking around out there who are 60, 80 pounds overweight but have normal blood sugar and normal blood pressure. Their joints are fine. They don't have gallbladder disease. There doesn't seem to be a greater risk for cancer.

"Why? I think it's because they have another set of genes that protects them from these adverse effects of being fat."

—S.V.

---

searchers have identified the genes of obesity, they must find out how the genes interact with a person's environment.

The revolution in obesity research began less than five years ago with the landmark discovery of a gene for leptin, the weight-regulating hormone found in both mice and people. Fat mice and skinny mice flashed across TV screens around the world when scientists could finally say that the only difference between them was a single gene. Since then geneticists have uncovered many more weight genes. One, a gene mutation that is also associated with red hair, causes severe obesity. In its normal form, the gene produces a hormone that inhibits eating and also influences hair pigmentation. A mutation in the gene produces a damaged version of the hormone, or no hormone at all. In one case, researchers noticed that both a five-year-old boy and a three-year-old girl who had each inherited two copies of the faulty gene were obese by the age of five months.

Another newly discovered family of genes makes compounds called uncoupling proteins, which allow people to convert excess fat into heat instead of storing it. Researchers have shown that animals with high levels of these proteins do not gain weight as easily as those with lower levels.

Obesity-related genes affect different aspects of weight control. For example, some genes might determine how quickly the gut lets the brain know that it is full. Others might dictate how effectively the body turns extra calories into body fat. There's a genetic component to how much fuel muscles need just to get through a sedentary day. And genes also lie behind a tendency that some people have toward spontaneous physical activity—fidgeting, toe tapping, hair twirling—which burns up a substantial number of calories.

It is now widely accepted among weight researchers that a person's particular complement of genes determines what activities make him or her susceptible to weight gain as well as how strong that susceptibility is. The bottom line is that genes alone don't make people fat. All of us simply have a greater or lesser genetic tendency to gain weight. Those with the strongest tendency—the worst combination of genes—are almost guaranteed to join the minority of people who weigh 300 pounds and up. The rest lie somewhere on a continuum that extends all the way down to those lucky people who can eat all the doughnuts they want and never need to punch a new hole in their belts.

> **People with the same weight and height may burn vastly different amounts of energy**

WHY DIETS DON'T WORK

Despite the role genes play in making people fat against their will, diet and exercise remain significant factors. As any dieter knows, losing pounds is never easy. That's because the body uses a remarkably efficient set of tricks to keep fat at a stable level. Researchers refer to this level as the set point. When people successfully lose weight, their bodies undergo a change in metabolic rate that may seem counterintuitive. For example, participants in one study who held their weight at 10 percent below their set point showed a 15 percent drop in daily energy expenditure. Their bodies slowed down energy use to counteract the pounds they had lost. Researchers find this shift in metabolism to be just as marked after a weight gain too. In the same study, subjects who increased their weight showed 10 to 15 percent increases in metabolism.

So if our bodies are so good at maintaining a set point, why do people get fat at all? William Ira Bennett, a doctor at Cambridge Hospital in Massachusetts, wrote in the *New England Journal of Medicine* that although our bodies continue to defend their set points, external factors, such as habitual levels of physical activity and the composition and tastiness of diets, can reset them. Bennett believes that over time a sedentary life and the mere availability of rich, palatable food will slowly increase the weight the body is geared to defend. Because of genes, some people are more susceptible to a change in set point than others. They will always have more trouble keeping off any weight they lose through dieting.

—S.V.

What's more, even if two people seem to have roughly the same tendency to gain weight, they may do so for different reasons, simply because of genetic variety. In 14 years of work at the National Institute of Diabetes and Digestive and Kidney Diseases in Phoenix, obesity researcher Eric Ravussin (now at Eli Lilly in Indianapolis) recently uncovered some fascinating examples. He looked at the differences in how people burn energy and how those differences contribute to weight gain. The work made him appreciate how widely metabolic rates can vary.

In a study of more than 500 volunteers, Ravussin and his colleague Pietro Tataranni analyzed resting metabolic rates—how much energy the body uses when it's just trying to maintain the status quo. The researchers gathered this information using a clear plastic ventilated hood that looks like something out of a viral-scare movie. It fits snugly around a subject's neck, continuously drawing in and siphoning off air. The wearer must lie awake for 40 minutes without moving. By measuring how much oxygen he consumes and how much carbon dioxide he breathes out, researchers can determine how much energy the subject spends on such basic functions as temperature control and involuntary muscle activity. Ravussin and Tataranni found that some of their volunteers burned as few as 1,067 calories a day, while others burned as many as 3,015.

Contrary to what many people think, a slow metabolism doesn't necessarily go hand in hand with weight gain, Ravussin says: "Most obese patients will tell you, 'I have something wrong with my metabolism.' And I believe that something is wrong. But it may not be their metabolic rate." When Ravussin has measured rates, he has found that people with the same physical characteristics—same weight, same height, same basic shape—may nevertheless burn dramatically different amounts of energy each day.

Other researchers have shown that exercise has remarkably different effects on different people. When peo-

CAN A VIRUS MAKE YOU FAT?

Although the idea sounds more like the premise of a B movie than scientific theory, two scientists at the University of Wisconsin in Madison believe they've found a virus that causes some people to get fat. Nikhil Dhurandhar and Richard Atkinson reported recently that when they injected a virus known as AD36 into mice and chickens, the animals' body fat increased. Because humans were unlikely to volunteer for such experimentation, the scientists decided to test for the presence of antibodies to the virus. Of 154 people tested, about 15 percent of those who were obese had the antibodies. None of the lean people did.

However, the findings don't necessarily prove that the virus caused obesity in the test group. As several virologists have pointed out, obese people may simply be more susceptible to such a virus. Still, in recent years researchers have been surprised to find that viruses can be linked to so many diseases that had been thought to have other origins. For example, viruses are now implicated in several types of cancer, hardening of the arteries, and even mental disorders such as depression. In addition, five viruses besides AD36 have already been shown to cause obesity in animals. The good news is that the same methods that produce flu shots each year could ultimately be used to create an antiobesity injection.--S.V.

---

ple exercise regularly for three to four months, their bodies can change dramatically: their hearts and muscles get stronger, and they can exercise harder for longer periods. But that is not true for everyone. When exercise physiologist Claude Bouchard of Laval University in Sainte-Foy, Quebec, put a group of 47 young men on a training program for 15 to 20 weeks, he found that some showed 100 percent improvement in their maximal oxygen uptake—a measure of how efficiently lungs, heart, and circulation can dispense oxygen to tissues crying out for it.

Other men, however, showed almost no change. Bouchard has seen the same lack of effect on other measurements of how people adapt to exercise, such as heart size, muscle fiber size, and how much work people can perform in 90 minutes. "We believe that it is quite remarkable," he says, "that for all the determinants that have been considered in a series of investigations performed in our laboratory, one can find nonresponders—even after 20 weeks of regular exercise at a frequency of five times a week over the last several weeks of the program."

When it comes to weight, it has long been our habit to group heavy people together as if they all suffer from the same condition and should respond to the same cure. Every diet-and-exercise program is pitched as a one-size-fits-all remedy. As scientists begin to understand how different bodies control weight, they are learning to characterize various types of obesity and treat people accordingly. To many researchers and pharmaceutical companies, that treatment means drugs. By one recent count, 62 new compounds for treating obesity are in various stages of testing and development. "I expect we'll see something like one or two new drugs being submit-

ted to us every year for the next five to ten years," says Leo Lutwak, a medical officer with the FDA's Center for Drug Evaluation and Research.

These include the family of so-called exercise pills, drugs designed to boost the rate at which bodies burn fat and dissipate the energy as heat—an effect that would provide many of the benefits of regular mild exercise. Other pharmaceutical approaches use leptin and related molecules to tell the body that its fat stores are already ample, or to target brain chemicals that control appetite. Other pills prevent our bodies from absorbing some of the fat that we eat.

But even without new drugs, knowledge of the differences between bodies can lead to more thoughtful ways of dealing with weight. For example, some people tend to burn less fat than others. As a result, when they're exposed to a high-fat diet, they gain weight more readily. For them, cutting down on fatty foods might be a far easier and more effective way to maintain weight than, say, embarking on a vigorous exercise program. Ultimately we will be forced to accept that each person's weight is as much a mark of his individuality as his face. And that could make weight really interesting.

The great weight debate

A major medical journal says people should worry less about their weight. The government says worry more. Here's what we say.

Last January, The New England Journal of Medicine published an editorial with the blasphemous title "Losing Weight—An Ill-Fated New Year's Resolution." The editors suggested that "the cure of obesity may be worse than the condition." That triggered a flood of media coverage, including a U.S. News & World Report cover story called "The New Truth About Fat." The story elaborated on the suggestion that most people don't need to worry about their weight since the risks of fat are overblown, efforts to lose weight futile.

Five months later, the government flatly contradicted that message by issuing new guidelines that lowered the threshold for being overweight—and pushed 30 million Americans over the line from fit to fat. The guidelines classify as overweight anyone with

The percentage of people who are obese has risen, especially in the past decade.

a body mass index (BMI) of 25 or more. Someone who's 5-feet 8-inches tall and weighs 165 pounds, for example, has a BMI of 25. The previous threshold for overweight, 27, allowed that person to hit 180 pounds or so before sounding an alarm. (To calculate your BMI, see the flowchart *Do you really need to lose weight?*)

The government took that step partly to underscore its concern about the fattening of America: The percentage of people who are obese, with a BMI of 30 or more, has risen considerably in the last 30 years, mainly in the past decade. More important, the government claims that excess weight can harm, and that shedding pounds can help.

Whom should you believe?

Teasing out the truth

The New England Journal editorial was right on several counts. It *is* hard to lose weight permanently. America does have an obsession with thinness, which drives millions of people, including many with no weight problem, to spend big bucks on dangerous or worthless drugs and fads. And certain people probably don't need to worry if they gain a few pounds.

But the editorial understated the risks of excess weight. The government guidelines, created by an expert panel after a comprehensive research review, provide solid evidence that weight matters. And the guidelines clarify *when* excess weight poses a significant threat by considering factors beyond just pounds: your health, the location of the fat, and, to a lesser extent, the proportion of fat versus muscle and bone.

Your health

As the Journal editorial acknowledged, the risk of hypertension, coronary heart disease, and diabetes rises as people get heavier, even if they're only moderately overweight, with a BMI of at least 25 but less than 30. Weaker evidence suggests that the risk of other disorders—breast cancer in postmenopausal women, colon cancer, infertility, thrombotic stroke (the kind caused by blood clots), gallstones, and osteoarthritis—also rises with BMI. Increasing weight may be similarly linked to increased mortality.

Dozens of clinical trials have shown that *losing* weight can reduce certain risk factors for disease, such as high blood pressure, high cholesterol levels, and a high blood-sugar level. There's not much direct evidence on how weight loss affects either the risk of disease itself or the overall death rate. However, some research suggests that slimming down

The skinny on how to lose weight

Losing weight and keeping it off is hard—but hardly impossible. And dropping even a few pounds can reduce certain major risk factors for major diseases (see story). Here's how to maximize the chance of success.

■ **Work it off.** To slim down permanently, you need to keep exercising. Strength training—using weights, machines, or elastic bands—builds muscle and bone; aerobic exercise, such as bicycling or brisk walking, can at least help preserve them. That's important, since muscle burns lots of calories, even when you're resting. And exercise, particularly aerobic exercise, burns calories during the workout and at a slightly elevated rate for a few hours afterwards.

Moderately paced activities may be better than intense workouts for losing weight, because the average overweight person can't do vigorous exercise long enough, at least at first, to burn enough calories. Aim for at least four weekly sessions of at least 45 to 60 minutes each. (Of course, building up to a faster pace will let you burn more calories.) Two or preferably three times a week, devote some of those minutes to strength training. That regimen may be all you need if you're only a little overweight.

Older people who need to lose should focus more on exercise—especially strength training and other weight-bearing exercises—than on diet. That's partly because they need to bolster their muscles and bones, partly because many of them are already eating an inadequate diet. Young and old alike should take a similar approach if their only body-fat problem is a chubby belly plus a weak physique.

Whatever your approach, try to make it fun. If you can't stand walking a treadmill or logging laps, choose workouts that don't seem like work, such as sports, hiking, or bird watching. At the very least, vary your regimen. (For more ways to make exercise enjoyable, see our April 1997 report.)

■ **Cut your calories.** To lose more than just a little weight, you'll almost surely have to eat less. A reasonable goal is to cut your daily intake by 300 to 500 calories. That step, combined with regular exercise, should help you lose about a pound a week. More drastic diets are less likely to yield long-lasting weight loss—and may be harmful.

Eating less fat is a simple, healthful way to cut calories. But it won't help if you compensate by consuming more calories overall, as many people do. (Note that "low-fat" foods often contain as many calories as regular versions, since manufacturers often adjust for the loss of tasty fat by adding extra sugar and other carbohydrates.) The most reliable way to reduce both calories and fat is to replace sugary or fatty foods with whole grains, beans, and produce. Of course, you could also eat smaller portions.

To stick with that leaner approach, keep looking for new foods, recipes, and restaurants that minimize the calories while maximizing the taste. Try to distinguish physical hunger from psychological appetite—and substitute interests and rewards that don't involve eating. Finally, set modest, reasonable goals, and don't obsess about your weight: Eating wisely and exercising regularly will improve your health whether or not it trims your waistline as much as you'd hoped. (For further tips on sticking with a healthful diet, see our May 1998 issue.)

■ **Think twice about fat pills.** Over-the-counter drugs and supplements that supposedly burn fat have little if any value. Prescription drugs may help some obese individuals, but the two most popular ones—dexfenfluramine (*Redux*) and fenfluramine (*Pondimin*)—were yanked off the market last year over concerns about possible heart-valve damage. That leaves only two drug options. One, the stimulant phentermine (*Fastin, Ionamin*), has only limited efficacy, and it often causes strong side effects, including agitation and insomnia. The other drug, sibutramine (*Meridia*), must be taken under close supervision, since it can cause potentially dangerous increases in heart rate and blood pressure.

The FDA may soon approve another medication, orlistat (*Xenical*), which inactivates certain intestinal enzymes needed to absorb fat from food. As a result, users may experience bloating, gas, and loose stools if they consume lots of fat. It may also block absorption of fat-soluble vitamins, including vitamins A, D, and E, so users should take a multivitamin supplement.

In addition to the short-term risks of those drugs, their long-term safety won't be known until they've been used extensively. You and your doctor shouldn't even consider such medication unless you're extremely obese and have truly tried and failed to lose weight without drugs.

---

may prolong life, both in obese people and in certain moderately overweight individuals. For example, a study of some 44,000 overweight women linked weight loss with a 20 percent lower death rate—but only in those who had at least one weight-related risk factor or disease. A similar study in overweight men suggested that shedding pounds may lengthen life only in those with diabetes.

Anyone whose BMI is 30 or more clearly needs to lose weight. The government advises people with a BMI of at least 25 but less than 30 to slim down if they have two or more risk factors—including some that have little to do with weight—or weight-related diseases (see flowchart for list). However, it's probably wise for moderately overweight people to shed pounds if they have even one of those factors or one weight-linked disease. Moderately heavy people who have *no* such factors or ailments—especially those with a BMI of 27 or more—may also want to lose weight, though the benefits are less clear. At the very least, anyone with a BMI of 25 or more should try to avoid gaining weight.

Where's the fat?

Fat on the belly is more metabolically active than fat on the hips or thighs. And when belly fat is metabolized, the byproducts can raise blood-cholesterol levels and reduce the

Do you really need to lose weight?

To answer that question, first determine your body-mass index (BMI), using this formula: Multiply your weight in pounds by 705. Divide the result by your height in inches. Then divide by your height in inches again to arrive at your BMI.

Next, assess how much abdominal fat you have. If your BMI is 25 or more, simply measure your waist. The threshold for concern is 35 inches in women, 40 inches in men. That method doesn't work if your BMI is less than 25. Instead, measure your waist at its narrowest point and your hips at their widest; then divide the waist measurement by the hip measurement. Men are at increased risk if their waist-to-hip ratio exceeds 0.95, women if it exceeds 0.80.

Now follow the flowchart to see if you should lose weight.

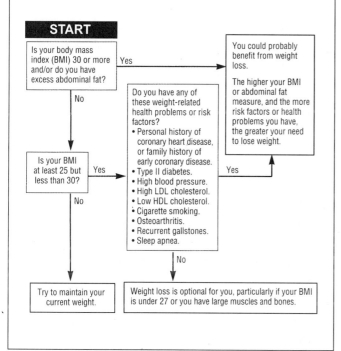

body's sensitivity to the hormone insulin. That reduced sensitivity causes blood-sugar levels to rise, which the body tries to control by churning out more insulin. Rising insulin levels may then increase blood pressure and, in theory, also trigger cancerous changes in colon cells. Moreover, abdominal fat produces more estrogen—which fuels the growth of breast cancer—than hip or thigh fat does.

All that may help explain why observational studies have linked big bellies with an increased risk of hypertension, coronary disease, diabetes, and, to a lesser extent, colon cancer and postmenopausal breast cancer. Many studies have found that a big tummy

may pose greater risks than an elevated BMI does. In fact, a pot belly appears to threaten even people who aren't overweight at all. Note that the opposite case—being somewhat "overweight" due to big muscles and bones rather than a flabby belly—typically poses no threat to health. (To assess your abdominal fat, see flowchart.)

Does age matter?

That controversial New England Journal editorial was inspired by a study suggesting that the link between BMI and death rates grows progressively weaker as people grow older. In a subsequent study, moderately overweight people actually had the lowest mortality after age 55.

But those studies had several major weaknesses. First, some of the volunteers may have had a low BMI because they were wasting away from some serious disease, not because they were trim and fit. Further, older people tend to lose muscle and bone and to put on fat, particularly abdominal fat. But BMI doesn't distinguish fat from other tissue. So a substantial number of older people with a seemingly favorable BMI may actually have too little lean tissue and too much total and belly fat—a decidedly unhealthy combination. The loss of muscle and bone increases the risk of deadly falls and fractures. And excess abdominal fat, unlike BMI, remains strongly correlated with increased mortality in old age.

So the criteria for who needs to lose weight are probably still the same for young and old alike. But the best *approach* to slimming down does depend partly on age (see "The skinny on how to lose weight").

Summing up

Obese people, with a BMI of 30 or more, clearly need to lose weight. So do those with lots of belly fat, regardless of their BMI.

There's no definitive proof that losing weight helps people who are only moderately overweight, with a BMI of 25 to 30. But the risks clearly do rise as people get heavier. Slimming down improves key risk factors, and it seems to cut mortality, at least in susceptible people. So virtually all moderately heavy people should at least consider losing weight. Those at greatest risk—due to health, health habits, or family history—should start trying to slim down.

Simplifying the Advice for Slimming Down

How to avoid the pitfalls of fad diets

IT'S KIND OF IRONIC. Weight Watchers, TOPS (Take Off Pounds Sensibly), Jenny Craig, and other weight-loss organizations that already promote sensible eating without too much hype have voluntarily adopted a code of stricter standards. That is, they have joined the Federal Trade Commission (FTC) Partnership for Healthy Weight Management, agreeing to disclose to consumers:

- any risks associated with their plans
- cost of the plans
- qualifications of the staff who administer the plans
- advice about the difficulty of maintaining weight loss once the pounds come off.

On the other hand, the creators of popular diets that need the *most* policing—because they promote unhealthful practices that promise much more than they can deliver—are free to ignore the guidelines' call. Among the plans rife with dietary imbalances and false promises: those espoused in *Sugar Busters!, Dr. Atkins' New Diet Revolution, Enter the Zone, The Five Day Miracle Diet, The New Beverly Hills Diet,* and *Protein Power.* Their sponsors are staying away even though the FTC's partnership is open to individuals as well as weight-loss companies (and has also been joined by health-promoting organizations such as The American Dietetic Association and the Centers for Disease Control and Prevention).

Though the lack of participation by the sponsors of the unsound plans is ironic, it's not surprising, because these diets do not live up to some of the major tenets of the Partnership for Healthy Weight Management. Among those tenets subscribed to by the Partnership:

- Products and programs that promise quick and easy results are misleading, since successful weight loss is a gradual process that requires focus on many fronts, including food choices, activity level, and how likely you are to eat in response to stress.

- Any ad that says you can lose weight without paying attention to calories "is selling fantasy and false hope."

- Any plan that eschews one or more food groups is setting people up for a lack of balance and potential nutrient deficiencies.

Just how far short do many of the popular plans fall? Tufts researchers Jeanne Goldberg, PhD, RD, and Julie Smith, MS, RD, have taken a systematic look at 10 of the popular diet books out there and found an alarming gap between the healthful eating promoted by the partnership guidelines and the food plans these books offer. For instance, the "induction phase" of *Dr. Atkins' New Diet Revolution* contains less than 60 percent of the fiber, copper, magnesium, manganese, and potassium that Americans should be consuming—no doubt because the diet is low in complex carbohydrates as well as fruits and vegetables.

Enter the Zone is lacking in fiber and vitamin D, while *The Five Day Miracle Diet* and *The New Beverly Hills Diet,* both low in dairy foods and starches, are deficient in calcium, carbohydrates, and zinc. *Sugar Busters!,* too, is low in calcium, in addition to fiber—and potentially high in unhealthful saturated fat.

All of this is to say nothing of the false promises made in the books espousing these plans. *Sugar Busters!* and *Enter the Zone,* for example,

From the *Tufts University Health & Nutrition Letter,* April 1999, pp. 4-5. © 1999 by Tufts University Health & Nutrition Letter. Reprinted by permission.

wrongly suggest that calories don't count. And all of the books tend to make weight loss sound much easier than it actually is.

Are the Diets Dangerous, or Just Useless?

Jane Kirby, RD, author of The American Dietetic Association's *Dieting for Dummies* (IDG Books Worldwide, Foster City, CA, 1998, $19.99), a sensible guide to weight loss that includes advice on spotting a fraud diet, says that for people in decent health, the biggest problem with going on fad diets is not nutrition status. Rather, it's "quality of life."

"Most unhealthful diets [that focus on just one food or eliminate whole food groups] are not going to harm you because they're so boring and impossible to stick with for too long," Ms. Kirby comments. "Just how much cabbage soup can you eat?" she asks rhetorically, referring to one of many diets that limits food choices.

It's the same with high-protein, low-carbohydrate diets that call for giving up everything from bread to bananas. You'll lose weight on such plans, Ms. Kirby says, because of the limited choices. But, she adds, "it can't work over the long term because we need flavor and texture diversity. We're hard-wired for it by nature. So you'll go off the diet. **You'll eventually realize that you really *do* want a bagel. This egg-white thing is not going to cut it.**"

Tufts's Dr. Goldberg agrees with Ms. Kirby that people tend not to stick to any one of these diets for too long. But, she says, many people go from one poor diet to another, and that's where nutrient deficiencies become a concern.

For instance, she points out, the low-carbohydrate, high-protein diets that are currently popular—*Atkins, Sugar Busters!*—are "remarkably consistent with respect to their nutrient deficiencies." All have too little calcium. "Women take in too little calcium to begin with," she says. "On these diets, they get even less.

"And then there's very little vitamin D, so they don't adequately absorb the calcium they do take in. So what happens when they go from the *Zone* to *Sugar Busters!* to *Atkins*? I'm concerned that it magnifies the problem.

"You can always find a few people who went on a fad diet, lost weight, and kept it off because after they slimmed down, they told themselves they would start to eat reasonably," Dr. Goldberg says. "I'm sure they're out there. But that's very atypical. More often what you'll find is the chronic dieter who goes from one diet to the next to the next."

The funny thing about all these diets, Dr. Goldberg says, is that "the pitfalls have been pointed out." People know what they are.

They also know the choices they *really* have to make—more fruits and vegetables, few fatty and sugary treats, more exercise. As the Partnership for Healthy Weight Management says, "Be sure to include at least five servings a day of fruits and vegetables, along with whole grains, lean meat, and low fat dairy products. It may not produce headlines, but it can reduce waistlines."

Unfortunately, Dr. Goldberg points out, "I don't think people are paying attention. They want the quick fix. They are going to some tropical island in two weeks. They don't want someone telling them that the weight loss on a high-protein diet is going to be all water and that the minute they go off the diet, they're going to gain it all back and more."

Getting around the quick-fix mentality

For people who really want to get off the diet merry-go-round and lose a significant amount of weight once and for all, Dr. Goldberg suggests paying attention to some of the lessons coming out of the National Weight Control Registry. The Registry, maintained by researchers at the University of Pittsburgh School of Medicine and the University of Colorado Health Sciences Center, is a record of hundreds

of people who have lost weight (at least 30 pounds) and kept it off (for at least one year).

"This is information for the real world," Dr. Goldberg says. "It's a compilation of techniques people really are living with" as opposed to advice being used to sell a diet program. She boils down the experience of the Weight Control Registry participants to five messages:

1 **To lose weight, combine different methods.** Some people start to lose weight using a structured plan such as Weight Watchers, Dr. Goldberg says. But then they might go off the plan and tailor a diet and exercise routine more to their own liking. The commercial plan may have just been what they needed to get started. As long as it works and doesn't exclude any foods or food groups, switching around or using a variety of methods at the same time is fine.

Likewise, Dr. Goldberg says, successful weight losers may have at different points paid more attention to total fat intake than to total calories. They weren't afraid to use what worked for them at a particular time.

What very few of them did, however, was follow a diet in which they restricted their intake to a very narrow group of foods, which Dr. Goldberg says was crucial to their loss of weight over the long term. Less than 5 percent of Registry participants succeeded that way.

2 **Identify a weight-loss trigger.** The Registry members were able to identify a particular aspect or point in their lives that was "overwhelmingly important" in getting started on the road to permanent weight loss, Dr. Goldberg says.

"You don't have to wait for the trigger to hit you over the head unexpectedly," she adds. "Hit *yourself* over the head. Make a proactive search. Don't wait to wake up one day and suddenly be inspired to diet."

For men, she points out, the trigger more often is about health. For women, it tends to involve an emotional consideration. Thus, a man may want to ask himself, "do I want to get rid of my blood pressure medication?" For a woman, the triggering question might be, "is there something about the way I carry myself that I really would feel more comfortable about if . . . ?"

3 **Exercise.** The members of the Weight Control Registry exercise a lot, Dr. Goldberg says. In fact, they walk an average of four miles a day, or 28 miles a week.

4 **Forget all-or-nothing.** People tend to say, "you've got to do it all or it isn't worth doing," Dr. Goldberg remarks. But that's not true. If you can't exercise the equivalent of walking 28 miles a week, it doesn't mean you shouldn't exercise at all. Make a start. Do what you *can* do. Something is always better than nothing. Nothing is exactly that—nothing.

It's the same with food restriction, Dr. Goldberg says. If you're eating 3,000 calories a day, maybe it's not realistic to try to cut back to 1,500 calories, or even 2,000 calories. **Maybe it makes more sense to acclimate yourself**

to weight loss by cutting out only 200 to 300 calories at first and going from there. By cutting out 200 calories daily, you'll lose about 20 pounds in the first year (more if you walk a little, too).

5 **Monitor yourself.** "When you look at the histories that successful weight losers provide," Dr. Goldberg says, "it's clear that they get on the scale at least once a week, on average." And they count calories, or fat, or both. In other words, they use at least one kind of concrete system for making sure that they're adhering to the plan.

Weight Loss Diets and Books

by J. Anderson and K. Wilken[1]

Approximately 30 percent of Americans are over-weight. Carrying too much weight increases risk of health problems such as hypertension, heart disease, gall bladder disease and diabetes. Losing weight—and keeping it off—can be challenging. Controlling fat intake, exercising and changing behavior are the keys to weight management.

Fat Intake

At 9 calories per gram, fat contains more than twice the calories of protein and carbohydrates (4 calories/gram each). Limiting your total daily fat intake to 30 percent or fewer calories from fat not only reduces fat and calories, but also reduces a risk factor for cardio-vascular disease.

You can estimate your desirable fat intake with the following rules of thumb: To maintain your weight, divide your current weight in pounds by two. If you want to lose weight, divide your current weight in pounds by three. This is your daily fat gram goal.

Watching your fat intake doesn't mean you must give up your favorite foods. Choose lean meats and dairy products. Use oils and spreads sparingly. Be aware of hidden fats in foods such as bakery products, crackers, nuts and salad dressings. Learn to modify recipes and use substitutions to lower the fat content.

Weight Loss Diets

Fad diet books often promise quick weight loss. The diets usually are difficult to continue for a long period and are not nutritious. Although people may lose weight initially, they easily regain it. At two-year follow-ups, fad diets have a very low success rate.

Safe and more effective weight loss plans have the following characteristics:

Quick Facts . . .

- The most effective way to lose and maintain weight is to limit fat intake, follow a healthy balanced diet and exercise regularly.

- Weight loss strategies should encourage setting realistic goals and making permanent changes in eating habits.

- Recommend no more than 1 to 2 pounds weight loss per week.
- Do not go below 1,200 calories per day.
- Refer to the Food Guide Pyramid and Dietary Guidelines.
- Focus on limiting fat intake rather than calories.
- Encourage exercise.
- Include a variety of nutritionally balanced foods from all food groups.
- Do not have a list of forbidden foods.
- Minimize hunger.
- Do not require special foods or vitamin supplements.
- Encourage setting realistic weight loss goals and making slow, moderate changes.
- Establish lifelong habits.
- Fit into your lifestyle.

Sample Weight Loss Diets and Books

Dr. Atkins' New Diet Revolution
1992—Robert C. Atkins, M.D. Another book: *Health Revolution*

From Reprinted with permission from Colorado State University Cooperative Extension, Fact Sheet 9.364, December 1998, *Nutrition Quackery*, J. Anderson, L. Patterson, and B. Daly, Dept. of Food Science and Human Nutrition. © 1998 by Colorado State University.

- **Characteristics:** High protein, high fat, low carbohydrate. Claims diet may help people with food intolerances or allergies, heart disease, diabetes, yeast infections. Megavitamin and mineral supplements daily.
- **Weaknesses:** Nutritionally unbalanced. Recommends as little as 15 grams carbohydrate a day. No bread, pasta or cereal. Low fruits and vegetables. Ketoacidosis is encouraged.
- **Comments:** Does not teach good eating habits. Can be dangerous. Claims are not nutritionally sound. May initially lose water weight.

Breaking the Behavior Chain

Behavior modification techniques can help alter poor eating habits. Begin by recording your eating habits to identify places, emotions or activities that lead to inappropriate eating.

To change those habits, use simple modification techniques. For example, make a rule to not eat when watching television. When you feel stressed, go for a walk or call a friend instead of eating cookies.

Taking personal responsibility for losing weight, believing you can succeed and having support from family and friends also are important factors in losing weight.

Eat More, Weigh Less
1993—Dean Ornish, M.D.

- **Characteristics**: Life Choice vegetarian diet. Low in fat, high in complex carbohydrates and fiber. Believes large changes are easier to make than moderate ones. Includes over 250 appetizing recipes. 10 percent of calories from fat.
- **Strengths:** Heart healthy diet. Does not limit amounts of food (no counting calories). Encourages moderate exercise.
- **Weaknesses**: Advocates giving up all meat, poultry, fish, oils, margarine, sugar, dairy (except nonfat) and products exceeding 2 grams of fat per serving.
- **Comments:** May be difficult to follow long-term, especially for non-vegetarians.

Fasting
- **Characteristics:** Often claimed to detoxify the body and lead to quick weight loss. Often followed by very low-calorie diets.
- **Weaknesses:** May feel weak, light-headed and shaky. Can lead to ketosis, kidney stones, nausea, fatigue and elevated uric acid levels. Life-threatening (especially thin people and over 75).

- **Comments**: Weight loss from water and muscle loss, then fat loss. When eating resumes, weight gain is primarily fat. Exercise accentuates the problems.

Fit for Life
1985—Harvey and Marilyn Diamond.

- **Characteristics:** Based on the erroneous theory of "detoxification." Toxic wastes build up and lead to obesity. Certain foods or food combinations detoxify the body.
- **Weaknesses:** Contains misinformation; nutritionally unbalanced; no dairy; deficient in calcium, zinc, vitamin D and B-12; low protein.
- **Comments:** Probably not dangerous but potentially unhealthy. Unsafe for children, adolescents, pregnant and lactating women. Will lead to weight loss as food intake is restricted.

The Fit-or-Fat Woman
1989—Covert Bailey. Other books: *The New Fit or Fat, The Fit-or-Fat Target* Diet

- **Characteristics**: Recommends aerobic exercise, balanced diet and weightlifting/body building. Focuses on body fat percentage, not weight loss. Covers stress, eating disorders, PMS, gaining weight.
- **Strengths:** Emphasis on exercise and balanced diet with more fiber and less fat and sugar. Warns against vitamin and mineral megadoses.
- **Weaknesses:** Recommends only 10 to 15 grams fat per day for obese women with 36 percent or more body fat.
- **Comments:** Straightforward, sound approach to reducing body fat.

The G-Index Diet
21-day diet. 1993—Richard N. Podell, M.D.

- **Characteristics:** Classifies foods based on how they affect blood sugar response (glycemic index). Claims eating high G-Index (GI) foods at one meal causes overeating at the next meal. Claims low GI foods lower insulin levels and rev up metabolism so you burn an extra 200 calories.
- **Strengths:** Emphasizes whole grains, low sugar, low fat. Recommends regular exercise.
- **Weaknesses:** Restricts nutrition-rich foods like baked potatoes, pineapple, raisins and carrots. True glycemic index of many foods is unknown.
- **Comments:** Eating a combination of high and low glycemic foods should avoid big blood sugar swings.

The McDougall Program
12-day program. 1990 - John McDougall.

- **Characteristics**: High complex carbohydrates and fiber, low fat. Unlimited amounts of "the right food" such as rice, potatoes and pasta. Restricts animal-derived foods and refined plant foods (white flour). High fat or sugar foods (honey, maple syrup, soybeans, nuts) for special occasions.
- **Strengths**: Reduction in sugar, salt and fat.
- **Weaknesses**: No meat, dairy, mayonnaise or oils, sugar, salt, coffee, cola, chocolate.
- **Comments**: Extremely low fat intake (5 to 6 percent of calories). If followed for a long time, potential for nutrient deficiencies in protein, calcium, zinc, vitamins D and B-12, and riboflavin. Unbalanced.

Exercise

People are more successful in losing weight when they alter eating habits and exercise regularly. Physical activity burns calories, raises metabolism, and helps you lose body fat (increasing the percentage of lean body mass). Exercise also promotes a sense of well-being and has beneficial effects on HDL cholesterol.

Contrary to popular belief, moderate activity does not increase your appetite. Find an activity that you enjoy. If you are very overweight or have other health problems, consult with your doctor before beginning an exercise program. Start slowly, then work up to at least 15 minutes a session, three to five times a week.

Outsmarting the Female Fat Cell
1993—Debra Waterhouse, M.P.H., R.D.

- **Characteristics**: OFF Plan focuses on exercise, changing eating habits—eat only when hungry, stop dieting, don't overeat, control night snacks, eat small frequent meals, choose low-fat foods (20 percent of calories from fat).
- **Strengths**: Emphasizes slow and permanent body fat loss. Uses behavior modification techniques. No restriction of foods.
- **Weaknesses**: Encourages eating only the first 12 hours of the day.
- **Comments**: Realistic plan for weight control. Allows individual tailoring of plan. Deals with emotional eating.

The New Pritikin Program
1990—Robert Pritikin

- **Characteristics**: Designed for lifelong nutrition, weight loss, and prevention of diseases such as heart disease, high blood pressure, cancer and diabetes. High in fiber and complex carbohydrates, low in fat. Low in cholesterol, sugars, salt, alcohol, coffee, tea. Foods categorized as "Go," "Caution," or "Stop." Includes stress management.
- **Strengths**: Exercise is encouraged. Variety of foods daily. Adequate carbohydrates, emphasizing complex carbohydrates. May be beneficial for some disease states.
- **Weaknesses**: Only 10 percent of calories from fat. Recommends limiting low-fat dairy and avoiding whole dairy, animal fats, tropical oils, caffeine, salt products, etc. For fast weight loss, recommends 1,000 calories/day for women and 1,200 calories/day for men.
- **Comments**: May be difficult to follow long-term due to low fat intake.

The T-Factor Diet
21-days of menus. 1989—Martin Katahn.

- **Characteristics**: Initially count daily fat grams. Add fat-free foods to avoid feeling hungry. For faster weight loss, follow Quick Melt program (count calories and fat grams). Recommends physical activity to avoid regaining weight.
- **Strengths**: Focuses on low-fat, high-fiber foods. De-emphasizes calorie counting. No elimination of foods.
- **Weaknesses**: Claims people are overweight because they eat too much fat. Quick Melt meets RDAs but is low in calories (1,100-1,300/day for women, 1,600-1,800/day for men).
- **Comments**: Lower ranges of recommended fat gram intake are quite low. Lose weight too quickly on Quick Melt.

The Zone Diet
Barry Sears, Ph.D. 1995.

- **Characteristics**: "Enter the Zone" maintains that carbohydrates are bad because they raise your blood sugar level and cause the release of the hormone insulin—supposed monster hormone. Claims insulin makes it hard to become thin. Supposedly takes the high-carbohydrate food and stores it as fat rather than using it for energy.
- **Strengths**: Promotes eating regular meals low in calories. Restricts fat to no more than 30 percent of total calories.
- **Weaknesses**: Promotes diet higher in protein, lower in carbohydrates than recommended. Carbohydrates, not proteins, are the preferred source of energy. If protein is used for energy, nitrogen must be removed. This can overtax the kidneys. Metabolic pathways supposedly connecting diet, insulin-glucogen and eicosanoids sound impressive but do not exist.

Carbohydrates and insulin don't make you fat. Eicosanoids don't cause disease.

- **Comments**: The Zone is based on half-truths, mixed messages and theories, not grounded in peer-reviewed research. There is nothing magical about The Zone Diet, it's just a very low-calorie diet.

Sugar Busters

Edited by Stewart Leighton, 1998. By three physicians and a businessman.

- **Characteristics**: Sugars and foods high in sugar are claimed to be "toxic" and the root of all health problems, including obesity, diabetes and heart disease. These are attributed to insulin that regulates sugar. To "bust" sugar out of the diet, the book recommends avoiding foods with high glycemic index (fruits and vegetables) and compensating with protein (meat) and fat.
- **Strengths**: None.

- **Weaknesses**: Promotes foods high in cholesterol, saturated fat. Eliminates many foods that provide essential vitamins and minerals. Recommends not drinking "excessive" fluids (water) with meals. No basis to claim fluids "bypass proper chewing," "dilute digestive juices."

- **Comments**: Insulin plays essential role in energy balance. Carbohydrates are important in diet. No scientific evidence for claims made. Claims are false. Not recommended.

---

1. J. Anderson, Cooperative Extension food and nutrition specialist and professor; and K.Wilken, Cooperative Extension food and nutrition specialist food science and human nutrition.

Issued in furtherance of Cooperative Extension work, Acts of May 8 and June 30, 1914, in cooperation with the U.S. Department of Agriculture, Milan A. Rewerts, Director of Cooperative Extension, Colorado State University, Fort Collins, Colorado. Cooperative Extension programs are available to all without discrimination. No endorsement of products mentioned is intended nor is criticism implied of products not mentioned.

Americans Ignore Importance of Food Portion Size

Medical College of Wisconsin Physicians & Clinics—Milwaukee, Wisconsin

Most Americans believe the kind of food they eat is more important for managing weight than the amount of food they eat, according to a new survey.

In the survey, a surprising 78 percent of respondents said that eating certain types of food while avoiding others was more central to their weight management efforts than eating less food. The survey was commissioned by the American Institute for Cancer Research, a private cancer charity.

This finding troubles nutrition experts, who have long suspected that messages about "low-fat" eating may cause the public to lose sight of a more pressing concern: total calorie intake. They stressed that effective weight management strategies place equal focus on both the kind and amount of food consumed. They added, however, that there is an increasing American trend to ignore the issue of portion size.

Indeed, the survey suggests that Americans are seizing on 'quick-fix'

strategies with little regard for how much food they actually consume. "People are eating more and wondering why they're getting fatter, " said Melanie Polk, M.M.Sc., R.D., Director of Nutrition Education at the Institute. "One big reason is that their focus is too narrow."

Americans, she said, are concentrating too exclusively on cutting fat, or going on fad diets that restrict carbohydrates, sugar, or some other factor. Too often, such strategies fail to address the larger picture of total calories consumed, not to mention good nutrition.

Portion Size Linked to Weight Management

Almost 62 percent of those responding to the survey said they were currently above their ideal weight. Half of those who were above their ideal weight said they needed to lose six to 20 pounds, and another 13 percent said they needed to lose 21 to 30 pounds. Ten percent of those who

said they were above their ideal weight reported being over by 50 pounds or more.

These numbers are in accordance with recent figures from the National Institutes of Health attesting that for the first time in history, the majority of Americans—an estimated 55 percent—are clinically overweight, while one in every four Americans is obese (severely overweight). This means that most Americans are now at increased risk for obesity-related diseases like cancer, coronary heart disease, stroke, diabetes, high blood pressure, gallbladder disease and osteoarthritis.

Anecdotal evidence from several sources illustrates the steady increase in U.S. portion sizes over the past few decades. Foreigners coming to this country express amazement at the amount of food served up in American homes and eateries. Foods adopted from foreign countries like croissants and bagels have grown to double or triple their original size, and the native muffin has ballooned from a standard ounce-and-half to as much as eight ounces today.

Meanwhile, fast food outlets feature gigantic "value meals" and "supersizes." Even table-service restaurants have swapped 10-inch plates (once the industry standard) for 12-inch sizes.

USDA statistics show that American total daily caloric intake has risen from 1,854 kcal to 2,002 kcal over the last 20 years. That significant increase—148 calories per day—theoretically works out to an extra 15 pounds every year. (Ironically, the same studies show that the average American has lowered the percentage of fat in his or her diet from 40 percent to 33 percent over the same amount of time.)

According to the survey, however, most Americans are unaware that portions they consume have increased in size. Six in ten (62 percent) of survey respondents said that the portions served in restaurants are the same size or smaller compared to 10 years ago. Eight in ten said the portions they eat at home are the same or smaller. Americans under 35 years of age were more likely to recognize that their food portions have grown compared to baby-boomers aged 35 to 54 and Americans 55 or older.

Each year, Medical College of Wisconsin physicians care for more than 180,000 patients, representing nearly 500,000 patient visits. Medical College physicians practice at Children's Hospital of Wisconsin, Froedtert Memorial Lutheran Hospital, the Milwaukee VA Medical Center, and many other hospitals and clinics in Milwaukee and southeastern Wisconsin.

Dieting Disorder

THE STORY

Despite 15 years of media coverage of the physical and emotional ravages of eating disorders, an estimated 5 million Americans every year still battle anorexia, bulimia and related disorders. While awareness and treatment have improved, no one has yet defined what triggers the problem. In an attempt to understand more, Australian researchers recently followed nearly 2,000 teens for three years to look for common characteristics among those who eventually developed eating disorders. Though we still don't fully understand why eating disorders develop, the results confirm what many specialists already believed: Serious dieting is a powerful predictor that an eating disorder may emerge.

During any six-month period, girls who dieted severely were 18 times more likely to develop an eating disorder than nondieters; they had an almost one in five chance of developing an eating disorder within a year. Female moderate dieters (which included 60 percent of girls at the beginning of the study) were five times more likely to develop an eating disorder than nondieters and over 12 months had a 1 in 40 chance of developing a new eating disorder. Neither weight nor extent of exercise was associated strongly with developing an eating disorder, although psychiatric illness was. The findings, reported in the March 20 *British Medical Journal,* suggest that two-thirds of new

cases of eating disorders arise in females who have dieted moderately.

All the new cases were bulimia nervosa, which involves binge eating followed by purging (self-induced vomiting or use of laxatives) or excessive exercise to prevent weight gain. This is more common than the more visible anorexia nervosa, in which weight drops to an unhealthy level.

Eating disorders are serious: They can lead to stomach problems and tooth decay, bone loss, blood and endocrine abnormalities, infertility—and ultimately death from starvation, suicide or heart problems. Treatment described in an April 8 summary in the *New England Journal of Medicine* involves education about nutrition, medical supervision, and a combination of individual, group or family therapy. Fluoxetine (Prozac) and other antidepressants have been helpful, especially in bulimia.

Is it possible to identify early signs of an eating disorder and find help before the problem becomes serious?—*The Editors*

THE PHYSICIAN'S PERSPECTIVE

David Rosen, M.D.
Associate Editor

Anorexia nervosa and bulimia nervosa—the more severe eating disorders—affect approximately 3 percent of young women. More than twice that number have other forms of disordered eating, a precursor that includes

day-long preoccupation with food (counting calories and fat grams and planning or avoiding food), and weight loss or bingeing not severe enough to meet the official criteria for an eating disorder. Older adults, men and preadolescents are also susceptible.

Research over the last two decades has helped us recognize that disordered eating and the more severe eating disorders result from complex interactions among genetic predisposition, personal psychology, family dynamics and sociocultural influences. Several recent studies have added to the evidence that these disorders have some basis in brain chemistry and may be inherited. In one, women who had recovered from bulimia nervosa showed higher levels of by-products of the brain chemical serotonin. Three other studies confirm that the disorder occurs in some families at rates much higher than in the general population. Still, no one completely understands why or how disordered eating arises in certain people. This frustrates our efforts to predict who is at greatest risk for these conditions or to reliably prevent their occurrence.

The Australian study gives us an important clue. Whatever the underlying factors are, severe dieting seems to be an important gateway to the development of these conditions in teens. So identifying dieting teens becomes an extremely useful strategy in offering earlier intervention to those at high risk. We know that early intervention improves the prognosis for disordered eating. And it is at least

POSSIBLE SIGNS OF AN EATING DISORDER

- Arrested growth
- Marked weight change
- Inability to gain weight
- Fatigue
- Constipation or diarrhea
- Susceptibility to fractures
- Disrupted menstruation

- Change in eating habits
- Difficulty eating in social settings
- Reluctance to be weighed
- Depression or social withdrawal
- Absence from school or work
- Deceptive or secretive behavior
- Excessive exercise

Source: Adapted from the New England Journal of Medicine, *April 8, 1999.*

plausible (though not proven) that by preventing dieting behavior altogether, we might be able to interrupt the pathway by which these conditions develop.

Sadly, we know that dieting behavior sometimes begins as young as 6 or 7 years of age. By middle school, most girls say they've dieted at least once. So what can be done?

- Emphasize "healthy" bodies. The goal should be fitness, not thinness.

- Praise kids for the things they do, rather than for the way they look.
- Don't diet yourself. Commit to life-long healthy eating, rather than quick-fix diets.
- If a child insists on dieting, insist that the diet be medically supervised.
- Get rid of the scale.
- Prepare kids, especially girls, for the changes of puberty, which may be interpreted as "getting fat."
- Forbid teasing about appearance.

Even playful teasing has powerful negative effects.

- Encourage an active lifestyle. This needn't involve organized athletics, but rather any movement—walking, dancing, biking—that is pleasurable enough to do every day.

It is time to seek help when a teen— or adult—can't give up dieting. That person is at risk for an eating disorder and should be helped to see a health-care professional as soon as possible.

FOR MORE INFORMATION

▼ *Eating Disorders Awareness and Prevention, 800-931-2237, members.aol.com/edapinc*

The Effects of Starvation on Behavior: Implications for Dieting and Eating Disorders

by David M. Garner, PhD

One of the most important advances in the understanding of eating disorders is the recognition that severe and prolonged dietary restriction can lead to serious physical and psychological complications.[1] Many of the symptoms once thought to be primary features of anorexia nervosa are actually symptoms of starvation. Given what we know about the biology of weight regulation, what is the impact of weight suppression on the individual? This question is particularly relevant for health professionals who treat eating disorders, but is also important in obesity treatment, for dieters, and for others who have lost significant amounts of body weight.

Perhaps the most powerful illustration of the effects of restrictive dieting and weight loss on behavior is an experimental study conducted over 50 years ago and published in 1950 by Ancel Keys and his colleagues at the University of Minnesota.[2] The experiment involved carefully studying 36 young, healthy, psychologically normal men while restricting their caloric intake for 6 months. More than 100 men volunteered for the study as an alternative to military service; the 36 selected had the highest levels of physical and psychological health, as well as the most commitment to the objectives of the experiment. What makes the "starvation study," as it is commonly known, so important is that many of the experiences observed in the volunteers are the same as those experienced by patients with eating disorders as well as some people who have undergone weight loss programs.

During the first 3 months of the semistarvation experiment, the volunteers ate normally while their behavior, personality, and eating patterns were studied in detail. During the next 6 months, the men were restricted to approximately half of their former food intake and lost, on average, approximately 25 percent of their former weight. Although this was described as a study of "semistarvation," it is important to keep in mind that cutting the men's rations to half of their former intake (to an average of 1,570 calories) is precisely the level of caloric deficit used to define "conservative" treatments for obesity.[3] The 6 months of weight loss were followed by 3 months of rehabilitation, during which the men were gradually refed. A subgroup was followed for almost 9 months after the refeeding began. Most of the results were reported for only 32 men, because four men were withdrawn either during or at the end of the semistarvation phase. Although the individual responses to weight loss varied considerably, the men experienced dramatic physical, psychological, and social changes. In most cases, these changes persisted during the rehabilitation or renourishment phase.

Attitudes and behavior related to food and eating

One of the most striking changes that occurred in the volunteers was a dramatic increase in food preoccupation. The men found concentration on their usual activities increasingly difficult, because they became plagued by incessant thoughts of food and eating. During the semistarvation phase of the experiment, food became a principal topic of conversation, reading, and daydreams. Rating scales revealed that the men experienced increase in thoughts about food, as well as corresponding decreases in interest in sex and activity during semistarvation. The actual words used in the original report are particularly

> **Many of the symptoms that might have been thought to be specific to anorexia nervosa and bulimia nervosa are actually the result of starvation.**

revealing and the following quotations followed by page numbers in parentheses are from Keys et al. with permission from the University of Minnesota Press.

"As starvation progressed, the number of men who toyed with their food increased. They made what under normal conditions would be weird and distasteful concoctions, (p. 832) . . . Those who ate in the common dining room smuggled out bits of food and consumed them on their bunks in a long-drawn-out ritual, (p. 833) . . . Toward the end of starvation some of the men would dawdle for almost 2 hours after a meal which previously they would have consumed in a matter of minutes, (p. 833) . . . Cookbooks, menus, and information bulletins on food production became intensely interesting to many of the men who previously had little or no interest in dietetics or agriculture, (p. 833) . . . [The volunteers] often reported that they got a vivid vicarious pleasure from watching other persons eat or from just smelling food (p. 834) . . ."

In addition to reading cookbooks and collecting recipes, some of the men even began collecting coffeepots, hot plates, and other kitchen utensils. According to the original report, hoarding even extended to non-food-related items such as "old books, unnecessary secondhand clothes, knick knacks, and other 'junk.' Often after making such purchases, which could be afforded only with sacrifice, the men would be puzzled as to why they had bought such more or less useless articles" (p. 837). One man even began rummaging through garbage cans. This general tendency to hoard has been observed in starved anorexic patients and even in rats deprived of food.[4,5] Despite little interest in culinary matters prior to the experiment, almost 40 percent of the men mentioned cooking as one of their postexperiment plans. For some, the fascination was so great *that they actually changed occupations after the experiment;* three became chefs!

The Minnesota subjects often were caught between conflicting desires to gulp their food down ravenously and consume it slowly so that the taste and odor of each morsel would be fully appreciated.

They did much planning as to how they would handle their day's allotment of food (p. 833). The men demanded that their food be served hot, and they made unusual concoctions by mixing foods together, as noted above. There also was a marked increase in the use of salt and spices. The consumption of coffee and tea increased so dramatically that the men had to be limited to nine cups per day; similarly, gum chewing became excessive and had to be limited after it was discovered that one man was chewing as many as 40 packages of gum a day and "developed a sore mouth from such continuous exercise" (p. 835).

During the 12-week refeeding phase of the experiment, most of the abnormal attitudes and behaviors related to food persisted.

Binge eating

During the restrictive dieting phase of the experiment, all of the volunteers reported increased hunger. Some appeared able to tolerate the experience fairly well, but for others it created intense concern and led to a complete breakdown in control. Several men were unable to adhere to their diets and reported episodes of binge eating followed by self-reproach. During the eighth week of starvation, one volunteer flagrantly broke the dietary rules, eating several sundaes and malted milks; he even stole some penny candies. He promptly confessed the whole episode, [and] became self-deprecatory (p. 884). While working in a grocery store, another man suffered a complete loss of will power and ate several cookies, a sack of popcorn, and two overripe bananas before he could regain control of himself. He immediately suffered a severe emotional upset, with nausea, and upon returning to the laboratory he vomited . . . He was self-deprecatory, expressing disgust and self-criticism (p. 887).

One man was released from the experiment at the end of the semistarvation period because of suspicions that he was unable to adhere to the diet. He experienced serious difficulties when confronted with unlimited access to food: "He repeatedly went through the cycle of eating tremendous quantities of food, becoming sick, and then starting all over again" (p. 890). During the refeeding phase of the experiment, many of the men lost control of their appetites and "ate more or less continuously" (p. 843). Even after 12 weeks of refeeding, the men frequently complained of increased hunger immediately following a large meal.

"[One of the volunteers] ate immense meals (a daily estimate of 5,000 to 6,000 calories) and yet started snacking an hour after he finished a meal. [Another] ate as much as he could hold during the three regular meals and ate snacks in the morning, afternoon, and evening, (p. 846) . . . Several men had spells of nausea and vomiting. One man required aspiration and hospitalization for several days, (p. 843) . . ."

During the weekends in particular, some of the men found it difficult to stop eating. Their daily intake commonly ranged between 8,000 and 10,000 calories, and their eating patterns were described as follows:

Subject No. 20 stuffs himself and he is bursting at the seams, to the point of being nearly sick and still feels hungry; No. 120 reported that he had to discipline himself to keep from eating so much as to become ill; No. 1 ate until he was uncomfortably full; and subject No. 30 had so little control over the mechanics of "piling it in" that he simply had to stay away from food because he could not find a point of satiation even when he was "full to the gills . . . ," "I ate practically all weekend," reported subject No. 26 . . . Subject No. 26 would just as soon have eaten six meals instead of three. (p. 847)

After about 5 months of refeeding, the majority of the men reported some normalization of their eating patterns, but for some the extreme overconsumption persisted "No. 108 would eat and eat until he could hardly swallow any more and then he felt like eating half an hour later" (p. 847). More than 8 months after renourishment began, most men had returned to normal eating patterns; however, a few were still eating abnormal amounts. "No. 9 ate about 25 percent more than his prestarvation amount; once he started to reduce but got so hungry he could not stand it" (p. 847).

Factors distinguishing men who rapidly normalized their eating from those who continued to eat prodigious amounts were not identified. Nevertheless, the main findings here are as follows: *Serious binge eating developed in a subgroup of men, and this tendency persisted in some cases for months after free access to food was reintroduced; however, the majority of men reported gradually returning to eating normal amounts of food after about 5 months of refeeding.* Thus, the fact that binge eating was experimentally produced in some of these normal young men should temper speculations about primary psychological disturbances as the cause of binge eating in patients with eating disorders.

These findings are supported by a large body of research indicating that habitual dieters display marked overcompensation in eating behavior that is similar to the binge eating observed in eating disorders.[6–8] Polivy et al. compared a group of former World War II prisoners of war and noninterned veterans and found that the former prisoners who had lost an average of 10.5 kg while prisoners of war, reported a significantly higher frequency of binge eating than noninterned veterans according to a self-report questionnaire sent by mail.

Emotional and personality changes

The experimental procedures involved selecting volunteers who were the most physically and psychologically robust. "The psychobiologic 'stamina' of the subjects was unquestionably superior to that likely to be found in any random or more generally representative sample of the population" (pp. 915–916).

Although the subjects were psychologically healthy prior to the experiment, most experienced significant emotional deterioration as a result of semistarvation. Most subjects experienced periods during which their emotional distress was quite severe; almost 20 percent had extreme emotional deterioration that markedly interfered with their functioning. **Depression** became more severe during the course of the experiment. Mood swings were extreme for some of the volunteers:

> [One subject] experienced a number of periods in which his spirits were definitely high . . . These elated periods alternated with times in which he suffered "a deep dark depression." (p. 903)

Irritability and frequent outbursts of **anger** were common, although the men had fairly tolerant dispositions prior to starvation. For most subjects, **anxiety** became more evident. As the experiment progressed, many of the formerly even-tempered men began biting their nails or smoking because they felt nervous. **Apathy** also became common, and some men who had been moderately fastidious neglected various aspects of personal hygiene. During semistarvation, two subjects developed disturbances of **psychotic** proportions. During the refeeding period, emotional disturbance did not vanish immediately but persisted for several weeks, with some men actually becoming more depressed, irritable, argumentative, and negativistic than they had been during semistarvation. After 2 weeks of refeeding, one man reported his extreme reaction in his diary:

> I have been more depressed than ever in my life . . . I thought that there was only one thing that would pull me out of the doldrums, that is release from C.P.S. [the experiment] I decided to get rid of some fingers. Ten days ago, I jacked up my car and let the car fall on these fingers . . . It was premeditated. (pp. 894–895)

Several days later, this man actually did *chop off three fingers of one hand* in response to the stress.

Standardized personality testing with the Minnesota Multiphasic Personality Inventory (MMPI) revealed that semistarvation resulted in significant increases on the Depression, Hysteria, and Hypochondriasis scales. The MMPI profiles for a small minority of subjects confirmed the clinical impression of incredible deterioration as a result of semistarvation. One man scored well within normal limits at initial testing, but after 10 weeks of semistarvation and a weight loss of only about 4.5 kg (10 pounds, or approximately 7 percent of his original body weight), gross personality disturbances were evident on the MMPI.

Social and sexual changes

The extraordinary impact of semistarvation was reflected in the social changes experienced by most of the volunteers. Although originally quite gregarious, the men became progressively more withdrawn and isolated. Humor and the sense of comradeship diminished amidst growing feelings of social inadequacy. The volunteers' social contacts with women also declined sharply during semistarvation. Those who continued to see women socially found that the relationships became strained. These changes are illustrated in the account from one man's diary:

> I am one of about three or four who still go out with girls. I fell in love with a girl during the control period but I see her only occasionally now. It's almost too much trouble to see her even when she visits me in the lab. It requires effort to hold her hand. Entertainment must be tame. If we see a

*show, the most interesting part of it is contained in scenes
where people are eating. (p. 853)*

Sexual interests were likewise drastically reduced.
Masturbation, sexual fantasies, and sexual impulses
either ceased or became much less common. One subject
graphically stated that he had "no more sexual feeling
than a sick oyster." (Even this peculiar metaphor made
reference to food.) Keys et al. observed that "many of
the men welcomed the freedom from sexual tensions and
frustrations normally present in young adult men" (p.
840). The fact that starvation perceptibly altered sexual
urges and associated conflicts is of particular interest,
since it has been hypothesized that this process is the
driving force behind the dieting of many anorexia nervosa patients. According to Crisp, anorexia nervosa is an
adaptive disorder in the sense that it curtails sexual concerns for which the adolescent feels unprepared.[10] During
rehabilitation, sexual interest was slow to return. Even
after 3 months, the men judged themselves to be far from
normal in this area. However, after 8 months of renourishment, virtually all of the men had recovered their interest in sex.

Cognitive and physical changes

The volunteers reported impaired concentration, alert-
ness, comprehension, and judgment during semistarvation; however, formal intellectual testing revealed no
signs of diminished intellectual abilities. As the 6 months
of semistarvation progressed, the volunteers exhibited
many physical changes, including gastrointestinal discomfort; decreased need for sleep; dizziness; headaches;
hypersensitivity to noise and light; reduced strength;
poor motor control; edema (an excess of fluid causing
swelling); hair loss; decreased tolerance for cold temperatures (cold hands and feet); visual disturbances (i.e., inability to focus, eye aches, "spots" in the visual fields);
auditory disturbances (i.e., ringing noise in the ears); and
paresthesias (i.e., abnormal tingling or prickling sensa-
tions, especially in the hands or feet).

Various changes reflected an overall slowing of the
body's physiologic processes. There were decreases in
body temperature, heart rate, and respiration, as well as
in basal metabolic rate (BMR), the amount of energy (in
calories) that the body requires at rest (i.e., no physical
activity) to carry out normal physiologic processes. It accounts for about two thirds of the body's total energy
needs, with the remainder being used during physical
activity. At the end of semistarvation, the men's BMRs
had dropped by about 40 percent from normal levels.
This drop, as well as other physical changes, reflect the
body's extraordinary ability to adapt to low caloric intake by reducing its need for energy. More recent research has shown that metabolic rate is markedly
reduced even among dieters who do not have a history
of dramatic weight loss.[11] During refeeding, Keys et al.

found that metabolism speeded up, with those consuming the greatest number of calories experiencing the
greatest rise in BMR. The group of volunteers who received a relatively small increment in calories during refeeding (400 calories more than during semistarvation)
had no rise in BMR for the first 3 weeks. Consuming
larger amounts of food caused a sharp increase in the
energy burned through metabolic processes.

Significance of the "Starvation Study"

As is readily apparent from the preceding description of
the Minnesota experiment, many of the symptoms that
might have been thought to be specific to anorexia nervosa and bulimia nervosa are actually the result of starvation.[12] These are not limited to food and weight, but
extend to virtually all areas of psychological and social
functioning. Since many of the symptoms postulated to
cause these disorders may actually result from undernutrition, it is absolutely essential that weight be returned
to "normal" levels so that psychological functioning can
be accurately assessed.

The profound effects of starvation also illustrate the
tremendous adaptive capacity of the human body and
the intense biologic pressure on the organism to maintain
a relatively consistent body weight. This makes complete
evolutionary sense. Over hundreds of thousands of years
of human evolution, a major threat to the survival of the
organism was starvation. If weight had not been carefully modulated and controlled internally, early humans
most certainly would simply have died when food was
scarce or when their interest was captured by countless
other aspects of living. The "starvation study" by Keys
et al. illustrates how the human being becomes more ori-
ented toward food when starved and how other pursuits
important to the survival of the species (e.g., social and
sexual functioning) become subordinate to the primary
drive toward food.

Some researchers have indicated publicly that this
study could not be conducted today because of the strin-
gent ethical guidelines for research using human subjects. However, rarely have ethical concerns been raised
regarding the use of very low calorie diets that involve
a level of calorie restriction that is approximately one
half of that used in the "starvation study." In light of the
profound changes observed in the "starvation study," it
would seem mandatory to warn participants of these potentially untoward effects as well as to carefully study
the psychological and physical impact of these programs.

Providing patients with eating disorders with the
above account of the semistarvation study can be very
useful in giving them an explanation for many of the
emotional, cognitive, and behavioral symptoms that they
experience. Recommendations to use the findings of this
study, as well as other educational materials,[1] are based
on the assumption that patients with eating disorder

often suffer from misconceptions about the factors that cause and then maintain symptoms. It is further assumed that patients may be less likely to persist in self-defeating symptoms if they are made truly aware of the scientific evidence regarding factors that perpetuate eating disorders.

One of the most notable implications of the Minnesota experiment is that it challenges the popular notion that body weight is easily altered if one simply exercises a bit of "willpower." It also demonstrates that the body is not simply "reprogrammed" at a lower set point once weight loss has been achieved. The volunteers' experimental diet was unsuccessful in overriding their bodies' strong propensity to defend a particular weight level. Again, it is important to emphasize that following the months of refeeding, the Minnesota volunteers did not skyrocket into obesity. On average, they gained back their original weight plus about 10 percent; then, over the next 6 months, their weight gradually declined. By the end of the follow up period, they were approaching their pre-experiment weight levels.

References

1. Garner DM. Psychoeducational principles in the treatment of eating disorders. In: Garner DM, Garfinkel PE, eds. Handbook for treatment of eating disorders. New York: Guilford Press, 1997:145–177.
2. Keys A, Brozek J, Henschel A, et al. The biology of human starvation. Vols 1 and 2. Minneapolis: University of Minnesota Press, 1950.
3. Stunkard AJ. Introduction and overview. In: Stunkard AJ, Wadden TA, eds. Obesity: theory and therapy. 2nd Ed. New York: Raven Press, 1993:1–10.
4. Crisp AH, Hsu LKG, Harding B. The starving hoarder and voracious spender: stealing in anorexia nervosa. J Psychosom Res 1980; 24:225–231.
5. Fantino M, Cabanac M. Body weight regulation with a proportional hoarding response in the rat. Physiol Behav 1980; 24:939–942.
6. Polivy J, Herman CP. Dieting and bingeing: a causal analysis. Am Psychol 1985; 40:193–201.
7. Polivy J, Herman CP. Diagnosis and treatment of normal eating. J. Consult Clin Psychol 1987; 55:635–644.
8. Wardle J, Beinart H. Binge eating: a theoretical review. Br J Clin Psychol 1981; 19,20:97–109.
9. Polivy J, Zeitlin SB, Herman CP, Beal AL. Food restriction and binge eating: a study of former prisoners of war. J Abnorm Psychol 1994; 103:409–411.
10. Crisp AJ. Anorexia nervosa: let me be. London: Academic Press, 1980.
11. Platte P, Wurmser H, Wade SE, et al. Resting metabolic rate and diet-induced thermogenesis in restrained and unrestrained eaters. Int J Eat Disord 1996; 20:33–41.
12. Pirke KM, Ploog D. Biology of human starvation. In: Beaumont PJV, Burrows GD, Casper RC, eds. Handbook of eating disorders: Part I. Anorexia and bulimia nervosa. New York: Elsevier, 1987:79–102.

Adapted by the author from Garner and Garfinkel (ref. 1). David M. Garner, PhD, is the director of the Toledo Center for Eating Disorders and an adjunct professor of psychology at Bowling Green State University and of women's studies at the University of Toledo, Ohio. He is co-editor of the *Handbook of Treatment of Eating Disorders*. He can be reached at 419–843–2000 or by e-mail at garnerdm@aol.com.

Unit 5

Unit Selections

Key Points to Consider

❖ What are the main causes of food-borne diseases?

❖ What are some of the best methods for avoiding or minimizing disease from contaminated foods?

❖ How dangerous has the *E. coli* bacteria become?

❖ What are some of the pros and cons regarding the safety of genetically modified food?

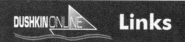 **Links**   **www.dushkin.com/online/**

These sites are annotated on pages 4 and 5.

Food-borne disease constitutes an important public health problem in the United States. The U.S. Centers for Disease Control has reported 76 million cases of food-borne illness each year out of which 5,000 end in death. The annual cost of losses in productivity ranges from 20 to 40 billion dollars. Food-borne disease results primarily from microbial contamination but also from naturally occurring toxicants, environmental contaminants, pesticide residues, and food additives.

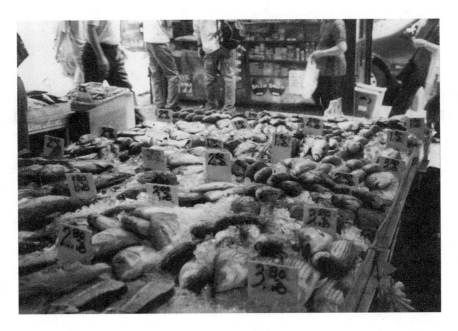

The first Food and Drug Act was passed in 1906 and was followed by tighter control on the use of additives that might be carcinogenic. In 1958, the Delaney Clause was passed and a list of additives that were considered as safe for human consumption (GRAS list) was developed. The Food and Drug Administration (FDA) controls and regulates procedures dealing with food safety, including food service and production. The FDA has established rules (Hazard Analysis and Critical Control Points) to improve safety control and to monitor the production of seafood, meat, and poultry. Even though there have been outbreaks of food poisoning traced to errors at the commercial processing stage, the culprit is usually mishandling of food at home, in a food service establishment, or other noncommercial setting. Surveys show that over 95 percent of the time people do not follow proper sanitation methods when working with food. The U.S. government, therefore, launched the Food Safety Initiative program to minimize foodborne disease and to educate the public about safe food handling practices. Additionally, for the first time this year, the newest edition of the U.S. government's *Dietary Guidelines* includes guidelines for food safety.

Some of the articles in Unit 5 review the seven highly effective habits that help cooks decrease food-borne illness as established by the Food Safety and Inspection Service (FSIS) and the U.S. Department of Agriculture (USDA). The most common foodborne illnesses come from bacterial infestation of food such as *Salmonella, Campylobacter,* hemorrhagic *E. coli* and *Listeria. Staphylococcus* and *Clostridium botulinum* produce toxins that cause illness. Outbreaks of food poisoning can be very serious and many times even deadly. Pasteurization and irradiation by the processing industry and using preventive techniques at home, such as avoiding cross-contamination, can prevent and contain these outbreaks. Still, people adopt many unsafe practices when it comes to preparing and storing food. The American Dietetic Association's (ADA) Nutrition Hot Line will provide you with reliable, timely, and objective answers to your questions and is staffed by registered dietitians.

The gravity of this subject is emphasized by *Campylobacter,* a bacterium that causes up to 4 million infections per year and its cousin, an antibiotic-resistant campylobacter that contributes to Guillain-Barré syndrome, which results in paralysis. Ninety percent of poultry test positive for the bacterium in studies conducted by the USDA. Use of antibiotics for poultry in the United States results in antibiotic-resistant strains of the bacterium. Concerns over the likelihood of drug resistance transferred from poultry to humans, creating a health problem, are being raised by the FDA.

E. coli 0157:H7 is particularly virulent and has been on the news because it causes 500 deaths per year. Children have died from hemolytic uremia and kidney failure by eating undercooked ground beef or drinking bacteria-infected unpasteurized apple cider and juice. Eliminating the presence of the bacterium is crucial to public health. In 1998 the FDA approved red meat product irradiation as a means to combat this public health problem.

The most current food safety controversy here and abroad is the genetic modification of crops and their unknown effects on health and the biosystem. Europeans are not willing to buy our GM crops because of these unanswered questions. Proponents argue that GM foods may alleviate hunger and disease in developing countries, and opponents argue that GM technology is not safe and is unpredictable and impossible to control. Additionally, the opponents contend that it is not restricted to the field in which the GM crop grows, but can be transmitted with toxic effects to endangered wildlife. Unit 7 will offer more information on this debate.

AMERICA'S DIETARY GUIDELINE ON FOOD SAFETY: A PLUS, OR A MINUS?

Kathleen Meister

KATHLEEN MEISTER, M.S., IS A FREELANCE MEDICAL WRITER
AND A FORMER ACSH RESEARCH ASSOCIATE.

Imagine a delicious, inexpensive convenience food that is low in fat, cholesterol, sodium, and calories—and provides all essential nutrients and dietary fibers in optimum quantities. This may seem the ideal food—but it would be far from ideal if it were contaminated with pathogenic bacteria.

The idea that a food must be microbiologically safe to be healthful may seem obvious. And addressing the issue of microbiological safety might seem integral to any guide to healthy eating. Until this year, however, the U.S. government's principal guide of this sort, the "Dietary Guidelines" document, did not so much as allude to the issue. The 2000 edition gives this issue a distinct Guideline, called "Keep food safe to eat."

WHAT ARE THE DIETARY GUIDELINES?

The Dietary Guidelines, which are issued as a brochure, are official recommendations concerning healthy eating for all Americans who are at least two years old. The document was first published in 1980, and groups of experts have updated it every five years. A draft of the latest edition was released in February 2000.

The Dietary Guidelines affect even Americans who don't know what they are—70 percent of the U.S. population. They represent a crucial federal policy statement—one that sets the nationwide agenda on food-related issues. Not only do they constitute the basis for federal food and nutrition programs; they are also in extensive educational use by nonfederal groups—including state and local-government agencies, voluntary organizations, professional associations, and food-industry groups.

> **The Dietary Guidelines affect even Americans who don't know what they are—70 percent of the U.S. population.**

FOODBORNE DISEASE

"Foodborne disease" refers to any disease that results from eating food contaminated with a pathogen, most often a bacterium. Such diseases constitute an important public health problem. The U.S. Centers for Disease Control and Prevention (CDC) has estimated that, each year in the U.S., there are 76 million cases of foodborne disease, with 325,000 cases involving subsequent hospitalization and 5,000 ending in death. Moreover, it has been estimated that the annual cost of related decreases in productivity ranges from $20 billion to $40 billion.

But, in the U.S., foodborne disease is almost always preventable. Most cases trace to improper handling of food between its initial production and its ingestion. In 1997 the U.S. government launched the Food Safety Initiative—a program whose goal is to minimize foodborne disease in the U.S. Integral to this program is educating the public about safe food-handling practices.

The emphasis on food safety has increased in recent years. One reason for this is that the proportion

Reprinted with permission from *Priorities*, Vol. 12, No. 2, 2000, pp. 18-22. © 2000 by the American Council on Science and Health, Inc., 1995 Broadway, 2nd Floor, New York, NY 10023-5860.

> **The U.S. Centers for Disease Control and Prevention (CDC) has estimated that, each year in the U.S., there are 76 million cases of foodborne disease. . . .**

of the American population especially vulnerable to foodborne disease, such as the elderly and persons whose immune systems are compromised, has increased. Another is that scientists have become aware that changes in how food is produced and distributed have led to changes in susceptibilities to mishandling and contamination.

Some foodborne-disease hazards have diminished in recent decades in the U.S.—for example, unpasteurized milk, improper home canning, and lack of a home refrigerator. But, meanwhile, the number of centralized, large-scale food-processing operations has increased considerably, and one slip in such an operation can result in the sickening of numerous consumers.

There have been changes in food handling at the end-user level as well. Half of every dollar that American consumers spend is spent on food prepared outside the home. Keeping such foods safe requires measures different from those that apply to dishes prepared at home.

THE CONSUMER'S PART IN FOOD SAFETY

The Dietary Guidelines document states: "Farmers, food producers, markets, and food preparers have a legal obligation to keep food safe, but we also need to keep foods safe in the home." For instance, although in the last few years the egg industry has impressively reduced *Salmonella enteritidis* contamination of whole chicken eggs, eating raw or undercooked eggs remains somewhat risky. Even the safest food purchase can quickly become unsafe. Foodservice establishments must try to ensure that takeout foods, such as roast chickens or prepared salads, are safe at purchase—but it is in any case incumbent on the buyer to ensure that, within two hours of its purchase, the food is eaten or appropriately refrigerated.

In recent years, several well-publicized outbreaks of food poisoning have been traced to errors at the com-

mercial-processing stage. For example, a large food-poisoning outbreak was traced to an ice-cream mix that had been transported in inadequately disinfected tankers previously used to transport shelled raw eggs. But most cases of foodborne disease in the U.S. result not from errors related to commercial processing, but from the mishandling of food in a foodservice establishment, at home, or in another noncommercial setting, such as a picnic.

While government regulation is crucial to keeping down foodborne disease in the U.S., it has little effect on the committing of food safety mistakes in noncommercial settings. No American governmental agency can pressure households to wash their cutting boards or to refrigerate the food in their doggie bags. The only non-intrusive way to improve food-handling practices in noncommercial settings is to instruct the public on food safety hows and whys. Therein lies the utility of the food safety aspect of the Dietary Guidelines document.

LOOKING OUT FOR NUMBER ONE

Although chemicals can cause foodborne disease, it is most commonly associated with microorganisms. As the food safety Guideline implies, in the U.S. at least, microbial food contamination is far more of a public health problem than is chemical food contamination. Yet many Americans evidently believe the fallacy that manmade additives and pesticides and other such chemicals make their food supply dangerous. The U.S. Food and Drug Administration has ranked diet-related hazards in descending order of dangerousness:

1. microbial contamination

2. naturally occurring toxicants

3. environmental contaminants (e.g., metals)

4. nutritional problems (i.e., malnutrition, undernutrition)

5. pesticide residues

6. food additives

By focusing on microbial contamination, the Dietary Guideline called "Keep food safe to eat" facilitates making it center stage in terms of public food-safety education.

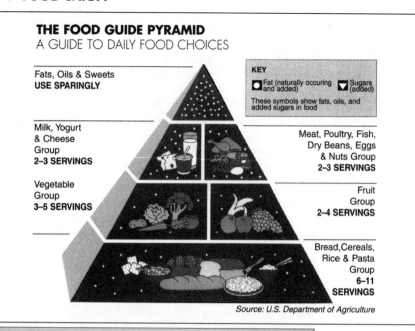

THE FOOD GUIDE PYRAMID
A GUIDE TO DAILY FOOD CHOICES

Fats, Oils & Sweets
USE SPARINGLY

KEY
◻ Fat (naturally occuring and added)   ▽ Sugars (added)
These symbols show fats, oils, and added sugars in food

Milk, Yogurt & Cheese Group
2–3 SERVINGS

Meat, Poultry, Fish, Dry Beans, Eggs & Nuts Group
2–3 SERVINGS

Vegetable Group
3–5 SERVINGS

Fruit Group
2–4 SERVINGS

Bread, Cereals, Rice & Pasta Group
6–11 SERVINGS

Source: U.S. Department of Agriculture

According to government surveys, behavior that is risky in terms of food-borne disease is common among Americans, of whom:

- 50 percent eat raw or under-cooked eggs,
- 23 percent eat undercooked hamburger,
- 17 percent eat raw clams or oysters,
- 28 percent leave perishable foods unrefrigerated for more than two hours,
- 26 percent do not wash cutting boards after they have cut raw meat or poultry on them, and
- 20 percent do not wash their hands after they have handled raw meat or poultry.

Each of the seven messages that amount to the food safety Guideline is consistent with established principles of food handling:

- Clean. Wash hands and surfaces often.
- Separate. Separate raw, cooked, and ready-to-eat foods while storing and preparing.
- Cook. Cook foods to a safe temperature.
- Chill. Refrigerate perishable foods promptly.
- Check and follow the label.
- Serve safely.
- When in doubt, throw it out.

CONTROVERSY OVER THE FOOD SAFETY GUIDELINE

No one can reasonably deny that the message of the food safety Guideline is scientifically well-grounded, but some qualified professionals have objected to the inclusion of this message in the Dietary Guidelines document. Some nutrition scientists say

> **[M]ost cases of foodborne disease in the U.S. result . . . from the mishandling of food in a foodservice establishment, at home, or in another noncommercial setting. . . .**

THE ALCOHOL GUIDELINE

Since its introduction, in 1980, the Dietary Guidelines document has called for moderateness in alcoholic-beverage consumption. Three changes in this Guideline, however, are present in the 2000 edition. Two of these are desirable: First, both the 1995 edition and the 2000 edition acknowledge that moderate alcohol consumption may reduce the risk of developing coronary heart disease (CHD), but unlike the previous edition, the 2000 edition states that this holds "mainly among men over age 45 and women over age 55." CHD is rare among young men and premenopausal women. Thus, moderate drinking is associated with lower death rates only among persons who are at least middle-aged.

Second, a mistake in the 1995 edition has been corrected. In that edition a list of "people who should not drink alcoholic beverages at all" included "individuals using prescription and over-the-counter medications." This was an overstatement: Some medications are quite compatible with alcohol. The new edition implies this and advises persons on medication to request "advice about alcohol intake" from their "health care professional."

But one of the three changes present in the 2000 edition is problematic: It states that "even one drink/day can slightly raise the risk of breast cancer." The claim that the positive statistical association of moderate alcohol intake and breast-cancer risk is causal is doubtful. The scientific evidence on this point is not consistent. Moreover, the possibility that this alcohol–cancer association is merely a result of confounders—in this event, non-alcohol related factors accompanying both drinking and the development of cancer—has not been ruled out. In any case, the association is weak, and if it proves causal, it would have to be weighed against the much stronger relationship between alcohol consumption and heart disease in women.

THE DIETARY GUIDELINES

NOW...

The U.S. Department of Agriculture (USDA) and the U.S. Department of Health and Human Services have jointly issued the Dietary Guidelines document every five years since 1980. The 2000 edition differs substantially from the 1995 edition. The number of Guidelines, for example, has increased from 7 to 10:

- Aim for a healthy weight.
- Be physically active each day.
- Let the Pyramid guide your food choices.
- Choose a variety of grains daily, especially whole grains.
- Choose a variety of fruits and vegetables daily.
- Keep food safe to eat.
- Choose a diet that is low in saturated fat and cholesterol and moderate in total fat.
- Choose beverages and foods to moderate your intake of sugars.
- Choose and prepare foods with less salt.
- If you drink alcoholic beverages, do so in moderation.

...AND THEN

The statements below represent the 1995 Guidelines.

- Eat a variety of foods.
- Balance the food you eat with physical activity—maintain or improve your weight.
- Choose a diet with plenty of grain products, vegetables, and fruits.
- Choose a diet low in fat, saturated fat, and cholesterol.
- Choose a diet moderate in sugars.
- Choose a diet moderate in salt and sodium.
- If you drink alcoholic beverages, do so in moderation.

that adding messages on new topics to the document may distract the public from the guide's thrust: discussion of food choices that are better in terms of specific food constituents. For example, the January 25, 2000, edition of *The New York Times* quoted Marion Nestle, Ph.D., of New York University: "What this has done is shift the focus of the guidelines from food to other factors. The deemphasis on food and increased emphasis on other factors is not a step forward."

Healthy eating entails many considerations—for example, energy intake versus energy expenditure, intakes of protein and essential nutrients, and intakes of saturated fat. It requires attention to the principles of moderation, variety, and balance. Above all, however, it requires that whatever is eaten be harmless with respect to bacterial and similarly acting pathogens. If it isn't, none of the other factors matter. Thus, the food safety Guideline is perhaps the most fundamental.

DON'T MESS WITH FOOD SAFETY MYTHS!

A food safety educator shares seven highly effective habits for food safety.

by Alice Henneman, M.S., R.D.

Alice Henneman is an extension educator with the University of Nebraska Cooperative Extension in Lancaster County. She is actively involved in developing and delivering consumer programs in the areas of food safety and nutrition. This article is adapted from information presented by Henneman in her international e-mail newsletter, Food-Talk *(http://www.ianr.unl.edu/ianr/lanco/ family/FoodTalk.htm), and her food safety game,* Don't Get Bugged by a Food-borne Illness. *Address correspondence to Alice Henneman, University of Nebraska Cooperative Extension in Lancaster County, 444 Cherrycreek Road, Lincoln, NE 68528-1507. Fax: (402) 441-7148. E-mail:ahenneman1 @unl.edu.*

True or false? The best way to decide if a food is safe to eat is to taste it.

That belief, and others like it, focuses our thoughts on food safety. Misconceptions about food safety abound and can make consumers sick! Once a food leaves the grocery store, the consumer becomes an important link in the food safety chain. Safely processed foods can become unsafe if mishandled in the home. Check your food safety savvy against the statements that follow. Have you—or consumers you know—been misled by any of the following food safety myths?

Three Myths That Make Consumers Sick

MYTH NO. 1

"If it tastes okay, it's safe to eat."

Fact: If you trust your taste buds to detect unsafe food, you may be in trouble.

Many consumers believe a food is safe to eat if it tastes, smells, or looks all right. The Council for Agricultural Science and Technology estimated in its 1994 report, Food-borne Pathogens: Risks and Consequences, that as many as 6.5 million to 33 million illnesses yearly are food related.[1]* You can't always rely on your sense of taste, smell, or sight to determine if a food is safe. Taking even a tiny bite to test the safety of a questionable food can be dangerous.

MYTH NO. 2

"We've always handled our food this way and nothing has ever happened."

Fact: If you use past experiences to predict whether a food is safe, you may have a food-borne illness in your future.

Many incidents of food-borne illness went undetected in the past. Food-borne illness signs and symptoms of nausea, vomiting, cramps, and diarrhea were often and still are blamed on the "flu." Also, both the nature of our food supply and the virulence of food-borne pathogens has changed.

In the past, the chicken served at night might have been walking around the backyard that afternoon! Today, your food may travel halfway around the world before it arrives at your table. Food often passes from producer to processor to retailer before it reaches you. The opportunities for mishandling are higher.

More potent forms of bacteria present further problems. For example, in 1990 the US Public Health Service cited *Escherichia coli* 0157:H7, *Salmonella*, *Listeria monocytogenes*, and *Campylobacter jejuni* as the four most serious food-borne pathogens in the United States. Twenty years ago, three of these—*Campylobacter*, *Listeria*, and *E. coli* 0157:H7—were not even recognized as sources of food-borne disease![2]

MYTH NO. 3

"I sampled it a couple of hours ago and never got sick, so it should be safe to eat."

Fact: Your timing may be way off if you believe this myth!

Although you may feel all right a few hours after eating a food, the food may still be unsafe for you and others to consume. A food-borne illness may develop within a half hour to a few days; some may occur as long as 2 or more weeks after a contaminated food is eaten. If sickness occurs

24 hours or longer after a food is eaten—which is often the case—it is frequently blamed on other causes.

Another consideration: While you might safely eat a food, someone with a weaker immune system could be more susceptible to a food-borne illness. Young children, older individuals, pregnant women, and persons with an illness are more vulnerable and would be more likely to get sick.

Finally, if you guess wrong about the safety of a food, you—and those you serve—may feel more than a few hours of discomfort! Some food-borne illnesses can last several weeks or longer and require hospitalization. Some can be fatal.

SEVEN HIGHLY EFFECTIVE HABITS FOR HOME FOOD SAFETY

How can food safety educators reach people with valid food safety information? One tactic cited by McNutt in Nutrition Today[3] for making food safety messages memorable is to use "a rap song or a 'little ditty' like the old Chiquita Banana song." This was one of several suggestions that consumers made as part of a focus group conducted by the Food Safety and Inspection Service (FSIS) of the US Department of Agriculture (USDA) in conjunction with the Food and Drug Administration.[3]

Based on my personal experience in providing consumer food safety information through an international e-mail newsletter, one of my most popular articles—according to reader response—used a ditty-type approach. Here are my seven highly effective habits for home food safety, based on recommendations of the USDA/FSIS.[4–8] These are offered as an example of one possible strategy to consider as you develop and deliver food safety messages.

These seven habits help cooks to do it right!

Habit 1: Hot or Cold Is How to Hold
Keep hot foods hot and cold foods cold. Avoid the "danger zone" between 40 and 140°F. Food-borne bacteria multiply rapidly in this zone, doubling in number in as little as 20 minutes.

Take perishable foods—such as meat, poultry, and seafood products—home immediately after purchase. Place them in the refrigerator (40°F or below) or freezer (0°F) on arrival. Buy a refrigerator/freezer thermometer at a variety, hardware, grocery, or department store. Monitor temperatures on a regular basis. When holding hot foods, keep them at an internal temperature of 140°F or higher. At events such as buffets at which food is set out for guests, serve smaller bowls of food and set out fresh food bowls as needed. For added safety, put foods on ice or over a heat source to keep them out of the temperature danger zone. Replace serving dishes with a new plate of fresh food; do not add fresh food to food that has been sitting out for a while.

Habit 2: Don't Be a Dope—Wash with Soap
Wash hands with soap and warm water for 20 seconds before and after handling food. This is especially important when handling raw meat, poultry, or seafood products. Bacteria can be spread all over your kitchen if you neglect to wash your hands properly.

Habit 3: Watch That Plate—Don't Cross-Contaminate
Cross-contamination occurs when bacteria are transferred from one food to another through a shared surface. Don't let juices from raw meat, poultry, or seafood come in contact with already cooked foods or foods that will be eaten raw. For example, when grilling, avoid putting cooked meat on the plate that held the raw meat. After cutting a raw chicken, clean the cutting board with hot, soapy water. Follow with hot rinse water before cutting greens for a salad. Place packages of raw meat, poultry, or fish on plates on the lower shelves of refrigerators to prevent their juices from dripping on other foods.

Habit 4: Make It a Law—Use the Fridge to Thaw
Never thaw (or marinate) meat, poultry, or seafood on the kitchen counter. It is best to plan ahead for slow, safe thawing in the refrigerator. Small items may thaw overnight. Larger foods may take longer—allow approximately 1 day for every 5 pounds of weight. For faster thawing, place food in a leak-proof plastic bag and immerse the bag in cold water. Change the water every 30 minutes to be sure it stays cold. After thawing, refrigerate the food until it is ready to use. Food thaws in cold water at a rate of approximately 1 pound per half hour. If food is thawed in the microwave, cook it right away. Unlike food thawed in a refrigerator, microwave-thawed foods reach temperatures that encourage bacterial growth. Cook immediately to kill any bacteria that may have developed and to prevent further bacterial growth.

Habit 5: More Than Two Is Bad for You
Never leave perishable foods at room temperature for longer than 2 hours. Perishable foods include raw and cooked meat, poultry, and seafood products. If perishable food is left at room temperature for longer than 2 hours, bacteria can grow to harmful levels and the food may no longer be safe. The 2-hour limit includes preparation time as well as serving time. Once fruits and vegetables are cut, it is safest to limit their time at room temperature as well. On a hot day with temperatures at 90°F or higher, your "safe use time" decreases to 1 hour.

Habit 6: Don't Get Sick—Cool It Quick
One of the most common causes of food-borne illness is improper cooling of cooked foods. Remember—bacteria are everywhere. Even after food is cooked to a safe internal temperature, bacteria can be reintroduced to food from

many sources and then can reproduce. Put leftovers in the refrigerator or freezer promptly after eating. As Habit 5 stresses, refrigerate perishable foods within 2 hours. Put foods in shallow containers so they cool faster. For thicker foods—such as stews, hot puddings, and layers of meat slices—limit food depth to 2 inches.

Habit 7: Cook It Right Before You Take a Bite

Always cook perishable foods thoroughly. If harmful bacteria are present, only thorough cooking will destroy them. Freezing or rinsing foods in cold water is not enough to destroy bacteria.

USDA recommends using a food thermometer to assure that meat and poultry reaches a safe internal temperature. There are many types of food thermometers. Some thermometers are inserted at the start of cooking and others are used for testing at the end. The depth of required penetration and the time it takes to register a temperature also vary. Although some thermometers are suitable for measuring the temperature of thin foods such as hamburger patties or chops, others are not. Read the manufacturer's instructions before selecting and using a food thermometer. In general, the thermometer should be placed in the thickest part of the food, away from bone, fat, or gristle. It may be necessary to insert the thermometer sideways for some foods. When the food being cooked is irregularly shaped, the temperature should be checked in several places. It is important to wash the thermometer probe with hot, soapy water after each insertion to prevent cross-contamination.

Cook beef, veal, and lamb to 160°F internally for medium doneness. Cook all cuts of fresh pork to 160°F. Large cuts of beef, veal, and lamb—like roasts and steaks—can be cooked to an internal temperature of 145°F (medium rare) if they have never been pierced in any way during slaughter, processing, or preparation, which can force surface bacteria into the center. Cook pierced beef, veal, and lamb to 160°F. It is especially important that ground meat, in which bacteria can spread during processing, is cooked thoroughly (160°F for ground red meat and 165°F for ground poultry). New research indicates that judging red meat by whether it is "brown inside" is not always a reliable indicator of a safe internal temperature.

Although "no pink in the juices" when you cut into a piece of meat is a visual sign of doneness, a consumer looking for a visual sign of doneness might continue cooking meat until it is overcooked and dry. Using a thermometer is an inexpensive way to help assure a safe and flavorful product.

Cook whole poultry to 180°F and poultry breasts and roasts to 170°F; cooked-out juices should appear clear rather than pink when poultry is pierced with a fork. Fish should be opaque and flake easily with a fork when done.

If raw meat and poultry have been mishandled (left in the danger zone too long—see Habit 1), bacteria may grow and produce heat-resistant toxins that can cause food-borne illness. Warning: If meat and poultry are mishandled when raw, they may not be safe to eat even after proper cooking.

WHEN IN DOUBT, THROW IT OUT!

Remember this phrase whenever you have a question about food safety and are unsure if the seven safe food habits have been followed.

AND FOR THOSE WHO STILL BELIEVE IN FOOD SAFETY MYTHS

Many people will not change their minds about food safety misconceptions until they—or a family member—become sick. This is somewhat like saying "I'll buy insurance after my house burns down." You only need an extra minute or two to wash hands, clean a cutting board, cook a food to a recommended temperature, and so on. This is a small price to pay to help ensure that you, family members, and friends avoid food-borne illness!

REFERENCES

1. *Food Safety from Farm to Table. Report to the President, Environmental Protection Agency, Department of Health and Human Services, and United States Department of Agriculture. May 1997:8.
2. The Partnership for Food Safety Education. Foodborne illness: a constant challenge (cited on the FightBAC Web site: http://www.fightbac.org/). November 1997.
3. McNutt K. Common sense advice to food safety educators. Nutr Today 1997;32:132.
4. USDA/FSIS. Basics for handling food safely (prepared by the Food Safety and Consumer Education Office). September 1997.
5. USDA/FSIS. Kitchen thermometers (prepared by the Food Safety Education and Communications Staff). October 1997.
6. USDA/FSIS. How Temperatures Affect Food (prepared by the Food Safety Education and Communications Staff). May 1997.
7. USDA/FSIS. Food safety in the kitchen: a "HACCP" approach (prepared by the Food Safety Education and Communications Staff). November 1996.
8. USDA/FSIS. The big thaw: safe defrosting methods (prepared by the Food Safety Education and Communications Staff). July 1996.

*AUTHOR'S UPDATE, 11/09/00
The Centers for Disease Control and Prevention estimated in their September 1999 article, *Food-Related Illness and Death in the United States,* that food-borne diseases cause approximately 76 million illnesses, 325,000 hospitalizations, and 5,000 deaths in the United States each year.[1a]

1a. Mead PS, Slutsker L, Dietz V, McCaig LS, Bresce JS, Shapiro C, Griffin PM, Tauxe RV. Food related illness and death in the United States. Emerg Infect Dis 1999;5(5). Available online at: http://www.cdc.gov/ ncidod/cid/vol5no5/mead.htm.

Bacterial Food-Borne Illness

by P. Kendall

P. Kendall, Colorado State University Cooperative Extension foods and nutrition specialist and professor, food science and human nutrition.

Quick Facts . . .

Bacterial food-borne illness is the result of mishandling food. It includes food infection and food intoxication.

Salmonella, Campylobacter, E. coli and *Listeria* bacteria in food cause food infection.

Staphylococcus and *Clostridium botulinum* bacteria produce a toxin (or poison) as a by-product of growth and multiplication in food and cause food intoxication.

Clostridium perfringens can multiply in foods to sufficient numbers to cause food poisoning.

Sanitation and proper heating and refrigeration practices will help prevent food-borne illness.

Food-borne infection is caused by bacteria in food. If bacteria become numerous and the food is eaten, bacteria may continue to grow in intestines and cause illness. *Salmonella, Campylobacter,* hemorrhagic *E. coli* and *Listeria* all cause infections.

Food intoxication results from consumption of toxins (or poisons) produced in food by bacterial growth. Toxins, not bacteria, cause illness. Toxins may not alter the appearance, odor or flavor of food. Common kinds of bacteria involved are *Staphylococcus aureus* and *Clostridium botulinum.* (See fact sheet 9.305, *Botulism,* for more information on its prevention.) In the case of *Clostridium perfringens,* illness is caused by toxins released in the gut when large numbers of vegetative cells are eaten.

Salmonellosis

Salmonellosis is a form of food infection that may result when foods containing *Salmonella* bacteria are

consumed. Once eaten, the bacteria may continue to live and grow in the intestine, set up an infection and cause illness. The possibility and severity of the illness depends in large part on the size of the dose, the resistance of the host and the type of organism causing the illness.

The bacteria are spread through indirect or direct contact with the intestinal contents or excrement of animals, including humans. For example, they may be spread to food by hands that are not washed after using the toilet. They also may be spread to raw meat during processing so that it is contaminated when brought into the kitchen. Because of this, it is important to make sure hands and working surfaces are thoroughly washed after contact with raw meat, fish and poultry before working with foods that require no further cooking.

Salmonella bacteria thrive at temperatures between 40 and 140 degrees F. They are readily destroyed by cooking to 165 F and do not grow at refrigerator or freezer temperatures. They do survive refrigeration and freezing, however, and will begin to grow again once warmed to room temperature.

Symptoms of salmonellosis include headache, diarrhea, abdominal pain, nausea, chills, fever and vomiting. These usually occur within 12 to 36 hours after eating contaminated food and may last two to seven days. Arthritis symptoms may follow three to four weeks after onset of acute symptoms. Infants, the elderly or people already ill have the least resistance to disease effects.

Preventive measures for campylobacter infections include pasteurizing milk; avoiding post-pasteurization contamination; cooking raw meat, poultry and fish; and preventing cross-contamination between raw and cooked or ready-to-eat foods.

Foods commonly involved include eggs or any egg-based food, salads (such as tuna, chicken or potato), poultry, pork, processed meats, meat pies, fish, cream desserts and fillings, sandwich fillings, and milk products. These foods may be contaminated at any of the many points where the food is handled or processed from the time of slaughter or harvest until it is eaten.

Campylobacteriosis

Campylobacteriosis or campylobacter enteritis is caused by consuming food or water contaminated with the bacteria *Campylobacter jejuni*. Considered a pathogen principally of veterinary significance until recently, this bacteria is now thought to be responsible for 2.5 times more food poisoning outbreaks per year than *Salmonella*.

C. jejuni commonly is found in the intestinal tracts of healthy animals (especially chickens) and in untreated surface water. Raw and inadequately cooked foods of animal origin and non-chlorinated water are the most common sources of human infection (e.g. raw milk, undercooked chicken, raw hamburger, raw shellfish). The organism grows best in a reduced oxygen environment, is easily killed by heat (120 F), is inhibited by acid, salt and drying, and will not multiply at temperatures below 85 F.

Diarrhea, nausea, abdominal cramps, muscle pain, headache and fever are common symptoms. Onset usually occurs two to five days after eating contaminated food. Duration is two to seven days, but can be weeks with such complications as urinary tract infections and reactive arthritis. Meningitis, recurrent colitis, acute cholecystitis, and Guillain-Barre syndrome are rare complications. Deaths, also rare, have been reported.

> *Preventive measures for listeriosis include maintaining good sanitation, pasteurizing milk, avoiding post-pasteurization contamination and cooking foods thoroughly.*

Listeriosis

Prior to the 1980s, listeriosis, the disease caused by *Listeria monocytogenes*, was primarily of veterinary concern, where it was associated with abortions and encephalitis in sheep and cattle. As a result of its wide distribution in the environment, its ability to survive for long periods under adverse conditions, and its ability to grow at refrigeration temperatures, *Listeria* has since become recognized as an important food-borne pathogen. *L. monocytogenes* is frequently carried by humans and animals. The organism grows in the pH range of 5.0 to 9.5. It is salt tolerant and relatively resistant to drying, but easily destroyed by heat. (It grows between 34 F and 113 F.)

Listeriosis primarily affects newborn infants, pregnant women, the elderly and those with compromised immune systems. In a healthy non-pregnant person, listeriosis may occur as a mild illness with fever, headaches, nausea and vomiting. Among pregnant women, intrauterine or cervical infections may result in spontaneous abortion or stillbirth. Infants born alive may develop meningitis. The mortality rate in diagnosed cases is 20 to 35 percent. The incubation period is a few days to three weeks. Recent cases have involved cole slaw, raw milk and cheeses made with raw milk.

> *Foods commonly involved in staphylococcal intoxication include protein foods such as ham, processed meats, tuna, chicken, sandwich fillings, cream fillings, potato and meat salads, custards, milk products and creamed potatoes. Foods that are handled frequently during preparation are prime targets for staphylococci contamination.*

Staphylococcal Intoxication

Staphylococcus bacteria are found on the skin and in the nose and throat of most people; people with colds and sinus infections are special carriers. Infected wounds, pimples, boils and acne are generally rich sources. *Staphylococcus* also are widespread in untreated water, raw milk and sewage.

When *Staphylococcus* get into warm food and multiply, they produce a toxin or poison that causes illness. The toxin is not detectable by taste or smell. While the bacteria itself can be killed by temperatures of 120 F, its toxin is heat resistant; therefore, it is important to keep the staph organism from growing. Keep food clean to prevent its contamination, keep it either hot (above 140 F) or cold (below 40 F) during serving time, and as quickly as possible refrigerate or freeze leftovers and foods to be served later. (See Figure 1.)

Symptoms include abdominal cramps, vomiting, severe diarrhea and exhaustion. These usually appear within one to eight hours after eating staph-infected food and last one or two days. The illness seldom is fatal.

> *Foods commonly involved in clostridium illnesses include cooked, cooled, or reheated meats, poultry, stews, meat pies, casseroles and gravies. Holding foods at warm (110 F) rather than hot (140 F) temperatures and cooling foods too slowly are the primary causes of perfringens contamination.*

Clostridium Perfringens Food-Borne Illness

Clostridium perfringens belong to the same genus as the botulinum organism. However, the disease produced by *C. perfringens* is not as severe as botulism and few deaths have occurred. Spores are found in soil, nonpotable water, unprocessed foods and the intestinal tract of animals and humans. Meat and poultry are frequently contaminated with these spores from one or more sources during processing.

Spores of some strains are so heat resistant that they survive boiling for four or more hours. Furthermore, cooking drives off oxygen, kills competitive organisms and heat-shocks the spores, all of which promote germination.

Once the spores have germinated, a warm, moist, protein-rich environment with little or no oxygen is necessary for growth. If such conditions exist (i.e., holding meats at warm room temperature for several hours or cooling large pots of gravy or meat too slowly in the refrigerator), sufficient numbers of vegetative cells may be produced to cause illness.

Symptoms occur within eight to 24 hours after contaminated food is eaten. They include acute abdominal pain and diarrhea. Nausea, vomiting and fever are less common. Recovery usually is within one to two days, but symptoms may persist for one or two weeks.

> *Preventive strategies for* E. coli *infections include thorough washing and other measures to reduce the presence of the microorganism on raw food, thorough cooking of raw animal products, and avoiding recontamination of cooked meat with raw meat. To be safe, cook ground meats to 160 F.*

E. Coli Hemorrhagic Colitis

Escherichia coli belong to a family of microorganisms called coliforms. Many strains of *E. coli* live peacefully in the gut, helping keep the growth of more harmful microorganisms in check. However, one strain, *E. coli* 0157:H7, causes a distinctive and sometimes deadly disease.

Symptoms begin with nonbloody diarrhea one to five days after eating contaminated food, and progress to bloody diarrhea, severe abdominal pain and moderate dehydration. In young children, hemolytic uremic syndrome (HUS) is a serious complication that can lead to renal failure and death. In adults, the complications sometimes lead to thrombocytopenic purpura (TPP), characterized by cerebral nervous system deterioration, seizures and strokes.

Ground beef is the food most associated with *E. coli* 0157:H7 outbreaks, but other foods also have been implicated. These include raw milk, unpasteurized apple juice and cider, dry-cured salami, homemade venison jerky, sprouts, and untreated water. Infected food handlers and diapered infants with the disease likely help spread the bacteria.

Preventing Food-Borne Illness

Food-borne illness can be prevented. The following food handling practices have been identified by the Food Safety Inspection Service of USDA as essential in preventing bacterial food-borne illness.

Purchase and Storage

- Keep packages of raw meat and poultry separate from other foods, particularly foods to be eaten without further cooking. Use plastic bags or other packaging to prevent raw juices from dripping on other foods or refrigerator surfaces.
- Buy products labeled "keep refrigerated" only if they are stored in a refrigerated case. Refrigerate promptly.
- Buy dated products before the label sell-by, use-by or pull-by date has expired.

Preparation

- Wash hands (gloved or not) with soap and water for 20 seconds before preparing foods and after handling raw meat or poultry, touching animals, using the bathroom, changing diapers, smoking or blowing your nose.
- Thaw only in refrigerator, under cold water changed every 30 minutes, or in the microwave (followed by immediate cooking).
- Scrub containers and utensils used in handling uncooked foods with hot, soapy water before using with ready-to-serve foods. Use separate cutting boards to help prevent contamination between raw and cooked foods.
- Stuff raw products immediately before cooking, never the night before.
- Don't taste raw meat, poultry, eggs, fish or shellfish. Use pasteurized milk and milk products.
- Do not eat raw eggs. This includes milk shakes with raw eggs, Caesar salad, Hollandaise sauce, and other foods like homemade mayonnaise, ice cream or eggnog made from recipes that call for uncooked eggs.
- Use a meat thermometer to judge safe internal temperature of meat and poultry over 2 inches thick (160 F or higher for meat, 180 F or higher for poultry). If your microwave has a temperature probe, use it.
- For meat or poultry less than 2 inches thick, look for clear juices as signs of "doneness."
- When using slow cookers or smokers, start with fresh rather than frozen, chunks rather than roasts or large cuts, and recipes that include a liquid. Check internal temperature in three spots to be sure food is thoroughly cooked.

Figure 1: Temperature of food for control of bacteria.

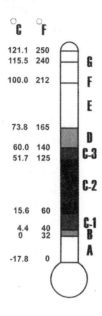

A. Freezing temperatures stop growth of bacteria, but may allow bacteria to survive. Set freezer to 0 F.

B. Cold temperatures permit slow growth of some bacteria. Do not store raw meats for more than five days or poultry, fish or ground meat for more than two days in the refrigerator.

C. DANGER ZONE.

C-1. Some growth of food poisoning bacteria may occur.

C-2. Temperatures in this zone allow rapid growth of bacteria and production of toxins by some bacteria. Do not hold foods in this zone for more than two hours.

C-3. Some bacterial growth may occur. Many bacteria survive.

D. Warming temperatures prevent growth but allow survival of some bacteria.

E. Cooking temperatures destroy most bacteria. Time required to kill bacteria decreases as temperature increases.

F. Canning temperatures for fruits, tomatoes and pickles in water-bath canner.

G. Canning temperatures for low-acid vegetables, meat and poultry in pressure canner.

• Avoid interrupted cooking. Never partially cook products, to refrigerate and finish later. Also, don't put food in the oven with a timer set to begin cooking later in the day.

• If microwave cooking instructions on the product label are not appropriate for your microwave, in-crease microwave time to reach a safe internal temperature. Rotate, stir and/or cover foods to promote even cooking.

• Before tasting, boil all home-canned vegetables and meats 10 minutes plus one minute per 1,000 feet.

Serving

• Wash hands with soap and water before serving or eating food. Serve cooked products on clean plates with clean utensils and clean hands.

• Keep hot foods hot (above 140 F) and cold foods cold (below 40 F).

• In environmental temperatures of 90 F or warmer, leave cooked food out no longer than one hour before reheating, refrigerating or freezing. At temperatures below 90 F, leave out no more than two hours.

Handling Leftovers

• Wash hands before handling leftovers and use clean utensils and surfaces.

• Remove stuffing before cooling or freezing.

• Refrigerate or freeze cooked leftovers in small, covered shallow containers (2 inches deep or less) within two hours after cooking. Leave airspace around containers to help ensure rapid, even cooling.

• Do not taste old leftovers to determine safety.

• If reheating leftovers, cover and reheat to appropriate temperature before serving (a rolling boil for sauces, soups, gravies, "wet" foods; 165 F for all others).

• If in doubt, throw it out. So they cannot be eaten by people or animals, discard outdated, unsafe or possibly unsafe leftovers in the garbage disposal or in tightly-wrapped packages.

References

Buchanan, R. L., and Doyle, M. P. Foodborne disease significance of Escherichia coli 0157:H7 and other enterohemorrhagic Escherichia coli. Food Technology, 51(10)69–76, 1997.

USDA. Food Safety Inspection Service. A Margin of Safety: The HACCP Approach to Food Safety Education. Government Printing Office, Washington, D.C. June, 1989.

Issued in furtherance of Cooperative Extension work, Acts of May 8 and June 30, 1914, in cooperation with the U.S. Department of Agriculture, Milan A. Rewerts, director of Cooperative Extension, Colorado State University, Fort Collins, Colorado. Cooperative Extension programs are available to all without discrimination. No endorsement of products mentioned is intended nor is criticism implied of products not mentioned.

Most Frequently Asked Questions

ABOUT FOOD SAFETY AND SPOILAGE

Carolee Bildsten, R.D.

Since December 1991, The American Dietetic Association (ADA) has operated the Consumer Nutrition Hot Line to provide objective and timely answers to food and nutrition questions from consumers. Below are some of the more frequently asked questions about food safety and the answers provided by registered dietitians who staff the hot line.

IS THE GREEN UNDER THE POTATO SKIN TOXIC? Yes, if eaten in amounts that exceed safety guidelines. The substance that appears as a green shade under the skin and in the eyes of potatoes is an alkaloid called solanine. It is a natural pesticide that protects the potato plant as it grows. Potatoes normally contain trace amounts (15 mg) of solanine. According to FDA regulations, 20 mg of solanine per 100 g of potato renders it unfit to eat. Solanine has a bitter taste and its level is increased in potatoes that are sunburned or blighted. Eyes of the potato and green patches on and below the skin should be trimmed away. Consequences of solanine toxicity can range from a minor upset stomach to serious illness.

CAN I EAT FOODS THAT HAVE MOLD ON THEM, SUCH AS FRUIT OR CREAM CHEESE? Most food items that have mold growing on them should be discarded because some types of mold are toxic and some are carcinogenic. One exception is hard cheese (such as Cheddar or Swiss); few of the molds that grow on hard cheeses produce toxins. However, just to be on the safe side, you should cut away the mold on cheese to a depth of 1 inch, then rewrap it with fresh, clean wrap to store. On the other hand, soft cheeses such as cream cheese, brie, and cottage cheese should be discarded because unseen mold spores may have spread throughout the cheese.

To differentiate between harmless molds on moldripened cheeses, such as blue, Gorgonzola, Roquefort, and Stilton, and potentially toxic molds, check the color and pattern. If they are different from the usual blue or green veins and you see furry spots or specks of other colors, discard the cheese.

All moldy fruit, vegetables, and breads should be tossed. As with soft cheeses, mold spores can spread easily throughout these foods. Cooking will not destroy the toxins that can make you sick.

ARE ALL GRILLED FOODS POSSIBLE CARCINOGENS? The charring—or "black stuff"—on grilled meats contains possible cancer-causing compounds called heterocyclic aromatic amines or HAAs. Although the research is inconclusive, it is best to avoid charring meat, poultry, and fish on the grill.

Cook meat to medium doneness, rather than well done, to an internal temperature of 160 degrees. An exception is hamburgers, which should always be cooked until well done. Grill poultry and fish until just done but before the surface becomes blackened. Scrape off any charred areas before serving.

Fat dripping on hot coals causes smoke that contains other possible cancer-causing compounds called polyaromatic hydrocarbons. Here again, the research is not conclusive. However, it is wise to trim visible fat from meat before cooking, catch additional fat in a drip pan, drain any high-fat marinades, and have a spray bottle with water for flare-ups.

SHOULD I USE WOOD OR PLASTIC CUTTING BOARDS? A 1993 study measuring the survival rate of bacteria on plastic and wooden cutting boards created quite a stir among food safety experts when the researchers recommended wood rather than plastic. This led to a number of subsequent studies comparing wooden and plastic cutting boards. Finally, a comprehensive review by the US Department of Agriculture (USDA) confirmed the conventional belief that plastic is safer than wood for cutting meat and poultry.

Here are the recommendations issued by USDA's Meat and Poultry Hot Line for cutting-board safety:

> Avoid cross contamination: Use plastic or glass surfaces for cutting raw meat and poultry. However, wooden cutting boards used exclusively for raw meat and poultry are acceptable. Use a different board for cutting other foods such as bread and produce. Any bacteria that remains after washing and is transferred to raw meat would be destroyed by cooking.
>
> Wash all cutting boards thoroughly: Use hot, soapy water to wash cutting boards after each use; then rinse and air or pat dry with fresh paper towels. Nonporous acrylic, plastic, or glass boards can be washed in an automatic dishwasher, as can solid (nonlaminated) wooden cutting boards.
>
> Sanitize cutting boards occasionally: Both wooden and plastic cutting boards can be sanitized with a solution of 2 teaspoons of liquid chlorine bleach (Clorox(TM))per quart of water. Flood the surface with the bleach solution and allow it to stand for several minutes, then rinse and air or pat dry with fresh paper towels.
>
> Replace battered cutting boards: Even plastic boards wear out over time. Once cutting boards become excessively worn or develop hard-to-clean grooves, they should be discarded.

HOW SHOULD I THAW MEAT AND POULTRY QUICKLY AND SAFELY?   The safest way to thaw meat, fish, and poultry is in the refrigerator. It should first be placed in a plastic bag or covered pan on the lowest shelf in the refrigerator to prevent juices from dripping onto other foods. This method requires some planning, because large, dense foods could take up to several days to thaw.

For quick thawing, use the microwave oven according to the manufacturer's directions and then cook defrosted food right away. Thawing in the microwave is safe if food is promptly cooked after thawing.

A third method is to thaw meat, fish, and poultry under cold water in an airtight plastic wrapper or bag, changing the water every 30 minutes until the food is thawed. For example, this is useful for thawing a turkey.

SHOULD I BE CONCERNED ABOUT MERCURY IN FISH? According to the Food and Drug Administration (FDA), which has regulatory authority over the seafood industry, the only two species that may exceed safe levels of mercury are shark and swordfish. Pregnant women and women of childbearing age who may become pregnant should limit consumption of shark and swordfish to no more than one serving per month. Other individuals should limit intake to 7 ounces per week.

You should also heed local advisories that accompany sport-fishing licenses warning people not to eat certain species of recreationally caught fish because of chemical concerns. Look for warnings posted at water's edge or listed in newspapers.

IS ALUMINUM COOKWARE SAFE TO USE?   More than half of all cookware sold today is made of aluminum, according to the Cookware Manufacturers Association. Most pieces of aluminum cookware are coated with nonstick finishes or processed to harden the metal's structure. The amount of aluminum leached in food from cookware is relatively minimal compared with the amount we ingest from other sources such as baked goods containing baking powder, plant and animal foods, and medications. Because it is the third most abundant element in the earth's crust, it is naturally present in air, water, and soil. Aside from its presence in the plants and animal products we consume, many over-the-counter medicines contain aluminum. Antacids are the largest carrier of aluminum.

The hypothesis that aluminum overload may cause Alzheimer's disease emerged in the 1970s when researchers found what they believed to be high concentrations of aluminum in the brain tissues of Alzheimer's patients. But subsequent studies failed to support this theory. Today, most experts conclude that either the aluminum in the earlier studies was a laboratory contaminant, or that its presence in brain tissue was a result, rather than a cause, of the disease. The FDA maintains that the normal intake of aluminum from all sources is not harmful. Nevertheless, cookware manufacturers advise against storing highly acidic or salty foods in aluminum pots and pans because this will cause surface pitting.

FOR MORE INFORMATION TO SHARE WITH CLIENTS AND PATIENTS

ADA/NCND: For food and nutrition information and a referral to a registered dietitian in your area, call the Consumer Nutrition Hot Line at (800) 366-1655 (no charge). For customized answers to your nutrition questions, call (900) CALL-AN-RD [(900) 225-5267]. Calls are $1.95 for the first minute plus $.95 for each additional minute.

REFERENCES

1. Safe Food for You and Your Family by the American Dietetic Association. Minneapolis, MN: Chronimed; 1996.
2. Duyff RL. The American Dietetic Association's Complete Food and Nutrition Guide. Minneapolis, MN: Chronimed; 1996.

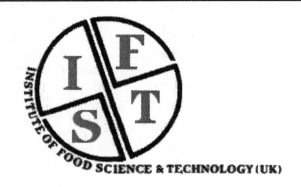

Avoiding cross-contamination in the home

The Institute of Food Science & Technology, through its Public Affairs and Technical & Legislative Committees, has authorised this paper, dated 25 May 1999, and prepared by its Professional Food Microbiology Group, as an IFST contribution to the 7th Foodlink National Food Safety Week which runs from 7–13 June 1999.

SUMMARY

Cross-contamination is a major cause of food poisoning. Food poisoning is preventable—avoiding cross-contamination is simple. Here we offer ten pointers for avoiding cross contamination in the home.

Where can germs be found?

Germs (food-poisoning organisms) exist harmlessly in many natural environments, for example farmyards and farm animals, poultry and wild birds and on fields that are fertilised with 'organic' manure. People and animals suffering from food-poisoning can also shed large numbers of germs, either through sickness or diarrhoea.

Insects, rodents and other pests ('vermin') as well as domestic pets can also harbour germs and transfer them from one place to another.

Germs may therefore be found in foods that are to be cooked. If the cooking is thorough, many types of germs (though not all) are killed, so their presence in raw foods such as meat, poultry, fish, eggs and vegetables may not be important provided these foods are cooked properly. However, these raw foods may spread contamination to other, unpackaged, ready-to-eat foods such as cheese, sandwiches, salad vegetables, cooked meats, pies and desserts.

What is cross-contamination and why must it be avoided?

Cross-contamination is the transfer of germs from their natural habitat to uncontaminated, ready to eat food.

Germs do not always cause food-poisoning, although for some people even low numbers may constitute a risk. The risk of food-poisoning increases greatly if germs are allowed to multiply ('breed'), either in the food itself or in a dirty place that can contaminate the food with large numbers of germs. Foods that not eaten immediately after thorough cooking should be stored in the 'fridge.

How does cross-contamination occur?

Cross-contamination, is its simplest form, occurs, for example, if blood from raw meat drips directly onto a ready-to-eat dessert placed at the bottom of the 'fridge, or in the shopping bag if the food is not properly wrapped.

Almost anything that is dirty can also transfer germs indirectly from a source of contamination to uncontaminated foods. Here are a few examples of common routes of cross-contamination:-

- hands
- dishcloths, teatowels, handtowels, aprons and floor cloths (especially if allowed to become dirty or remain wet)
- work surfaces
- packaging used for raw foods
- pets (especially if allowed to walk on the worktop)
- pets' bowls
- vermin
- dirty rinse water and washing up bowls
- waste bins and dustbins
- children's toys that have been in the garden
- dirty utensils or utensils that have been in contact with raw egg, meat or vegetables, for example chopping boards, knives, bowls and food processors.

Ten points for avoiding cross-contamination in the home

1. Remember that raw foods come from farms. Germs exist naturally even on the most hygienic farms so we must assume that raw food might be contaminated and keep it separate from ready-to-eat-food. This applies to **all** raw foods, even if 'free-range' or 'organic' and whether you have bought them in the village store or from the supermarket. Therefore **choose foods that have been processed for safety.** The World Health Organisation recommends that consumers should, for example:
   ■ always buy pasteurised milk
   ■ thoroughly wash certain foods eaten raw, such as lettuce, other salad vegetables and fruit.
2. **Keep raw and cooked foods apart during storage,** either in the refrigerator, the freezer or the larder. Store ready-to-eat food above raw meat and poultry. Commodities such as salad vegetables may be placed in the middle. Cover all food and place on a plate any food that is likely to drip.
3. **Use different utensils for preparing raw and cooked foods.** Don't, for example, prepare a raw chicken and then use the same unwashed cutting board and knife to carve the cooked bird. After preparing raw foods in a food processor, clean the parts thoroughly using hot water with detergent or in the dishwasher. Remember that using separate utensils is just as important when cooking on the barbeque!
4. **Wash hands, including finger-tips,** thoroughly with soap and water for at least 20 seconds and dry them thoroughly before you start preparing food. Do this **repeatedly** during food preparation—after every interruption and **always** if you have had to change the baby's nappy or have been to the toilet. After preparing raw foods such as fish, meat, or poultry, wash again before you start handling other foods. Rings can harbour germs—remove them before preparing food!
5. **Keep all kitchen surfaces meticulously clean** because every food scrap, crumb or spot is a potential reservoir of germs. The most important aspect of cleaning is physical removal of germs using hot water, a detergent and 'elbow grease' to remove food residues, especially fat. Disinfectants only work at their best on a surface that is already clean!
6. Frequently change cloths that come into contact with plates and utensils and wash in very hot water before re-use. **After use, dry dishcloths, teatowels, handtowels and aprons rapidly to stop any germs from breeding.** Don't use floorcloths for cleaning plates and utensils. Wash and dry floorcloths after use on floors!
7. **Dry the washing by allowing the items to drain naturally and rapidly or by using a dishwasher!** These are the most hygienic methods.
8. **Protect foods from domestic pets, insects and rodents. Do not allow domestic pets to walk on kitchen worktops!** Remember, too, that smaller pets such as birds and especially turtles often harbour germs.
9. **Always use clean, drinkable water for food preparation and for washing up.** After washing foods that are to be cooked, change the water before washing ready-to-eat foods.
10. **Do not prepare food for others if you are sick or have a severe skin infection.** Cover cuts with waterproof plasters.

Additional precautions

If you suspect cooked, or ready-to-eat/food might be contaminated, don't eat it!

Take the same precautions with cutting boards, utensils and other items that contain an antibacterial as with ordinary ones. Germs breed less quickly on those with built-in antimicrobial, but if they become contaminated they are just as liable to transmit contamination.

Remember:

Food-poisoning is preventable—avoiding cross-contamination is simple!

Also visit Foodlink at
http://www.curryhouse.co.uk/cw/foodlink.htm

The Institute of Food Science & Technology (IFST) is the independent professional qualifying body for food scientists and technologists. It is totally independent of government, of industry, and of any lobbying groups or special interest groups. Its professional members are elected by virtue of their academic qualifications and their relevant experience, and their signed undertaking to comply with the Institute's ethical Code of Professional Conduct. They are elected solely in their personal capacities and in no way representing organisations where they may be employed. They work in a variety of areas, including universities and other centres of higher education, research institutions, food and related industries, consultancy, food law enforcement authorities, and in government departments and agencies. The nature of the Institute and the mixture of these backgrounds on the working groups drafting IFST Position Statements, and on the two Committees responsible for finalising and approving them, ensure that the contents are entirely objective.

IFST recognises that research is constantly bringing new knowledge. However, collectively the profession is the repository of existing knowledge in its field. It includes researchers expanding the boundaries of knowledge and experts seeking to apply it for the public benefit.

Campylobacter

Low-Profile Bug Is Food Poisoning Leader

by Audrey Hingley

When it comes to food poisoning, big outbreaks make headlines. E. coli in apple juice and alfalfa sprouts. *Listeria* in cheese and hot dogs. *Salmonella* in eggs and on poultry. But the most frequently diagnosed food-borne bacterium rarely makes the news. The name of the unsung bug? *Campylobacter.*

"Most *Campylobacter* infections are sporadic and not associated with an outbreak, but we know it causes up to 4 million human infections a year," says Frederick J. Angulo, D.V.M., an epidemiologist with the national Centers for Disease Control and Prevention.

Federal and state health experts have long recognized that *Campylobacter* causes disease in animals. Conclusive proof that the bacteria also causes human disease emerged in the 1970s, and by 1996, *Campylobacter* was sitting atop the bacterial heap as the number one cause of all domestic food-borne illness.

In addition, with the emergence of antibiotic-resistant *Campylobacter,* "the true magnitude of the problem is becoming clearer," says Angulo, who also heads the CDC arm of the National Antimicrobial Resistance Monitoring System.

Campylobacter is commonly found in the intestinal tracts of people or animals without causing any symptoms of illness. But eating contaminated or undercooked poultry or meat, or drinking raw milk or contaminated water, may cause *Campylobacter* infection, or campylobacteriosis.

Symptoms of campylobacteriosis usually occur within two to 10 days of ingesting the bacteria. Children, the elderly, and people with weakened immune systems are particularly at risk. The most common symptoms include mild to severe diarrhea, fever, nausea, vomiting, and abdominal pain.

Most people infected with *Campylobacter* can get well on their own without treatment, though antibiotics may be prescribed for severe cases. But complications can occur, such as urinary tract infections or meningitis. The bacteria also is now recognized as a major contributing factor to Guillain-Barré syndrome, the most common cause of acute paralysis in both children and adults.

Concerns About Chicken

Although found in many farm animals, *Campylobacter* in poultry is causing experts the most con-

From *FDA Consumer,* September/October 1999, pp. 14-17. Reprinted by permission of *FDA Consumer,* the magazine of the U.S. Food and Drug Administration.

cern. There have been several studies pointing to high levels of *Campylobacter* present on poultry at the retail level, including a recent two-year Minnesota Department of Health study that found that 88 percent of poultry sampled from local supermarkets tested positive for the bacteria.

"The retail study was in collaboration with the Minnesota Department of Agriculture; their inspectors went to supermarkets throughout the St. Paul/Minneapolis Twin Cities area to cover a variety of supermarket types, from big chains to mom-and-pop stores," says Kirk E. Smith, D.V.M., a Minnesota state epidemiologist who participated in the study.

Many prior surveys have found *Campylobacter* contamination rates of between 40 and 60 percent, he says. "But 88 percent—this degree [of contamination] surprised even me," he admits.

In studies conducted by the U.S. Department of Agriculture's poultry microbiological safety research unit, more than 90 percent of poultry tested positive for *Campylobacter,* in levels ranging from one cell to over a million cells per bird.

Norman J. Stern, Ph.D., research leader for the unit, says the infection of poultry broiler flocks typically occurs at week three in the six-week growing cycle. It's not unusual, he says, for *Campylobacter* to infect the entire flock.

Things only get worse by the time the chickens reach the processing plant, he says. USDA studies have found a hundredfold increase in bacteria amounts on the birds' exterior from that detected on the farm. "The exterior contamination represents consumer exposure," he explains.

To help reduce that exposure, Stern says the poultry industry is currently participating in a USDA-led study that will cover "every element of production where chickens can become infected, from . . . shells to farmers' boots to wild bird droppings. When we're done . . . we will be able to genetically fingerprint the organism so we can ascribe a relationship between various environmental sources and the

spread of pathogens." The study was slated to end in September.

Resistance to Antibiotics

According to the Minnesota Department of Health study, the number of *Campylobacter* infections that are resistant to a class of antibiotics called fluoroquinolones has been on the increase since 1992. While most Americans acquired the resistant infections while on foreign travel, Kirk explains, "we have been seeing a significant increase in domestically acquired resistant cases as well." The Food and Drug Administration approved the use of fluoroquinolones in food animals in 1995. The study concluded that antibiotic use in U.S. poultry is contributing to antibiotic resistance.

Resistance to fluoroquinolones, not only by *Campylobacter* but by other bacteria as well, is a concern, explains Jesse Goodman, M.D., chief of the division of infectious diseases at the University of Minnesota, "because fluoroquinolones are commonly used to treat severe infectious diarrhea, often before the specific cause has been identified. Fluoroquinolones are very important drugs for treating a variety of serious human infectious diseases."

CDC studies also show an increase in resistance to fluoroquinolones and this can be correlated to fluoroquinolone use in poultry, according to Angulo. In addition, "We did a case control study in 1997, comparing people with [nonresistant] *Campylobacter* infections with fluoroquinolone-resistant infections, and found that those with resistant infections [were] more likely to have severe infections, bloody diarrhea, and be hospitalized."

Because of the concern over antibiotic resistance, FDA is considering whether, before it reviews a new animal drug for approval, manufacturers must assess the likelihood that use of a certain drug in food animals will transfer resistance and create a public health problem. In addition, new procedures for monitoring antibiotic use and resistance after approval also are being considered.

"FDA believes a new regulatory framework is needed to address resistance concerns raised by the food animal use of antibiotics," says Goodman, who also serves as a deputy medical director for FDA.

The Animal Health Institute, a national trade association representing manufacturers of animal health products, says it also is concerned about the possibility of antibiotic use in food animals causing resistant bacteria to develop. But the organization believes that the requirements FDA is proposing may have "unintended negative consequences on animal health . . . and risk sending unhealthy animals into the food chain."

Hollinger says, "At this time we are not taking action toward withdrawal of these products from the market. We have asked the sponsors of poultry fluoroquinolone products to provide data that would describe the prevalence of resistance in poultry flocks and identify possible actions to prevent the emergence of disease in treated flocks."

Calling it a "farm to plate" approach, Hollinger says that the *Campylobacter* problem can be addressed "at any number of points" along the food chain. "They all need to be reviewed and evaluated for new methods to deal with the problems."

USDA's Stern says he believes the poultry industry is "trying very hard" to move toward enhanced food safety for economic as well as safety benefits. For example, he explains, a company could use extensive microbiological criteria to ensure safety as a marketing tool. Just as consumers are willing to pay more for "gourmet" coffees or specialty food items, an increasingly health-conscious consumer could be wooed by a health emphasis when it comes to safer poultry products, he says.

Vaccine on the Horizon

A team of Navy, Army, and drug industry researchers is also moving ahead in the development of a prototype vaccine for *Campylobacter.* The vaccine has shown promise in animal models and currently is undergoing clinical trials.

Capt. Louis A. Bourgeois, director of the enteric diseases program at the Naval Medical Research Center in Bethesda, Md., says the Navy has been involved in *Campylobacter* research since the early 1980s.

"Historically, the military has had longstanding diarrheal problems with troops deploying overseas," he explains. "*Campylobacter* was an emerging pathogen in the early '80s, and by the mid-1980s, we began doing more directed studies towards a vaccine development."

Bourgeois and his fellow researchers say an approved vaccine is likely "several years away" but they remain optimistic. Bourgeois says private companies are interested in a vaccine due to its possible application in "traveler's diarrhea," a common ailment.

"We know from animal model work that we can protect animals against *Campylobacter* colonization," says colleague Daniel Scott, M.D., deputy director of the Navy's enteric diseases program. "We have also gained an increasing amount of knowledge in the clinical and preclinical development of this product, especially in terms of what happens with the actual infection. We are already seeing some evidence that term protection can occur, which allows for a lot of optimism."

The Consumer's Role

While researchers, regulatory agencies, and scientists grapple with *Campylobacter,* what can you do to protect yourself?

"Consumers go to the supermarket thinking everything [there] is clean, and that is just not true," says Donald H. Burr, Ph.D., a research microbiologist in FDA's Center for Food Safety and Applied Nutrition. "People can't assume that anymore. Consumers have a responsibility in food safety."

Those responsibilities include prompt refrigeration, thorough cooking, avoiding cross-contamination, and washing hands and surfaces often. In addition:

- Don't let raw foods such as uncooked poultry touch other food, since bacteria can spread.
- Thaw raw poultry on a bottom shelf in the refrigerator so that blood or juices don't drip onto other foods.
- Do not reuse marinades from raw meat or poultry.
- Never put cooked poultry or meat back on the plate that held the raw product.
- Wash your hands frequently, especially after handling raw meat and poultry.
- Wash kitchen surfaces and cutting boards often, especially after they have come in contact with raw meat or poultry.

Audrey Hingley is a writer in Mechanicsville, Va.

Tracking Down Trouble

Bacteria That Cause Food-Borne Illness

Bacteria	Cases of Food-Borne Illness
Listeria	77
Vibrio	51
Yersinia	139
E. coli O157:H7	340
Shigella	1,263
Salmonella	2,207
Campylobacter	3,974
Total	8,051

Campylobacter was the culprit in an overwhelming number of cases detected by the FoodNet system in 1997. FoodNet, a joint project of FDA, the national Centers for Disease Control, and USDA's Food Safety and Inspection Service, tracks cases of food-borne infections at early-warning sites in several states. The numbers are combined totals from California, Connecticut, Georgia, Minnesota, and Oregon.

E. Coli 0157:H7—How Dangerous Has It Become?

Escherichia coli 0157:H7 is now recognized as an important cause of bloody diarrhea; it causes hemorrhagic colitis, which begins with watery diarrhea and severe abdominal pain and rapidly progresses to passage of bloody stools. It is the leading cause of postdiarrheal hemolytic-uremic syndrome (HUS), characterized by acute kidney failure, among children in the U.S. and Canada. Infection with *E. coli* 0157:H7 results in a disturbingly high frequency of serious complications. Data from outbreak investigations in the U.S. suggest 5%–10% of infected children develop HUS. Approximately 25,000 cases of food-borne illness can be attributed to *E. coli* 0157:H7 each year, resulting in as many as 100 deaths.

Among the identified dietary risk factors, foods of bovine origin, particularly undercooked ground beef, have been the most frequently implicated source. Other foods, such as apple cider and mayonnaise-containing sauces, have also been implicated in outbreaks. However, the original source of contamination in these cases was suspected of being of bovine or other animal origin. Nondietary risk factors include person-to-person transmission in daycare settings or swimming in contaminated water.

L. Slutsker et al. reported on a two-year case-control study in the U.S. in which 118 cases of *E. coli* 0157:H7 were found in 30,463 persons examined. Case questionnaires were completed by 93 patients. Eighty-six did not develop HUS, but 100% had diarrhea, 92% had abdominal cramps, 90% had bloody diarrhea, 45% had nausea, 45% had subjective fever, and 37% had vomiting. The seven patients with HUS ranged in age from one to 82 years. Vomiting within three days of diarrhea onset was the only symptom significantly associated with HUS. Those patients younger than 13 years old who developed HUS were more likely to have received an antimicrobial agent within three days after onset of their diarrhea. Other than hamburg-ers and hot dogs, no other foods were positively associated with illness, including other beef, poultry, or dairy products. (See *J Infect Dis,* 1998; 177:962.)

Consumption of visibly undercooked ground beef was the only dietary factor independently associated with *E. coli* 0157:H7-related diarrhea. The findings of the current study are supported by two Canadian studies that linked sporadic *E. coli* 0157:H7 infection with consumption of undercooked meat and under-cooked ground beef at picnics or special events. The fact that undercooked ground beef rather than ground beef *per se* was a risk factor for infection underscores the importance of proper cooking for prevention of *E. coli* 0157:H7 infection.

Recently, outbreaks of *E. coli* 0157:H7 have been linked to fresh produce, specifically leaf and iceberg lettuce and unpasteurized apple cider and juice. Local unchlorinated water sources such as rural wells are also potential sources. Prevention of sporadic infection requires recognition and modification of risk factors. In addition, since the infectious dose for this pathogen is low and person-to-person spread not uncommon, it is important to identify cases to prevent secondary transmission in households and in the community.

The Source of *E. Coli* 0157:H7

How did the relatively innocuous bacterium *Escherichia coli* found in human and animal intestines become the deadly strain of *E. coli* 0157:H7? It is theorized that this deadly strain was created from a dysentery epidemic in Central America. Scientists believe that a virus, which invades cells like bacteria to reproduce, carried a toxin-producing gene from *Shigella,* the bacteria that were causing the epidemic, over to *E. coli.*

The resultant *E. coli* 0157:H7 is surprisingly tough and virulent. Most bacteria do not produce disease unless a person is exposed to millions of them, but as few as 10 *E. coli* 0157:H7 can produce illness—far too few to see or smell. While most bacteria, including those which cause botulism, cannot live in acidic environments, *E. coli* 0157:H7 is able to grow in foods like unpasteurized apple cider and commercial mayonnaise. This acid tolerance may also signal the pathogen's resistance to other protective measures such as heat, radiation, and antimicrobials. Successful prevention strategies must focus on eliminating the presence of the microorganism, rather than on preventing pathogen growth as is traditionally done.

Dairy cows and other cattle seem to be the "Typhoid Marys" of the epidemics, carrying the bacteria harmlessly in their feces. From there, the bacteria enter the food supply. A single contaminated carcass can be ground up with scores of other cows to produce hamburgers. *E. coli* 0157:H7 has gotten into apple cider possibly because farmers fertilized their crops with cow manure or cows grazed in the orchard. The same may be said for the lettuce and alfalfa sprouts. Washing prepackaged salad mixes and vegetables, even if the label says they are prewashed, would help prevent this source of contamination.

Preventive Measures

To kill any disease-causing bacteria, the following procedures are recommended. For whole cuts of meat, sear the entire surface; the interior of a whole cut is generally safe. Cook ground beef, veal, lamb, and pork to an internal temperature of 160° F; 165° F for ground poultry; and 180° F for whole poultry. Washing hands with soap and hot running water while rubbing hands together for 20 seconds is an effective preventive recommendation for all food handlers.

The FDA wants the food industry to take more responsibility. It is working on voluntary guidelines to encourage safer handling of fruits and vegetables, similar to the HACCP guidelines in place for fish, meats, poultry, dairy, and eggs.

Is It Safe to Eat?

■ *Like water and oil, food has become a hot international political issue. Europe and the U.S. risk trade wars over beef and bananas, while British consumers are up in arms over genetically modified food, and tainted animal feed, contaminating the food chain, has brought down the Belgian government.*

It all began in a California strawberry patch. An American biotechnology company, Advanced Genetic Sciences, applied for permission to spray the strawberries with genetically modified bacteria to protect the plants against frost damage. For four years, environmentalists fought in the courts against the company's proposals. On April 24, 1987, they lost the battle, but the war against genetically modified (GM) crops had just begun.

A decade ago, deliberately releasing GM life forms into the open environment caused the sort of furor in America that they are now creating in Britain. Another 1987 GM experiment in the U.S.—this time in a potato patch—was vandalized within a month. Things suddenly turned ugly between the anti-GM activists and the scientific establishment.

The row resurfaced in Britain this May with the leaking of a letter from the government's chief scientific adviser, Robert May, in which he said he could not contemplate the commercial growing of GM crops until at least 2003. Yet ministers have refused to agree to a moratorium, saying that commercial production may begin after the first year of farm-scale field trials.

There are fewer than 200 small experimental plots in Britain—many no bigger than a suburban lawn—where GM plants are grown. Most of them are on the land of research institutes or universities and are strictly for research purposes. Three licenses have been issued for larger, farm-scale trials to assess the full impact of growing GM crops for commercial purposes. Further licenses are expected to be issued over the next year.

Between 1996 and 1997, the area of land in the world planted with commercial GM crops quadrupled from 6.9 million acres to 31 million acres—equivalent to an area the size of England. In the U.S., the war against GM crops and food has largely been lost. The U.S., China, Canada, and Argentina are now the main countries where GM crops are grown commercially. The battleground has shifted to Britain and Europe, where environmental activists have been prepared to go to jail for digging up GM crops.

The environmentalists are opposed to the release of any GM organism into the environment on the grounds that the risks are too great and can never be eliminated. Douglas Parr, scientific campaigner for Greenpeace, says that it is effectively impossible for scientists to make genetic engineering safe because the technology is inherently unpredictable. "Genetic engineering crosses a fundamental threshold in the human manipulation of the planet, changing the nature of life itself," says Parr.

Parr's fears were in fact voiced 10 years ago by the British government's previous chief scientist, William Stewart, who was a key figure in Britain's first and, so far, most authoritative inquiry into the release of GM organisms, published in 1989. Stewart said there are genuine concerns about deliberately releasing into the environment new life forms whose genes are tweaked by the hand of man.

"Unlike chemicals, biological agents can multiply in the environment. There is therefore a risk that, once released, it will be impossible to control them," he said at the time of the report. Yet Stewart and May oppose an indefinite moratorium. Indeed, a moratorium was considered and rejected 10 years ago by experts, who thought it would prevent exploiting the "enormous potential" GM crops offer.

In the past 10 years, the debate has become a political football. Prime Minister Tony Blair wants to be seen promoting the potential benefits of the new science. Meanwhile, the Conservatives have taken every opportunity to question the safety and usefulness of new foods and crops, detecting that the government is vulnerable to public opposition on GM.

Scientists argue that GM food offers new ways to alleviate hunger and disease. A type of rice engineered with genes for iron enrichment could alleviate the suffering of thousands of children in Southeast Asia, and crops resistant to pests could boost food production worldwide.

Supporters of GM technology argue that virtually every food we eat is the product of human manipulation of genes by selective breeding. The government's Advisory Committee on Novel Foods and Processes says GM technology could be less risky than conventional breeding because scientists can define exactly which genes they are manipulating and the end products have to go through extensive tests.

Recent monarch butterfly research [see box] is the hardest evidence yet to suggest that the influence of a GM crop may go beyond the actual field in which it grows. It strikes at the heart of the debate over GM crops because it shows that pollen can transmit toxic effects to endangered wildlife.

—Steve Connor, "The Independent" (centrist), London, May 21, 1999.

Biotech's Moral Imperative

In the time it takes to read this sentence, the world population will have grown by about five. There will be another 170 people in the world at the end of the next minute. This is because more babies are being born and fewer old people are dying each year. There are about 240,000 more people in the world today than there were yesterday. The planet's population grows by about 87 million every year. A science watchdog, the Nuffield Council on Bioethics, has warned that there is a "moral imperative" to develop genetically modified (GM) crops—higher yielding, better nourishing, more resistant—to feed the extra billion mouths expected in the next three decades.

Consider the problem. There are three needs for a harvest: acreage, fertile topsoil, and fresh water. The consensus is that it takes 1.25 acres to provide a sufficient and varied diet for an adult human. Right now, the world average per person is just over two thirds of an acre.

For a while during the so-called green revolution, food production outpaced population. Yields per acre grew, and the areas under cultivation increased. But the area of harvested cropland reached its peak in 1981 and has been falling ever since. With more people, there is more demand for places to live, which consumes farmland. In addition, farmland is being destroyed by being overworked.

The minimum amount of grain needed to keep a vegetarian supplied with bread, rice, or cornmeal for a year is 1,080 pounds. How much grain you can grow depends on sunlight, soil, and water. The depth of topsoil is critical. The latest estimate, from David Pimentel of Cornell University, is that farmers are losing 24 billion tons of topsoil every year to wind

Monarchs in GM Tumbrils

FINANCIAL TIMES

Concern about the environmental impact of genetically modified (GM) crops is likely to be fueled by new research showing that a popular variety of modified corn can kill butterflies. The crop, known as Bt-corn, is genetically engineered to produce a bacterial toxin that protects against corn pests. Researchers from Cornell University found that its pollen can kill monarch butterfly larvae.

"These results have potentially profound implications for the conservation of monarch butterflies," the scientists say. With the amount of Bt-corn planted in the U.S. projected to increase, they say it is imperative that more research be done on the environmental risks posed by biotechnology.

Bt-engineered corn was one of the first commercial successes of the GM industry. Last year, 7 million acres of the crop were planted in the U.S. to protect against the European corn borer, which causes annual losses of about $1.2 billion. The Bt-corn contains genes from the *Bacillus* *thuringiensis* bacteria, which produces a toxin that kills the pest.

Up to now, the corn was thought to be toxic only to the corn borer and harmless to non-target organisms, such as bees and ladybugs. But Cornell researchers have focused on the corn's pollen, which has been found to contain the Bt toxin. The wind can carry this pollen more than 60 miles, allowing it to be ingested by insects feeding off other plants.

In laboratory tests, the scientists found that nearly half of the monarch larvae that ate leaves dusted with the pollen sickened and died.

Monarch butterflies are not an endangered species, but their migratory behavior is threatened by disruption of their habitat. The scientists say more research is needed before the risks posed by the crops can be weighed against benefits, such as reduced pesticide use.

—John Losey, "Financial Times" (centrist), London, May 20, 1999.

and water erosion. At this rate, one third of the world's arable land will be depleted within the next 20 years.

The forests are home to millions of as yet undescribed and unnamed species, many of which could provide tomorrow's foods and drugs, and many of which will be extinct in the next few decades. But even as humans colonize new soils, they use them for things other than food. About half of all humans will be city dwellers by the year 2000. New homes need new bricks, new tiles, new roads, and sewers.

Human beings have become the biggest single earth-moving force on the planet, shifting more soil even than rainfall and rivers. According to Roger Hooke of the University of Maine, rivers wash 24 billion tons of silt into the sea each year, but humans now shift 35 billion tons of soil each year just to make roads, build houses, and mine ores.

The green revolution was achieved by new rice, wheat, and corn hybrids watered by newly engineered irrigation systems, fed by artificial fertilizers, protected by pesticides, and tilled by oil-burning machines. Although yields are still high, there has been no increase in record yields for 20 years, and grain output per person is falling.

Farmers use 150 million tons of phosphate each year: The world's supplies could run out in 2050. Oil demand will outstrip supply in about 2020, says John Edwards, once chief geologist with Shell Oil. And, far more ominous, there are already water problems. It takes 1,000 tons of water to grow a ton of wheat. But cities and heavy industry are consuming more water than ever.

Gretchen Daily of Stanford University in California calculates that humans use one quarter of all the rain that falls from heaven and is taken up by plants. The other 10 million species that share the planet divide the remaining three quarters. About 17 countries face "absolute" water scarcity. That is why the Nuffield Council on Bioethics wants the government to race ahead with research on new drought-tolerant, salt-tolerant, pest-resistant, protein-rich crops.

Prince Charles calls this argument "emotional blackmail" [see box]. The charity Christian Aid condemns it, arguing that today's hungry are surrounded by plenty and that distributing resources fairly is a more urgent problem. This is true. The Worldwatch Institute in Washington recently calculated that if people in the U.S. simply wasted one third less food each day, there would be enough to feed 25 million people, roughly equivalent to the population of North Korea, which has been in the grip of a severe famine.

But in just under four months, the world would be home to another 25 million people, and four months after that, another 25 million, and so on. Two hundred years ago, Thomas Malthus wrote: "The power of population is so superior to the power in the earth to produce subsistence for man that premature death must in some shape or form visit the human race." —*Tim Radford, "The Guardian" (liberal), London, June 3, 1999.*

Royal Protest

FINANCIAL TIMES

The response from Britain's food industry to the attack by the Prince of Wales on genetically modified crops has been largely delivered through gritted teeth. Stephen Smith of Novartis, the Swiss life-sciences group, says he is undismayed. "It's not for us to criticize the beliefs the prince holds so strongly," he says.

Christopher Haskins of Northern Foods was prepared to open his jaw a little wider. "His views are somewhat predictable. As an enthusiastic organic farmer, he comes at it with a closed mind—it's rather like asking the pope for his views on the Church of England," he says.

Even before the prince's intervention in the debate, the British food industry had virtually surrendered to public pressure on the issue of genetically altered foods. Almost every food manufacturer, fast-food chain, and large supermarket chain intends to eliminate genetically modified ingredients as far as possible.

Many say they remain committed to the technology and believe it will bring benefits for consumers, especially in parts of the world where food is in short supply. But the entry of Prince Charles into the controversy will make it harder for the biotechnology industry to persuade food companies to stand up for foods with genetic modifications, even if they regard the technology as progress.

In expressing his views on biotechnology, the prince believes he is able to voice public concerns that find no outlet elsewhere. But the prince's forays into controversy are frustrating for the businesses affected.

"He is a nice man, but utterly confused and a terrible philosopher," says political philosopher Alan Ryan of New College, Oxford. "He has very primitive ways of thinking."

—*John Willman and Vanessa Houlder, "Financial Times," London, June 2, 1999.*

Unit Selections

Key Points to Consider

❖ How can consumers protect themselves from misinformation in the nutrition field?

❖ How do you interpret the different types of research studies so that you can get at the truth of health claims?

❖ What are some of the positive and negative aspects of the information available on the Internet?

❖ What are some of the truths about the effect of herbs in a person's diet?

❖ What are some of the dangers of using nutrition supplements to improve athletic performance?

❖ What are the values of using dietary supplements?

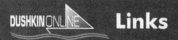 **Links**   **www.dushkin.com/online/**

These sites are annotated on pages 4 and 5.

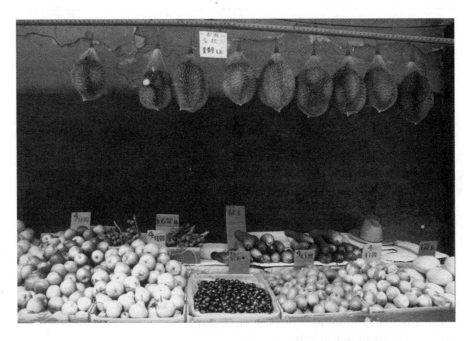

Americans spend approximately $25 billion on alternative treatments. According to an American Dietetic Association (ADA) Survey, 90 percent of consumers polled get their nutrition information from television, magazines, and newspapers.

Nutrition is a field that is vulnerable to quackery. The Food and Drug Administration (FDA) defines quackery as misinformation about health. Quacks abound in our culture, from health food store salespeople to popular talk show hosts, to self-proclaimed "nutritionists" with no background in nutrition or credentials from accredited schools. Quacks also pretend to be able to cure a health problem or a disease. Nutritionists and dietitians have worked hard through the years to set the record straight and distribute reliable and valid information.

Most quacks will claim that Americans are addicted to "junk" food and attempt to sell their vitamin supplements instead. They also allege that processing and storage of food removes most of the nutrients and that our soil is depleted so our foods are not nutritious. Some of the articles in this unit deal with nutrition quackery. Targets are groups of people who are not able to interpret information critically: the naïve, who look for a magic cure; the desperate, who have a fatal disease; and the alienated who are disappointed with the medical profession.

A new source of information is the Internet, which allows distribution and promotion of just about anything. About 29 percent of Americans turn to the Internet for information. We need to be vigilant as to the type of information we get from different Web sites. How to judge the validity of information and guidelines for recognizing and avoiding unreliable sites is described in the article entitled "The Mouse That Roared."

Herbs and nutrition supplements are the subjects of two articles. Herbs have been used for medicinal purposes in the East for thousands of years. The World Health Organization reports that 70 percent of the world uses herbal medicines for some aspect of health care. In the United States, herbal supplement sales exceed $3 billion per year. Since the FDA classifies herbs as dietary supplements, they are not tested for safety or efficacy. Only when it is proven that an herbal product has produced ill effects or death can the FDA take regular action. Even though many herbs have documented health benefits, many more are toxic. Herbs have not had the rigorous testing that pharmaceuticals have. Their active ingredients are not standardized and their safety and long-term effects have not been studied in well-controlled trials. Presently the herbal industry is attempting to resolve the issue of standardization. The recently formed consumer lab (CL) assays products for purity, identity, activity, and consistency.

Among the population groups that are most vulnerable to using megadoses of herbs, vitamin/mineral supplements, and ergogenic aids are athletes. Selective ergogenic aids and dietary supplements, including the health risks involved, are presented in the article, "Nutrition Supplements: Science vs. Hype."

Foods rich in soy protein have been popular among vegetarians and health conscious individuals for quite a while. More recently, health claims about soy lowering the risk of heart disease has increased soy sales. Some data are controversial and confusing. Concerns revolve around isoflavones, individual soy components sold as dietary supplements, which may increase risk of breast cancer. Since evidence is far from conclusive, consumers would be wise to add some form of soy protein to their diet, but avoid over-the-counter isoflavone supplements. The article "Food for Thought About Dietary Supplements" dispels any myths and answers questions pertinent to vitamin supplementation. Vitamins in megadoses may have pharmacological effects as they may be potentially toxic, can adversely affect the bioavailability of another nutrient, and could precipitate a deficiency.

This unit concludes with an article that questions whether health food stores are better than traditional supermarkets. Actually, buying from a health food store does not automatically guarantee that you are getting a healthful product and the nutrition expert at the health food store may not be an "expert" at all!

Nutrition Quackery

by J. Anderson, L. Patterson and B. Daly[1]

Each year Americans spend an estimated $25 billion on alternative treatments in search of short cuts or simple solutions to better health. Health fraud can be defined as misinformation about health, ranging from a self-proclaimed medical expert who has discovered a miracle cure, to a food supplement or drug that is promoted with unproven health claims.

10 Red Flags for Consumers

1. Recommendations that promise a quick fix.

2. Dire warnings of danger from a single product or regimen.

3. Claims that sound too good to be true.

4. Simplistic conclusions drawn from a complex study.

5. Recommendations based on a single study.

6. Dramatic statements that are refuted by reputable scientific organizations.

7. Lists of "good" and "bad" foods.

8. Recommendations made to help sell a product.

9. Recommendations based on studies published without peer review.

10. Recommendations from studies that ignore differences among individuals or groups.

A person who pretends to be able to cure a disease or health problem is defined as a quack. Problems that help promote quackery include:

- Lack of laws to prevent someone from selling anything as long as it is called a dietary supplement.
- Almost anyone can call himself or herself a nutritionist. Thousands of people who call themselves nutritionists have dubious credentials from nonaccredited schools.
- Research scientists who go public with their findings before their study has been published in a peer-reviewed journal or duplicated, thus causing consumer confusion about what to believe.

A product may state that you can eat all you want and still lose weight, or that it can help overcome the aging process, arthritis and even cancer. These products usually do nothing to improve health and often are expensive. Even worse, they can be harmful or delay necessary medical treatment.

Targets of Questionable Treatments

Alternative treatments are designed to appeal to anyone, but certain populations are likely targets:
- The unsuspecting who are unable to question things critically. To them, all health claims seem to make sense.
- The naive who are looking for a magic cure. They believe that printed or spoken claims must be true.
- The desperate who have incurable or potentially fatal diseases and are hoping for a cure that medical science has not yet been able to provide.
- The alienated who feel animosity toward medicine or the scientific community.

Aging

A Congressional subcommittee study revealed 60 percent of victims of alternative treatments are older people. The normal aging process is fertile ground for questionable treatments. Many products claim to reverse or delay conditions associated with aging. Cosmetics and creams are said to erase wrinkles or cure baldness. Vitamins and minerals are said to cure or prevent disease or even lengthen life. A healthy lifestyle may help delay conditions associated with aging, but no preparation or process can stop the process.

Arthritis

Individuals who suffer from chronic illnesses often turn to questionable treatments. Arthritis is a painful and sometimes debilitating disease that has no cure. However, it can go into spontaneous remission, meaning that pain and swelling can disappear for days, weeks, months or even years. When people experience such a remission, they are easily convinced that whatever they have been doing brought the relief. Thus, unproven miracle cures for arthritis flourish.

Examples of unproven remedies include vibrating chairs, sitting in abandoned uranium mines, unapproved drug treatments and questionable diets such as gin-soaked raisins. Since there is no cure for arthritis, these treatments not only are ineffective, but they can do considerable harm in addition to delaying proper diagnosis and treatment. People who suffer from arthritis should see a physician for therapy tailored to their needs.

Cancer

Alternative treatments often are attractive to people who are seriously ill. Cancer patients spend millions of dollars each year on treatments that do nothing to relieve their illness or suffering.

> By trying alternative treatments instead of getting effective medical help, cancer patients may allow the disease to progress beyond the treatable stage.

Cancer is not a single disease, so no one device or remedy will diagnose, treat or prevent all types of cancer. Effective treatment depends on early diagnosis and treatment. By trying alternative treatments instead of getting effective medical help, cancer patients may allow the disease to progress beyond the treatable stage.

Autoimmune Disorders (HIV/AIDS)

Incurable, highly publicized autoimmune disorders have brought a boom in the sale of unproven products or treatments. People who are HIV positive or who have AIDS spend millions of dollars abroad or illegally in this country to obtain unproven drugs and

therapy. These drugs provide little, if any, benefit and are often toxic. People who are HIV positive or who have AIDS may delay effective treatment by using alternatives.

Not all unapproved AIDS treatments are motivated by profit. An underground network of "guerilla clinics" provides unapproved drugs free to patients. However good their intentions may be, the drugs are still ineffective and sometimes dangerous.

The fear generated by the disease has created a potentially unlimited market for products aimed at AIDS prevention. Unsubstantiated claims may create a false sense of security or may lead consumers to avoid precautions that are known to prevent the disease.

Weight Loss

Weight loss schemes and devices probably are the most popular form of quackery. Millions seek a painless, effortless way to shed unwanted pounds. Weight loss is a multibillion-dollar industry that includes books, fad diets, drugs, special foods and clinics. Some products or treatments can produce weight loss, but the effect usually is temporary. The weight is quickly regained and may be even more difficult to lose when the next diet is attempted. Fad diets may not provide adequate calories or nutrients and can be harmful.

> The only way to lose weight effectively and safely is to increase activity while decreasing food intake.

The only way to lose weight effectively and safely is to increase activity while decreasing food intake. Weight loss should be gradual, 1 to 2 pounds per week, to allow for the development and maintenance of new dietary habits. Prior to beginning any weight loss program, see your doctor to be certain that you need to lose weight. Consult a registered dietitian to determine a safe and effective weight loss program. Some weight loss may be unnecessary. The key is to assess your health status and act accordingly.

Adolescence

Teenagers, too, are consumers of alternative treatments. Young shoppers may have money from part-time jobs or access to mom and dad's credit card. It is estimated that teens spend about $80 per month on personal items. Adolescence often brings feelings of insecurity about physical development. Teens may be drawn to experiment with products that promise to enhance appearance or speed their development. A number of products that may appeal particularly to teens include:

Questionable Diagnostic Methods

Kinesiology

This process involves placing a substance in the mouth or elsewhere on the body. A reaction to it is determined by measuring resistance in muscle groups. Kinesiology has been proven to be ineffective.

Cytotoxic Testing

Food extracts are mixed with a drop of the patient's blood to diagnose food allergies. Cytotoxic testing is not reproducible.

Hair Analysis

Hair testing can be used to determine the status of a few minerals. However, hair minerals are influenced by pollution, age, race and hair products. Hair analysis is ineffective in determining vitamin deficiencies. The technique is often misused to sell unnecessary dietary supplements.

Herbal Crystallization Analysis (HCA)

A drop of saliva and a drop of copper chloride are placed on a glass slide and left to dry. The spot is visually analyzed to see if any crystals form "curative patterns." Based on the patterns, consumers are prescribed an herb to get rid of their disease or illness. This method has never been proven.

Muscle Strength Testing

This method involves putting pressure on the patient's extended arm or leg. Any weakness indicates allergies or impaired function, and an appropriate nutritional supplement is prescribed to help the patient get better. This method is ineffective.

Live Cell Analysis

This diagnostic test claims to determine what nutrients you need. It involves having a drop of blood analyzed by an instrument called the Darkfield microscope to see if there are any unhealthy cells, cells with free radical damage, or cells that are not getting enough oxygen and nutrients. If unhealthy cells are present, you take an enzyme tablet (which costs over $100) and magically all your cells are now normal. This test is both unreliable and unproven.

- Breast developers. Creams or lotions do not work and are a waste of money. Breast developing devices strengthen muscle but do not increase breast size.
- Weight loss methods. As many as 75 percent of teen girls report they are dieting. Fad diets are especially dangerous for teens because they have high nutritional needs to support their rapid growth and development.
- Steroids and growth hormones. These dangerous and illegal drugs often are used by teens and other athletes to give them a competitive edge.
- Tanning products. Tanning beds, sun lamps or the sun itself promise to produce a healthy glow but instead cause aging of the skin. Exposure to ultraviolet radiation from any source is the leading cause of skin cancer.

Athletes

Athletes are highly susceptible to unsubstantiated claims for ergogenic aids as they attempt to gain a competitive edge. Ergogenics are substances or procedures that are reported to increase energy or otherwise enhance athletic performance. Athletes that already adhere to proper training, coaching and diet may look for an advantage by resorting to nutritional supplements. Nutritionally based ergogenic aids have increased in popularity with the ban of anabolic steroid use.

Other factors that have increased the popularity of ergogenic aids are:

1. Coaches, athletes and the public who have inadequate knowledge of sports nutrition. Athletes often take the advice of their coach, who may also be misinformed. Each athlete is different, and nutrition advice must be individualized.
2. Magazines constantly bombard us with nutrition information for athletes. Some of the more popular products include aspartic acid, bee pollen, brewer's yeast, choline, gelatin, ginseng, glycine, inosine, kelp, lecithin, protein supplements and wheat germ oil.

Some of the ways companies promote their product as worthwhile is by claiming it is university-tested when no research has been done and by using unauthorized endorsements by professional organizations. Little scientific evidence exists to support any performance-enhancing ability of these products. Some may also be harmful. Costs range from approximately $18 to $140 for a one-month supply.

Dietary Supplements

Americans spend billions of dollars per year on dietary supplements. For most healthy adults, supplements are an unnecessary expense. High doses of some supplements can be harmful. High-potency supplements can contain several times the Recommended Dietary Allowances (RDAs) and can function like a drug. Others, like vitamins A or D, can build up to toxic levels in the body.

The RDA is already set above the amount of vitamins and minerals we really need, so taking megadoses of them is not necessary. To arrive at the RDA, the Food and Nutrition Board of National Academy of Sciences–National Research Council first estimates the average daily requirement for each nutrient. People vary in their needs, so scientists increase the figures to account for the needs of people with high requirements.

The U.S. food supply provides an ideal source of nutrients. Eating a variety of food every day provides adequate nutrients for most people. Even if you do take a supplement, it should be just that, a supplement, not a substitute. A one-a-day multivitamin and mineral supplement that meets 100 percent of the RDA is adequate. Remember, pills do not provide a quick fix for a poor diet.

How Can You Protect Yourself?

Learn to protect yourself from questionable health products and services by being an informed consumer. Online service can be a reliable source for articles from consumer health publications and professional medical journals. But beware! Special bulletins or forums are not necessarily sources of accurate nutritional or medical advice. You do not know who is on the other line giving you advice. Question information that you see or read in advertisements. Question anyone selling products door to door or through the mail. Don't allow yourself to be rushed into buying. The following tips can help you evaluate questionable advertising and sales techniques:

- Does the seller promise immediate, effortless or guaranteed results?
- Does the advertisement contain words like "breakthrough," "miracle," "special" or "secret"? These are used to appeal to your emotions and are not scientific or medical words.
- Is the product or service a "secret remedy" or a recent discovery that can not be found anywhere else?
- Is the product recommended for stress, or being promoted as "natural," claiming it will help "detoxify," "revitalize" and "purify" your body?
- Does the manufacturer claim that the product is effective for a wide variety of ailments? The

broader the claims, the less likely they are to be true.
- Do the promoters offer testimonials or case histories of patients who have been "cured"?
- Are vitamin and mineral dose recommendations greater than the RDAs? Reliable sources will make only recommendations that are in line with the RDAs.
- Is the product being sold by a self-proclaimed "health advisor"? Insist on identification and professional credentials that are nationally accredited and recognized, such as a registered dietitian (RD) or a Master's degree in nutrition.
- Does the sponsor claim to have a cure for a disease (like arthritis or cancer) which is not yet understood by medical sources?
- Do the promoters use guilt or fear to sell the product?
- Does the advertisement claim Food and Drug Administration (FDA) approval? It is illegal to suggest FDA approval as a part of any marketing claim. However, all medical products sold across state lines must be registered with the FDA. Ask for the FDA proof of product listing if in doubt.
- Remember, if it sounds too good to be true, it probably is!

References

The following fact sheets are available from Colorado State University Cooperative Extension:

9.362, Nutrition for the Athlete.

9.363, Weight Loss Programs and Products.

9.364, Weight Loss Diets and Books.

9.368, Weight Management: It's All About You.

9.338, Food vs. Pills.

For further information and additional references, call Dr. Jennifer Anderson, Department of Food Science and Human Nutrition, Colorado State University, (970) 491-7334.

[1]J. Anderson, Colorado State University Cooperative Extension foods and nutrition specialist and professor; L. Patterson, graduate student intern; and B. Daly, undergraduate student food science and human nutrition.

Issued in furtherance of Cooperative Extension work, Acts of May 8 and June 30, 1914, in cooperation with the U.S. Department of Agriculture, Milan A. Rewerts, Director of Cooperative Extension, Colorado State University, Fort Collins, Colorado. Cooperative Extension programs are available to all without discrimination. No endorsement of products mentioned is intended nor is criticism implied of products not mentioned.

Yet Another Study—Should You Pay Attention?

How to know when to take health research news with a grain of salt

Hot Dogs Cause Cancer? Researchers Say Yes

New warnings revive fears about the danger of eating hot dogs, particularly among children

Study Links Hot Dogs, Cancer Ingestion by Children Boosts Leukemia Risk, Report Says

SO WENT headlines in the *Los Angeles Times,* the *New York Times,* and the *Washington Post* back in June of 1994. They came on the heels of three studies published simultaneously in a cancer research journal.

One of the studies found that children who eat more than 12 hot dogs a month have nine times the normal risk of developing childhood leukemia. The second suggested that children born to mothers who eat at least one frank a week during pregnancy have double the normal risk of developing brain tumors. The third traced brain tumors in children to *fathers* who ate hot dogs before conception. The risk of leukemia to children born of fathers who consumed hot dogs regularly was 11 times normal.

The problem: the three studies—and most certainly all the media commentary they attracted—were riddled with scientific holes.

To be sure, many of the reports in newspapers and other media outlets did point out weaknesses in the stud-

ies. But those weaknesses were strung between unnecessarily alarming headlines and warnings from researchers who, perhaps, had themselves experienced something of a knee-jerk reaction to the research. For instance, the concluding paragraph of the *New York Times* article leaves readers with this quoted advice about frankfurters from the former director of a cancer research center: "Reduce consumption of them as much as you can. They are a source of a possible cancer risk. I would not expose my children to it. It's like secondhand smoking."

Therein lies the difficulty at the heart of the matter. If scientists can't always look at research with a cool eye, how in the world are *you* supposed to? Following, **four questions to ask yourself as you read about study results or hear about them on the news.** They should help you put the latest reports into perspective as you try to make informed decisions about how to improve or maintain your lifestyle habits.

1 *What are the actual numbers as opposed to the relative numbers?* Let's say the hot dog research was airtight and children who eat franks more than a dozen times each month really are nine times (900 percent) more likely to get leukemia than children who eat them less often. The question is, how likely are children to develop leukemia to begin with?

They have a 0.3-in-1,000 chance. If you multiplied that number by nine to get the risk for children who have more than a dozen franks every month, the answer comes to roughly 2.5 in 1,000.

The point here is that even if something is many times more likely to happen under certain circumstances, that doesn't mean its potential influence is great enough to warrant changing the way you live your life.

Adding to the mathematical irrelevance of the findings is that there were only 17 children out of hundreds in the study who ate more than 12 franks each month—much too few to make any declarations about the dangers of hot dogs for the general population.

2 *What type of study was it?* There are three major types of human research—clinical trials, epidemiologic studies, and population-based intervention trials—and each has inherent strengths and limitations.

Clinical trials A clinical trial is an experiment conducted in a controlled setting, often a hospital, where researchers give a group of people treatment—such as a supplement, drug, or diet—and then measure their response.

Clinical trials are believed to yield very accurate results that can help establish cause-and-effect relationships between various substances or lifestyle activities and specific health outcomes. However, they tend to be conducted on restricted groups of people that include, for instance, just one age group, sex, or race. That allows the scientists to keep the study environment more "air-tight" so that variations within the population being studied don't confound the results. However, it means the results are not necessarily generalizable to all people. Clinical trials often need to be repeated in different groups with different genetic makeups and lifestyles before a recommendation for the general public can reliably be made.

Epidemiologic studies

Epidemiologic studies look at much larger groups of people than clinical trials—up to tens of thousands of subjects. These are not experiments in which researchers control a certain aspect of the subjects' lives but, rather, make *observations* of free-living populations in which they search for relationships between lifestyle or genetic factors and the risk for chronic diseases. Harvard University's Nurses' Health Study, which looks at the lifestyles of some 90,000 women, is an example of epidemiologic research.

Because epidemiologic research is generally conducted on large groups of people, the results tend to be more generalizable to the population at large. However, epidemiology virtually never proves cause and effect; it can only make *associations* on which other researchers might then decide to base a clinical trial to test whether "X" lifestyle actually leads to "Y" condition.

Granted, the more people in the study and the more tightly controlled it is for various lifestyle factors, the higher the chance that there really is something to any association found. But still, one can never automatically assume that an association proves a cause.

To show just how tenuous links brought to light in epidemiologic studies can be, scientists who published research on aspirin and heart disease in the prestigious journal *The Lancet* pointed out that according to one of their findings, people born under the signs of Gemini and Libra are likely to be harmed by taking aspirin rather than helped. If that piece of their research were serious science, the conclusion might be drawn by some that astrological influences directly affect health. The researchers highlighted the association specifically to point out the mistakes that could be made in viewing epidemiologic associations as fact.

Population-Based Intervention Trials Sort of a cross between an epidemiologic study and a clinical trial, a population-based intervention trial is a project in which large numbers of people live freely rather than in a controlled setting but are given either a treatment or a placebo and then observed to see whether a specific outcome occurs. A study of 29,000 male Finnish smokers that was released a few years ago, in which those who took beta-carotene turned out to be more likely to develop lung cancer than those who didn't, is an example of an intervention trial.

The strength of such studies is that, like epidemiologic research, they can observe thousands of people. The drawback is that they cannot be as well-controlled as clinical trials. Thus, it may not always be the treatment that's having the effect (or the full effect) but something in the subjects' lifestyles that the scientists didn't account for.

3 *Does the study stand alone, or are its results corroborated by other pieces of research?* A single study hardly ever tells the whole story. While the goal of the media is to turn a piece of research into news—or at least to make news sound exciting—the goal of scientists is to add *incrementally* to a body of knowledge. In fact, before a scientist makes a recommendation, there must be supportive evidence from a variety of approaches so that the strengths of all of them combined compensate for the weaknesses in any single one. Clinical and epidemiologic studies are not the only kinds of investigations necessary. There is also research conducted with tissue cultures and with laboratory animals—which often doesn't make the front page or the 6 o'clock news.

Consider the hot dog research. The scientists who conducted it commented that perhaps chemicals in hot dogs called nitrites cause leukemia. One way they could test that theory would be to "contaminate" normal cells in the laboratory with various doses of nitrites and see whether the cells mutated in such a way as to suggest that inside the body, the mutations would develop into leukemia.

They could also feed various doses of hot dogs—or of nitrites themselves—to laboratory animals and see if hot dog-nourished animals developed leukemia at a faster rate than those fed other meats. Cell culture studies and animal studies would also be necessary to help determine why hot dog-eating mothers raised their children's risk of developing brain cancer two-fold while hot dog-eating fathers raised the risk 11-fold. After all, for 9 months, a developing fetus is directly affected by everything its mother eats. Thus, without any clues to a plausible mechanism for how a father's frankfurter consumption could have so much more of an effect than a mother's, the numbers remain in the realm of fluke findings, and the hot dog hypothesis remains just that.

4 *Was the study published in a peer-reviewed journal?* Peer review is the process by which experts in a particular field review a study before it is accepted for publication in order to ensure that it was conducted appropriately. It is their express role to poke holes in the study's design or the researchers' interpretations. Only if they deem the study scientifically "clean" do the publication's editors print it. The journal in which the hot dog-leukemia research was published, *Cancer Causes and Control*, is not peer-reviewed. If it were, the research, riddled as it is with inconsistencies and faulty methodology, probably never would have made it into print.

Mini-Glossary of Research Terms

Placebo-controlled: If a clinical trial or population-based intervention trial is placebo-controlled, that means there is a group similar to the treatment group that is given a mock pill, or placebo. The effect on the placebo group allows researchers to tell whether the actual treatment is having an effect or whether it's just the fact that their subjects are being treated; sometimes just being given a "sugar pill" provides a psychological boost that yields beneficial results.

Double-blind: A double-blind trial is one in which neither the study participants nor the researchers heading the study know who is getting the real treatment and who is getting the placebo until the experiment is over. As a result, the subjects can't knowingly alter their lifestyles during the trial to make the treatment more or less effective, and the researchers are prevented from reading into findings in order to come up with "expected" results.

Prospective study: In a prospective epidemiologic study, scientists look at a group of people at a specific point (or points) in time and then wait to see who gets what diseases before making associations between lifestyle and risk of illness. Harvard's Nurses' Health Study is prospective.

Retrospective study: In a retrospective study, researchers compare people with a disease or other condition to a similar group of people who aren't affected and then look backwards in time to see what differences in their lifestyles might have contributed to the different outcomes in their health status. Some retrospective studies are designed better than others. In the retrospective study that looked at pregnant women's consumption of hot dogs, mothers with teenage children were asked to recall what they ate as many as 14 years ago. (Can you remember what you ate last week?)

The Mouse that Roared:

Health Scares on the Internet

The World Wide Web is a tremendous resource for consumers and others who want an additional outlet to help them take control of their health. "The Internet is full of important, even lifesaving, medical information," stated Randolph Wykoff, M.D., M.P.H., of the U.S. Food and Drug Administration (FDA). But, not all Internet information passes the test of the Hippocratic oath. Enter: Doctor Deception who now makes house calls.

On occasion, some not-so-sound information spoils a wealth of excellent information on the Internet. With a click of the mouse, a word-of-mouth phenomenon can be multiplied exponentially via the World Wide Web or electronic mail and result in questionable nutrition, food safety and health stories being sent directly to your computer. In the age of the Internet and instantaneous global communication—in tandem with an increasing interest in nutrition's relation to health—it is not surprising that anyone with a modem can send consumers and others into a food and health panic.

Most of us have heard at least a few of the following myths that have been started and perpetuated on the Web: the great kidney harvest caper; the antibacterial sponge made with agent orange; the fluorescent lights that leach vitamins from your body; the cancer-causing shampoo, and dozens, maybe hundreds more.

These would all be simply entertaining if everyone recognized them as practical jokes, the mantras of unhappy people, or simply misunderstandings given life on the Internet. But not everyone can recognize these tall tales as fiction.

The Bias Belt

Some of the most egregious myths come from legitimate sounding individuals who have fallen in love with their theories. They believe they are serving the public by warning them of dire health consequences as the result of touching, smelling, eating or drinking a perfectly safe product. Many consumers are confused and unwittingly oblige in the scam by forwarding the frightening electronic mail or referencing the site to family, friends and associates believing they are doing them a service. And, receiving one of these reports from a family member or friend adds to its alleged authenticity.

A recent *TIME Magazine* article (April 26, 1999) sums it up well: "The Web is praised as a wondrous educational tool, and in some respects it is. Mostly though, it appears to be a stunning advance in the shoring up of biases, both benign (one's own views) and noxious (other views)."

In most cases, there is no harm intended by those who position their opinions as facts. In other instances, the sly intent of the author may be relatively easy for health professionals, who have a strong science background, to detect. But, for some consumers with little frame of reference to tell fact from fiction, it can be misleading.

For example, an innocent Web surfer looking for information about dietary fats may stumble across one of several Web sites spreading fear and confusion about a frequently used cooking oil. With a masthead featuring a skull and crossbones, or the headline: "Canola Oil: Deadly for the Human Body!," such sites may cause baseless consumer concern. If the consumer does not seek unbiased information, he or she will miss the real story: canola oil, a safe, monounsaturated oil, can help lower blood cholesterol levels when substituted for saturated fats in the diet.

Where Did You Hear That?

"At one time, doctors were the primary source of health information for

From *Food Insight,* May/June 1999, pp. 1, 4-5. Reprinted with permission from the International Food Information Council Foundation.

consumers, but in the late 1990s the paradigm for securing this type of information changed," remarked Fergus Clydesdale, Ph.D., University of Massachusetts. Now, for both consumers and health professionals, the primary source of information is the news media. This information source replaces the traditional physician-patient relationship for consumers. For health professionals, media accounts now precede the medical journals and attendance at academic meetings. Often, a consumer first raises an issue with his or her health professional by asking about a story that ran in an on-line story, the local paper or on the evening TV news before health professionals have even received their journals.

A recent telephone survey conducted by Schwarz Pharma, Inc., and reported in the *American Journal of Public Health,* noted that approximately 29 percent of Americans have turned to the Internet for medical information—a number that, although not high compared to other media outlets, is likely to grow.

According to the *1997 Nutrition Trends Survey* conducted by The American Dietetic Association (ADA), 57 percent of consumers named television as their main source of nutrition information, followed by magazines at 44 percent and newspapers at 23 percent. Doctors and dietitians were at just 9 and 5 percent, respectively (see graph).

The same ADA survey, however, found that the tables were turned in terms of credibility. Information from doctors and dietitians/nutritionists was found to be "more valuable" (52%) than that from television news and newspaper articles (24% and 21%, respectively). The Internet may follow this same pattern of delivery versus credibility—the Internet or World Wide Web was found to be the least believable source of medical and health news according to respondents in the 1997 report, *Americans Talk About Science and Medical News* from the National Health Council. While the Internet can be a valuable source for scientifically accurate health information, it can also be a

frontier town with no sheriff for assuring the truth of the information presented.

John Renner, M.D., of the National Council for Reliable Health Information remarked, "There is a health information shock factor on the Internet because there is so much information, both good and bad, marvelous and terrible. We've moved from a small library of information with a friendly librarian, to a huge warehouse with lots of people offering information," he continued. Consumers have not faced this situation before. The problem is the public can be deceived—believing that because they have seen something on the Web, it must be true.

A perfect example of how the public can be misled is a recent Internet article by a Nancy Markle that has taken on a "cyberlife" of its own. The article alleges that aspartame (a sweetener found in food and beverages) causes lupus, multiple sclerosis (MS) and other diseases and conditions, none of which has any scientific validity. Highly respected health professional organizations were fraudulently associated with the story, and numerous vulnerable people were needlessly frightened by this scientifically false allegation.

One of the marvels of the Internet is that as easily as you can receive *inaccurate* information, you can search

for and find *accurate* information. If consumers were concerned about the alleged aspartame connection with MS, they could check the Multiple Sclerosis Foundation's Internet site for accurate information. David Squillacote, M.D., senior medical advisor of the MS Foundation wrote in his response to the Internet scare, "This series of allegations by Ms. Markle are almost totally without foundation. They are rabidly inaccurate and scandalously misinformative." Fortunately, numerous reliable organizations, Internet sites and publications have refuted this particular epidemic of hysteria and provided additional context for consumers.

The FDA's website is an excellent source for accurate information. Consumers wishing to counteract or confirm the aspartame story can find the following information from the FDA which could allay their fears: "After reviewing scientific studies, the FDA determined in 1981 that aspartame was safe for use in foods. . . . To date, the FDA has not determined any consistent pattern of symptoms that can be attributed to the use of aspartame, nor is the agency aware of any recent studies that clearly show safety problems."

What's a Cyber-Citizen to Do?

How can consumers judge the validity of information received via electronic

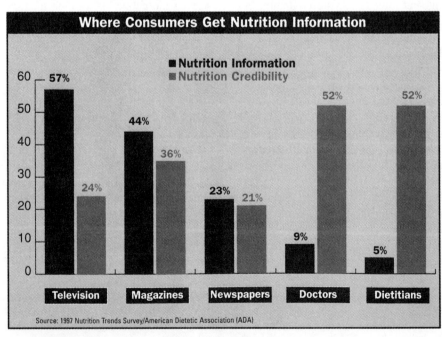

Where Consumers Get Nutrition Information

■ Nutrition Information
■ Nutrition Credibility

Television: 57%, 24%
Magazines: 44%, 36%
Newspapers: 23%, 21%
Doctors: 9%, 52%
Dietitians: 5%, 52%

Source: 1997 Nutrition Trends Survey/American Dietetic Association (ADA)

mail or popping up in a Web search? The foremost guideline for sorting the "trash" from the "treasure" is—just because something is printed on the Internet does not mean that it is true or credible.

Unfortunately for most of us, the best defense against nutrition misinformation and quackery on the Internet is in-depth scientific knowledge. Since not everyone has the level of scientific awareness or advanced degrees necessary to judge the validity of every story, the following tactics may be useful:

- Ask questions. Anecdotes and one individual's personal story are not scientific evidence.
- Look at the source of the information. A professional medical organization or government agency such as the American Academy of Family Physicians or the U.S. Department of Agriculture is more likely to have reliable information than an unknown person or group of people.
- If the story mentions a specific health condition, such as diabetes or breast cancer, search the Internet for reputable health professional organizations and foundations devoted to that disease. An example would be the American Diabetes Association or the American Cancer Society.
- Watch out for use of buzzwords like "conspiracy" and "poison."
- Don't take assertions at face value—give the other side of the issue the benefit of the doubt. Do your homework and call or e-mail appropriate health professional organizations to get a balanced picture.
- Consult with your doctor, a registered dietitian or other health professional.

The Internet has been a boon to consumers who want research and information on voluminous issues and topics at the tip of their fingers. It has also empowered many people to find health information to help them improve their well-being. Nevertheless, the ease of Web publishing has also given an unregulated forum to unreliable sources. Careful scrutiny and a healthy dose of skepticism are still necessary to determine what applies to you and what may need a second opinion.

Internet sources for sound nutrition and health information

- Tufts University Nutrition Navigator
  http://navigator.tufts.edu
- The American Dietetic Association
  http://www.eatright.org
- The International Food Information Council
  Foundation http://ificinfo.health.org
- Medline
  http://www.nlm.nih.gov/databases/freemedl.html
- National Institutes of Health
  http://www.nih.gov
- The U.S. Food and Drug Administration
  http://vm.cfsan.fda.gov
- Mayo Health Oasis (of the Mayo Clinic)
  http://www.mayohealth.org
- Johns Hopkins Health Information
  http://www.intelihealth.com/IH/ihtIH
- World Health Organization
  http://www.who.int
- Food & Agriculture Organization
  http://www.fao.org
- Government healthfinder
  http://www.healthfinder.gov

Herbals for Health?

by E. Serrano and J. Anderson[1]

[1]*E. Serrano, Colorado State University Cooperative Extension food and nutrition specialist, and J. Anderson, Cooperative Extension food and nutrition specialist and professor; food science and human nutrition.*

Quick Facts . . .

People take herbs for many reasons and many conditions.

Natural does not mean safe.

The Food and Drug Administration does not test herbs for safety or efficacy.

The best prescription for disease prevention is a healthy lifestyle.

Using herbs and plants for medicinal purposes has a long tradition. In India and China, these traditions date back thousands of years.

Once thought of as "traditional medicine" used by native or ancient cultures, herbal medicine has emerged as a popular alternative or supplement to modern medicine. According to the World Health Organization, 4 billion people, almost 70 percent of the world population, use herbal medicine for some aspect of primary health care.[1]

It is estimated that in the United States alone, botanical dietary supplements exceed $3 billion per year.[2] Herbal products can be found in grocery stores and on the Web, as well as natural food markets, their traditional source. Forty percent of Americans take dietary supplements. About half of these people take vitamin and mineral supplements, a third take some type of herbal product, and the rest take other ergogenic aids, such as amino acids or protein powders.[3] The herbal market is growing steadily at about 20 percent each year.[2] With this increase, however, come many questions.

The term herbs in this fact sheet refers to plants used for oral medicinal purposes, not herbs for cooking. It includes botanicals, herbs, herbals, herbal products, herbal medicines, herbal remedies and herbal supplements.

Why Take Herbs?

People take herbs for many reasons and many conditions. One of the biggest reasons is that herbs are considered natural and therefore healthier and gentler than conventional drugs. (Ironically, many prescription drugs are of herbal origin.) They are used for everything from upset stomachs to headaches. Some people take them for overall health and well-being, not for any specific condition. For others, herbal use is grounded in traditions passed down from generation to generation or recommended by folk healers.

Are Herbs Effective?

Many herbs have health benefits. Research has shown that echinacea cuts the length of colds and that powdered ginger is effective against motion sickness and nausea. Overall, however, research is lacking, especially well-controlled studies. There are many unanswered questions. At this point, our understanding is largely anecdotal. We don't know all of the short-term and long-term benefits and risks of many herbs, let alone all of their active or beneficial ingredients.

To address this uncertainty, federal law states that herbs cannot claim to *prevent, diagnose, treat,* or *cure* a condition or disease. Herbs may carry health-related claims about effects on the "structure or function of the body" or "general well-being" that may result from the product. This definition is very loose and gives rise to misleading health claims. Ultimately, the consumer is responsible for checking their validity and avoiding prod-

Reprinted with permission from Colorado State University Cooperative Extension, Fact Sheet 9.370, June 2000, *Nutrition Quackery,* J. Anderson, L. Patterson, and B. Daly, Dept. of Food Science and Human Nutrition. © 2000 by Colorado State University.

ucts with fraudulent claims. See fact sheet 9.350, *Nutrition Quackery.*

The best prescription for disease prevention is a healthy lifestyle. This includes a diet high in whole grains, fruits and vegetables, and low in fat. Physical activity also plays an important role. Finally, there is no data to suggest that herbs are more beneficial than conventional drugs for treating illnesses.

Are Herbs Safe?

Because herbs are natural, many people believe they are safe. Unfortunately, this is not always the case. While many herbs may be considered safe, some have hazardous side effects. In fact, in the past few years there have been several deaths related to herbal products. In some cases, small amounts of herbs, even those found in teas, have had devastating effects. To date, the following herbs are considered toxic and, given their side effects, should be avoided:[4,5]

- Chapparal—liver damage.
- Comfrey—liver damage.
- Ephedra/ma huang—rapid heart beat, heart attack.
- Germander—liver damage.
- Lobelia—breathing problems, rapid heartbeat, coma, death.
- Magnolia/stephania—kidney damage.
- Kombucha—linked to a possible death.
- Willow bark—Reye's syndrome in children.
- Wormwood—nerve damage, arm/leg numbness, delirium, paralysis.
- Yohimbe—anxiety, paralysis, gastro-intestinal problems, psychosis.

Herbs also may interact with prescription medications, over-the-counter drugs, vitamins and minerals. For example, ginkgo taken with aspirin may lead to spontaneous and/or excessive bleeding.[6] High doses of garlic may enhance the blood-thinning activities of anti-inflammatory medications and vitamin E.[6] Proceed cautiously. Herbs are not tightly regulated like drugs

If you do take herbs:

- *Follow the instructions on the label.*
- *If any unusual side effects arise, discontinue immediately.*

and other medications, even though they often are used for similar purposes. Advise your doctor, pharmacist and other health professionals of all herbs you are taking.

Medical professionals suggest taking herbs for only short periods. It is unclear if short-term benefits continue over a longer time or if long-term herb use could actually be detrimental to health. Follow the instructions on the label. If any unusual side effects

Medical professionals suggest taking herbs for only short periods. Do not take them in place of medical treatment or conventional medicine for chronic conditions or diseases. They are not recommended for people with certain medical conditions nor for children under 6.

arise, discontinue immediately. In addition, herbs are not recommended in place of medical treatment or conventional medicine for chronic conditions or diseases, such as severe depression, diabetes, hypertension and heart disease. Herbs also are not recommended for people who may be immuno-compromised, such as the elderly or those with HIV; people with kidney damage or liver disease; anyone who may be undergoing surgery or other invasive procedures; and pregnant or lactating women. Herbal products also are not recommended for children under 6.

How Are Herbs Regulated?

If herbs can be unsafe, why are they so readily available? This is because herbal products—like vitamin and mineral supplements—are classified by the U.S. Food and Drug Administration (FDA) as dietary

supplements, not drugs. As a result, they are not tested for safety or efficacy. Thus herbal products can be marketed at any time, without scientific research and without approval from the FDA. Drug companies, on the other hand, must conduct clinical studies to determine the effectiveness of the drugs, safety, possible interactions with other substances, and appropriate dosages. The FDA must review the data and authorize the drug's use before the product may be marketed. The FDA can take regulatory action on an herbal product only after it has received a sufficient number of reports of ill effects and can show the product is unsafe. At this point, the FDA can recommend the product be withdrawn from the market and/or labeled to reflect potential side effects. This system of regulation is always after the fact, not before.

Moreover, herbs—unlike drugs—are not standardized. When you buy a drug, even an over-the-counter one, you know that each capsule contains the same amount of active ingredient. Drug companies have to follow strict quality-control measures. Herb companies do not. Doses differ between herb capsules and from product to product. The active ingredients also vary depending on the plant part (flower, root, seeds, nuts, bark, branch), plant form (dried, extract, tincture, tea) and plant species. An independent test by *Consumer Lab* in early 2000 found that nearly a quarter of the 30 brands of ginkgo biloba they tested did not have the expected levels of active ingredients. Furthermore, every single product that failed their test claimed it was standardized.

The herbal industry is taking steps to address standardization. Much work is still needed. Currently, if manufacturers follow certain protocols for extracting or drying herbs, they can include USP (for the United States Pharmaceopia) or NF (for Natural Formulary) on their label. It does not ensure that doses are the same from one bottle to another, or that the product is safe. It does attempt to eliminate huge differences. The most rigorous stamp of approval is from

Table 1: Top ten most commonly used herbs.

Common name, source	Main uses	Apparent efficacy	Possible side effects	Comments
Echinacea (*Echinacea angustifolia*)	• Reduce duration of colds. • Boost immune system. • Heal wounds.	+ + +	• Minor GI symptoms, chills, short-term fever reaction, nausea and vomiting (uncommon and mild). • Allergic reactions (especially people allergic to the daisy/aster family).	
Evening primrose oil (*Oenothera biennis*)	• Reduce menopausal symptoms, sore breasts. • Treat allergic skin rash. • Prevent heart disease. • Treat rheumatoid arthritis, Raynaud's.	+/– +/– + +/–	• Headaches, GI distress at high doses.	• Clinical evidence of its safety is inconclusive. • Good source of cis-gamma-linolenic acid (GLA). • Anticoagulant, so may enhance effect of blood thinners.
Feverfew *Tanacetum parthenium*)	• Reduce migraines, headaches. • Treat arthritis.	+ +/–	• Mouth ulcers, inflamed mouth tissues from chewing leaf. • GI discomfort and dry mouth.	• Do not take with blood thinners—may inhibit platelet activity.
Garlic (*Allium sativum*)	• Prevent heart disease. • Lower high blood cholesterol. • Lower high blood pressure. • Improve blood clotting disorders. • Prevent cancer. • Used as antibiotic, antibacterial, antiviral.	+ + + + +/– +/–	• Breath and skin odor. • Possible nausea, heartburn, dizziness. • Topical garlic can cause skin irritation, blistering and burns.	• Fresh garlic is the best form. • Garlic contains allin and allicin. • If consuming high doses of garlic, do not take blood-thinning drugs, ginkgo or high-dose Vitamin E.
Ginger (*Zingiber officinale*)	• Improve motion sickness. • Reduce nausea. • Used as digestive aid.	+ + +	• No side effects observed at recommended dosages.	• People with gallstones should not take ginger without consulting a doctor.
Ginkgo biloba (*Ginkgo biloba*)	• Improve memory in Alzheimer's patients. • Improve blood flow. • Used as antioxidant.	+/– +/– +	• Allergic skin reaction. • Headaches. • Seed ingestion dangerous. • GI upset (rare).	• Do not take with other blood-thinning drugs or high doses of garlic or Vitamin E.
Ginseng (*Panax ginseng*)	• Improve fatigue. • Enhance physical performance. • Reduce stress.	+ – +/–	• Side effects rare. • Menstrual abnormalities, breast tenderness. • Insomnia.	• Not recommended for people with high blood pressure, hypoglycemia. • Do not take with stimulants, including excessive caffeine.
Kava kava (*Piper methysticum*)	• Lower anxiety, tension, restlessness. • Enhance sleep.	+ +	• Mild GI disturbances. • Red eyes, puffy face, muscle weakness. • Extended continuous intake can result in temporary yellow discoloration of skin, hair, nails. • Enlarged pupils. • Rare allergic skin reactions.	• Not recommended for depressed people. • Do not drive or operate machinery when taking kava kava. • Do not take with alcohol, other barbituates.
St. John's wort (*Hypericum perforatum*)	Internally: • Treat depression. • Improve premenstrual depression. • Treat seasonal affective disorder (SAD). Externally: • Used for wounds (inflammation), muscle aches, first-degree burns.	 + – +/– +	• Photosensitivity, especially in fair-skinned people. • May cause allergic reaction.	• Not recommended for severe or chronic depression. • May enhance effects of MAO inhibitors. • Do not take with anti-depressants or alcohol.
Saw palmetto *Serenoa repens*)	• Treat benign prostatic hyperplasia. • Improve overall prostate health. • Enhance sexual vigor, enhance breast size.	+ +/– –	• GI disturbances, headaches (rare). +/• Large amounts may cause diarrhea.	

+ Research supports efficacy/safety of this product when used appropriately. See disclaimer below.

+/– Clinical evidence is inconclusive.

– Research finds that it is ineffective/unsafe.

Except where noted in comments, research indicates these 10 herbs appear to be safe *when used appropriately*.

Disclaimer: What we know about herbs is constantly changing, so take any herb with caution. Herbs generally are not recommended for people suffering from autoimmune disorders or liver disease, people undergoing surgery or other invasive medical procedure, pregnant or lactating women, or infants and small children. Use herbs only for minor conditions and only for the short-term. Discontinue if you experience any adverse side effects.

the newly formed *Consumer Lab* (CL). CL conducts independent tests of products for identity and potency (proper labeling), purity (any contaminants), and consistency (the same identity, potency and purity from one batch to the next). Products that pass their tests are listed on CL's Web site.

Summary

The herb industry is growing. More herbs are available than ever before, and Americans are embracing their use. To date, however, herbs have not been well studied and are not well understood. Until we have a clearer picture, consumers must become informed in order to protect themselves from questionable health products and services. Here are some tips to do so:

- Determine whether you really need an herbal supplement.
- Be an informed consumer. Research the product to determine: safety, validity of claims, dosage, most effective form, plant part, species, how long to use it, side effects, any counterindications with other supplements or medications, and reasonable price.

- Inform your doctor, pharmacist and other health care professionals of any herbs you are considering or that you routinely use. Consult them with any questions.
- Pick brands that have been tested for consistency in dosage by looking for the USP or NF symbols.
- Read the product label and follow the instructions.
- Use herbal products only for minor conditions and only for the short-term. If a condition is serious or chronic, consult your doctor.
- Discontinue herbs if you experience *any* adverse side effects.
- Avoid herbal therapies if you suffer from certain conditions or under certain circumstances. (See Are Herbs Safe?, above.)
- Do not take herbal products known to be toxic. The list in this fact sheet may not include all potentially toxic herbs, so regularly check the resources listed in this fact sheet for additional toxic herbs.

Resources

The following are reliable resources for information on herbs and other dietary supplements:

Foster S., Tyler V.: Honest Herbal *(4th edition), Binghamton, N.Y., The Haworth Press, Inc. 1999*

Stephen Barrett, Quackwatch: *www.quackwatch.com.*

Healthcare Reality Check: www.hcrc.org/index.html.

Consumer Lab: www.consumerlab.com.

References

1. *Abramov, V. Traditional Medicine. N 134, 1–3. 1996. World Health Organization.*
2. *The U.S. Food and Drug Administration, Center for Food Safety and Applied Nutrition. Economic Characterization of the Dietary Supplement Industry Final Report. 1999.*
3. *Industry Overview.* Nutrition Business Journal. *1999, 4:1–5.*
4. *Foster S., Tyler V.:* Honest Herbal *(4th edition), Binghamton, N.Y., The Haworth Press, Inc. 1999.*
5. *SupplementWatch: www.supplementwatch. com. 2000.*
6. Herbal Medicine: Expanded Commission E Monographs. *Blumenthal, M., Goldberg, A., Brinckmann, J., eds. American Botanical Council. 2000.*

Issued in furtherance of Cooperative Extension work, Acts of May 8 and June 30, 1914, in cooperation with the U.S. Department of Agriculture, Milan A. Rewerts, Director of Cooperative Extension, Colorado State University, Fort Collins, Colorado. Cooperative Extension programs are available to all without discrimination. No endorsement of products mentioned is intended nor is criticism implied of products not mentioned.

Nutrition Supplements: Science vs Hype

In Brief: Aggressive marketing has led millions of recreational and elite athletes to use nutrition supplements in hopes of improving performance. Unfortunately, these aids can be costly and potentially harmful, and the advertised ergogenic gains are often based on little or no scientific evidence. No benefits have been convincingly demonstrated for amino acids, L-carnitine, L-tryptophan, or chromium picolinate. Creatine, beta-hydroxy-beta-methylbutyrate, and dehydroepiandrosterone (DHEA) may confer ergogenic or anabolic effects. Chromium picolinate and DHEA have adverse side effects, and the safety of the other products remains in question.

Thomas D. Armsey Jr, MD; Gary A. Green, MD

Nutrition supplements are a lucrative business in the United States. According to the Council for Responsible Nutrition,[1] the retail sale of dietary supplements generated $3.3 billion in 1990, and revenues increase each year. This enormous expenditure is largely the result of aggressive advertising aimed at high school, college, and recreational athletes, all eager for anabolic-steroid-like gains through dietary aids. Riding the crest of the fitness wave, nutrition supplements appeal to millions of consumers willing to pay billions of dollars for alleged benefits that are too good to be true.

Unfortunately, these supplements are subject to little regulation by the US Food and Drug Administration (FDA). Advertised claims to the contrary, many supplements have not been subjected to the scientific scrutiny required of prescription drugs. Furthermore, given the size and continued growth of the supplement industry, the FDA will probably never

be able to monitor its products effectively. The resulting lack of regulation can lead to unscrupulous advertising, impurities in manufacturing, and potentially dangerous reactions among supplement users.

Such potential outcomes obligate physicians to learn about current nutrition supplements so they can educate patients about the effects and risks of supplement use. Team physicians in particular can advise athletes, coaches, and administrators in these matters. Competing with slick advertisements and exaggerated claims can be difficult, but by using recent scientific research on commonly used supplements, their mechanisms of action, and possible adverse reactions, physicians can offer sound recommendations to patients who are either users or interested in trying these aids.

Creatine Monohydrate

Creatine, or methylguanidine-acetic acid, is an amino acid that was first identified in 1835 by Chevreul. It is synthesized from arginine and gly-

cine in the liver, pancreas, and kidneys and is also available in meats and fish.[2] Creatine was first introduced as a potential ergogenic aid in 1993 as creatine monohydrate and is currently being used extensively by athletes throughout the United States. A National Collegiate Athletic Association (NCAA) study, publication pending, revealed that 13% of intercollegiate athletes have used creatine monohydrate in the past 12 months (Frank Uryasz, personal communication, February 1997).

According to current theory, creatine supplementation increases the bioavailability of phosphocreatine (PCr) in skeletal muscle cells. This increase is thought to enhance muscle performance in two ways. First, more available PCr allows faster resynthesis of adenosine triphosphate (ATP) to provide energy for brief, high-intensity exercise, like sprinting, jumping, or weight lifting. Second, PCr buffers the intracellular hydrogen ions associated with lactate production and muscle fatigue during exercise. Therefore, creatine supplementation may provide an ergogenic effect by increasing the force of muscular contraction and prolonging anaerobic exercise.[3]

Numerous well-designed studies have demonstrated that creatine supplementation has an ergogenic potential. Greenhaff et al[4] showed that 5-day oral dosages of 20 g/day increased muscle creatine availability by 20% and significantly accelerated PCr regeneration after intense muscle contraction. Birch et al[5] and Harris et al,[6] in laboratory and field studies, demonstrated significant performance enhancement in male athletes, in both brief, high-intensity work and total time to exhaustion, using creatine supplementation of 20 to 30 g/day.

Recent data reveal that the mean creatine concentration in human skeletal muscle is 125 mmole/kg-dm (dry muscle), with a normal range between 90 and 160 mmole/kg-dm.[7] This wide spectrum of creatine concentration may explain why some of the published studies have not demonstrated significant ergogenic effects. In a study by Greenhaff,[7] approximately half of the tested athletic subjects exhibited concentrations lower than 125 mmole/kg-dm, with strict vegetarians substantially lower. These individuals exhibited the most significant increases in muscle creatine concentration, PCr regeneration, and performance enhancement with the use of creatine. On the other hand, athletes with elevated baseline levels of creatine showed little or no ergogenic effect when tested after ingesting creatine.

While creatine use has skyrocketed, no serious side effects have been scientifically verified in subjects using relatively brief (less than 4 weeks) creatine regimens. However, there are anecdotal reports of a dramatic increase in muscle cramping associated with the use of creatine monohydrate (J. Kinderknecht, MD, personal communication, June 1996). Future research will, we hope, clarify whether these adverse reactions are caused by creatine supplementation.

Chromium Picolinate

Chromium is an essential trace mineral present in various foods, such as mushrooms, prunes, nuts, whole grain breads, and cereals.[8] A normal American diet contains 50% to 60% of the recommended daily allowance (RDA) of chromium. It has an extremely low gastrointestinal absorption rate, so supplement manufacturers have bound chromium with picolinate (CrPic) to increase the absorption and bioavailability.

Chromium supplementation became popular after it was found that exercise increases chromium loss, raising the concern that chromium deficiency may be common among athletes[9]. Chromium seems to function as a co-factor that enhances the action of insulin, especially in carbohydrate, fat, and protein metabolism. Promoters of CrPic claim it increases glycogen synthesis, improves glucose tolerance and lipid profiles, and increases amino acid incorporation in muscle.

CrPic supplementation gained scientific credence in the early 1980s when researchers demonstrated anabolic-steroid-like effects with dosages of 200 micrograms/day. Evans[10,11] and Hasten et al[12] demonstrated a decreased percentage of body fat and increased lean mass among college athletes and students who took CrPic supplements and performed resistance exercise training. However, critical analysis of these studies reveals that imprecise measurement techniques, rather than CrPic supplementation, may account for these "ergogenic" results. More recent studies by Clancy et al[13] and Hallmark et al[14], using more precise measurement techniques, failed to demonstrate any significant improvement in percent body fat, lean body mass, or strength.

Most studies of CrPic supplementation reveal no side effects except gastrointestinal intolerance with dosages of 50 to 200 micrograms/day for less than 1 month. However, anecdotal reports of serious adverse

effects, including anemia,[15] cognitive impairment,[16] chromosome damage,[17] and interstitial nephritis[18] have been reported with CrPic ingestion in increased dosages and/or durations. Therefore, the use of chromium picolinate supplementation as an ergogenic aid should be strongly discouraged and considered potentially dangerous.

Amino Acids

Amino acids are the basic structural units of proteins, and one might expect that the more amino acids ingested, the greater the potential for building skeletal muscle. According to the 1989 RDA, an average adult must ingest 0.8 g/kg lean body mass/day of protein in order to fulfill the body's protein requirements. Athletes, however, have traditionally been assumed to need significantly more protein than the average individual, so they commonly use various protein supplements.

Theories suggest that increasing the bioavailability of amino acids promotes protein synthesis and attenuates the muscle loss that occurs during both strength and endurance exercise. These theories have gained support through scientific experimentation in protein metabolism. Fern et al[19] and Lemon et al[20] demonstrated that strength trainers increased protein synthesis with substantially increased protein ingestion during 4 weeks of resistance training. By tracking the nitrogen balance of these athletes, a new daily protein requirement (1.4 to 1.8 g/kg lean mass/day) was developed for strength athletes.

Amino acid supplementation also plays a role in endurance athletes. Lemon[21] and Gontzen et al[22] demonstrated that endurance athletes who train at moderate intensity (55% to 65% of VO[2] max) and high intensity (80% of VO[2] max) for more than 100 minutes significantly increase protein breakdown unless their protein intake equals 1.2 to 1.4 g/kg lean mass/day.

Several factors make the amount of amino acids that athletes need less clear. Although all of the cited studies demonstrate the advisability of protein intakes higher than the current RDA, no well-designed study has yet shown that amino acid supplementation enhances performance. In addition, no scientific evidence supports protein supplementation in dosages greater than 2 g/kg lean mass/day. Finally, the improved conditioning that occurs over a 4- to 8-week training period may decrease protein breakdown, which may result in a maintenance protein requirement much closer to the current RDA.

L-Carnitine

Carnitine is a quaternary amine whose physiologically active form is beta-hydroxy-gamma-trimethylammonium butyrate. This is found in meats and dairy products and is synthesized in the human liver and kidneys from two essential amino acids, lysine and methionine. L-carnitine is thought to be ergogenic in two ways. First, by increasing free fatty acid transport across mitochondrial membranes, carnitine may increase fatty acid oxidation and utilization for energy, thus sparing muscle glycogen. Second, by buffering pyruvate, and thus reducing muscle lactate accumulation associated with fatigue, carnitine may prolong exercise.

Early studies by Gorostiaga et al,[23] Wyss et al[24]), and Natalie et al[25] indirectly demonstrated an ergogenic effect of this compound. These studies showed a decreased respiratory exchange ratio (RER) with L-carnitine supplementation (2 to 6 g/day) during exercise, suggesting that fatty acids rather than carbohydrates were used for energy. However, these studies had several problems in methodology, including the use of the RER as the sole measure of enhanced fatty acid oxidation. The RER is an indirect measure of lipid utilization that is influenced by many factors, such as preexercise

diet, fitness level, and exercise intensity and duration.[26] These confounders were not controlled and may have influenced the results.

A more controlled study by Vuchovich et al[27] avoided these problems by directly measuring muscle glycogen and lactate levels through biopsy and serum analysis. This study failed to demonstrate any glycogen-sparing effect or reductions in lactate levels while supplementing with 6 g/day of L-carnitine. Furthermore, no study to date has confirmed performance enhancement with carnitine supplementation. Finally, many currently available supplements actually contain D-carnitine, which is physiologically inactive in humans but may cause significant muscle weakness through mechanisms that deplete L-carnitine in tissues. Therefore, carnitine should not be advocated as an ergogenic supplement.

L-Tryptophan

L-tryptophan, an essential amino acid, is not commercially available in its pure form but is found in many combination supplement products and reportedly remedies insomnia, depression, anxiety, and premenstrual tension.[28] Athletes in the past decade have taken L-tryptophan because of its advertised ergogenic effects. The theoretical mechanism for these effects is an increase in serotonin levels in the brain; these increases produce analgesia and reduce the discomfort of prolonged muscular effort, thereby delaying fatigue. This theoretical model gained scientific credence in 1988 when Segura and Ventura[29] demonstrated a 49% increase in total exercise time to exhaustion when subjects ingested a total of 1.2 g of L-tryptophan (four 300-mg doses within 24 hours of exercise) vs placebo. Such a profound improvement in performance is difficult to imagine, and these results have never been replicated. Two larger, well-designed studies by Seltzer et al[30] and Stensrud et al[31] failed to demonstrate any improvement in subjective

or obective outcome measures when supplementing with 1.2 g of L-tryptophan vs placebo. The results of these two studies are more consistent with current research data on exercise.

Physicians should be aware of two other developments that argue against supplementing with L-tryptophan. Its use has declined among elite athletes, possibly suggesting that they are recognizing its minimal ergogenic effects. More important, L-tryptophan ingestion was linked to multiple cases of eosinophilia myalgia syndrome and 32 deaths.[28] Though these cases were probably due to contamination of L-tryptophan produced by one Japanese manufacturer, and not to the amino acid itself, they illustrate the quality and purity questions regarding unregulated supplements.

Beta-Hydroxy-Beta-Methylbutyrate

One of the most recent additions to the nutrition supplement market is beta-hydroxy-beta-methylbutyrate (HMB). It is a metabolite of the essential branched-chain amino acid leucine and is produced in small amounts endogenously. HMB is also found in catfish, citrus fruits, and breast milk. In the early 1980s, researchers at Iowa State University hypothesized that HMB was the bioactive component in leucine metabolism that regulates protein metabolism. The exact mechanism of this process is unknown, but promoters hypothesize that HMB regulates the enzymes responsible for protein breakdown. They propose that high HMB levels decrease protein catabolism, thereby creating a net anabolic effect.

Research in livestock[32–36] and humans seems to suggest that supplementation with HMB may increase muscle mass and strength. Nissen conducted two randomized, double-blind, placebo-controlled studies[37,38] to evaluate the ergogenic potential of HMB in exercising men. In the first study, 41 untrained subjects

Table 1. Daily Dose Costs of Various Nutrition Supplements Used by Athletes.

Creatine

- 20–30 g/day (loading dose): $7.20/day for one week
- 10–15 g/day (maintenance dose): $3.60/day

Chromium
200 mg/day: $0.43/day

L-Carnitine
2.0 g/day: $2.67/day

Beta-Hydroxy-Beta-Methylbutrate

- 13 g/day: $3.48/day
- 11.5 g/day: $1.74/day

Dehydroepiandrosterone

- 150 mg/day: $0.67/day
- 1100 mg/day: $1.34/day

L-Tryptophan
Currently unavailable in pure form due to federal regulation

Sources: National Supplement Association and General Nutrition Centers

participated in a 4-week resistance training program. The subjects, whose diets were controlled, were given either HMB supplements of 1.5 or 3 g/day or a placebo. Those receiving HMB supplements showed significant improvements in muscle mass and strength as well as significant decreases in muscle breakdown products (3-methylhistidine and creatine phosphokinase) when compared with placebo subjects. The second study evaluated trained and untrained male subjects in a similarly designed weight training program. Relative to a placebo group, the subjects supplementing with 3 g/day demonstrated significant increases in muscle mass and one-repetition maximum bench press as well as decreases in percent body fat.

Further studies of HMB may continue to support the supplement's anabolic effects and elucidate its role in protein metabolism. No side effects of HMB supplementation have been reported, but the safety of this agent is still unknown. Therefore, it is premature to recommend its use as a safe and effective ergogenic aid.

Dehydroepiandrosterone

Attention focused on dehydroepiandrosterone (DHEA) in 1996 when the FDA banned its sale and distribution for therapeutic uses until its safety and value could be reviewed. The ensuing media attention popularized this supplement, and manufacturers began selling it as a nutritional aid rather than a therapeutic drug.

DHEA was identified in 1934 as an androgen produced in the adrenal glands. It is a precursor to the endogenous production of both androgens and estrogens in primates.[39] It is also available in wild yams, which are sold in many health food stores as a source of DHEA. As a precursor to androgenic steroids, DHEA may increase the production of testosterone and provide an anabolic steroid effect. Promoters claim that this compound slows the aging process and accordingly advertise it as the "fountain of youth."

Only a few randomized, double-blind, placebo-controlled studies on the effects of DHEA supplementation have been published. Two have demonstrated significant increases in androgenic steroid plasma levels, along with subjective improvements in physical and psychological well-being, while supplementing with 50 mg/day for 6 months[40] or 100 mg/day for up to 12 months.[41] Whether DHEA has any effect on body composition or fat distribution is still unclear. Its effect on healthy individuals younger than 40 years old is also virtually unstudied.

DHEA users have reported few adverse effects from the supplement, but one is irreversible virilization in women, including hair loss, hirsutism, and voice deepening.[42] In addition, men have reported irreversible gynecomastia, which may result from an elevation in estrogen levels. Because this supplement is so new, long-term adverse effects are unknown. Unlike most other nutrition supplements, DHEA may substantially increase the risk of uterine and prostate cancer that accompanies prolonged elevation in the levels of unopposed estrogen and testosterone. Therefore, the safety of this supplement must be questioned.

Of particular interest to competitive athletes is the effect that DHEA supplementation may have on the test used by the International Olympic Committee and NCAA in their screening for exogenous testosterone use. Using DHEA could alter the testosterone-epitestosterone ratio so it exceeds the 6:1 limit set by both groups (personal communication, Don Catlin, MD, 1997); thus DHEA

Table 2. Protein Supplements Cost Comparison: Daily Cost of 2 g Protein/kg for a 70-kg Individual

Brand name protein powder: $9.80/day
($0.07/g protein)
Generic Protein Powder: $2.80/day ($0.02/g protein)
Tuna: $2.80/day ($0.02/g protein)

Source: National Supplement Association

users could risk disqualification from international competition.

Given the lack of evidence that DHEA enhances athletic performance and its potentially devastating adverse effects, DHEA supplementation is not recommended.

Purity, Cost, and Final Thoughts

Although some of the supplements discussed here may have benefits, physicians should remain skeptical about the use of any supplement. The purity of agents available to consumers is in doubt, as we have seen with L-tryptophan. *The Medical Letter,* for example, analyzed several commercial preparations of melatonin and found unidentifiable impurities in four of six samples.[43] The supplements used for the research reported in this review were pure, but consumers in the largely unregulated marketplace cannot be assured of that same purity in the products they buy.

There is also the issue of cost (tables 1 and 2). At current rates, doses of the supplements discussed range as high as $7.20/day, the cost of a loading dose of creatine (20 to 30 g/day). It makes little sense to invest in supplements that offer minimal or no benefit, especially for athletic departments in this era of shrinking budgets.

The key word in nutrition supplements is nutrition. NCAA guidelines state that "there are no shortcuts to sound nutrition, and the use of suspected or advertised ergogenic aids may be detrimental and will, in most instances, provide no competitive advantage.[44]" Physicians need to educate athletes, parents, coaches, trainers, and athletic administrators in sound dietary practices or see to it that a nutrition professional does so. Then nutrition supplements can be put in proper perspective, and decisions regarding their use can be based on proper scientific study and proven benefit to the individual.

References

1. Cowart VS: Dietary supplements: alternatives to anabolic steroids? Phys Sportsmed 1992;20(3):189–198
2. Walker JB: Creatine: biosynthesis, regulation and function. Adv Enzymol Relat Areas Mol Med 1979;50:177–242
3. Maughan RJ: Creatine supplementation and exercise performance. Int J Sport Nutr 1995;5(2):94–101
4. Greenhaff PL, Bodin K, Soderlund K, et al: The effect of oral creatine supplementation on skeletal muscle phosphocreatine resynthesis. Am J Physiol 1994;266(5 pt 1):E725–E730
5. Birch R, Noble D, Greenhaff GL: The influence of dietary creatine supplementation on performance during repeated bouts of maximal isokinetic cycling in man. Eur J Appl Phys 1994;69(3):268–276
6. Harris RC, Soderlund K, Hultman E: Elevation of creatine in resting and exercised muscle of normal subjects by creatine supplementation. Clin Sci 1992;83(3):367–374
7. Greenhaff PL: Creatine and its application as an ergogenic aid. Int J Sport Nutr 1995;5(suppl):S100–S110
8. Clarkson PM: Do athletes require mineral supplements? Sports Med Digest 1994;16(4):1–3
9. Campbell WW, Anderson RA: Effects of aerobic exercise and training on trace minerals chromium, zinc, and copper. Sports Med 1987;4(1):9–18
10. Evans GW: The role of picolinic acid in metal metabolism. Life Chem Reports 1982;1:57–67
11. Evans GW: The effect of chromium picolinate on insulin controlled parameters in humans. Int J Biosocial Med 1989;11:163–180
12. Hasten DL, Rome EP, Franks ED, et al: Effects of chromium picolinate on beginning weight training students. Int J Sport Nutr 1994;2(4):343–350
13. Clancy SP, Clarkson PM, DeCheke ME, et al: Effects of chromium picolinate supplementation on body composition, strength, and urinary chromium loss in football players. Int J Sport Nutr 1994;4(2):142–153
14. Hallmark MA, Reynolds TH, DeSouza CA, et al: Effects of chromium and resistive training on muscle strength and body composition. Med Sci Sports Exerc 1996;28(1):139–144
15. Lefavi RG: Sizing up a few supplements. Phys Sportsmed 1992;20(3):190–191
16. Huszonek J: Over-the-counter chromium picolinate. [Letter] Am J Psychiatry 1993;150(10):1560–1561
17. Stearns DM, Wise JP, Patierno SR, et al: Chromium picolinate produces chromosome damage in Chinese hamster ovary cells. FASEB 1995;9(15):1643–1648
18. Wasser WG, Feldman NS: Chronic renal failure after ingestion of over-the-counter chromium picolinate. [Letter] Ann Int Med 1997;126(5):410
19. Fern EB, Bielinski RN, Schultz Y: Effects of exaggerated amino acid and protein supply in man. Experimentia 1991;47(2):168–172
20. Lemon PW, Tarnopolsky MA, MacDougall JD, et al: Protein requirements, muscle mass/strength changes during intensive training in novice bodybuilders. J Appl Physiol 1992;73(2):767–775
21. Lemon PW: Effect of exercise on protein requirements. J Sports Sci 1991;9 (special):53–70
22. Gontzen I, Sutzecu P, Dumitrache S: The influence of muscular activity on the nitrogen balance and on the need of man for proteins. Nutr Rep Int 1974;10:35–43
23. Gorostiaga EM, Maurer CA, Eclache JP: Decrease in respiratory quotient during exercise following L-carnitine supplementation. Int J Sports Med 1989;10(3):169–174
24. Wyss V, Ganzit GP, Rienzi A: Effects of L-carnitine administration on VO^2 max and the aerobic-anaerobic threshold in normoxia and acute hypoxia. Eur J Appl Physiol 1990;60(1):1–6
25. Natalie A, Santoro D, Brandi LS, et al: Effects of acute hypercarnitinemia during increased fatty substrate oxidation in man. Metabolism 1993;42(5):594–600
26. Krogh A, Lindhard J: The relative value of fat and carbohydrate as sources of muscular energy. Biochem J 1920;14(July):290–363
27. Vuchovich MD, Costill DL, Fink WJ: Carnitine supplementation: effect on muscle carnitine and glycogen content during exercise. Med Sci Sports Exerc 1994;26(9):1122–1129
28. Teman AJ, Hainline B: Eosinophilia-myalgia syndrome. Phys Sportsmed 1991;19(2):81–86

29. Segura R, Ventura JL: Effect of L-tryptophan supplementation on exercise performance. Int J Sports Med 1988; 9(5):301–305

30. Seltzer S, Stoch R, Marcus R, et al: Alterations of human pain thresholds by nutritional manipulation of L-tryptophan supplementation. Pain 1982;13(4):385–393

31. Stensrud T, Ingjer F, Holm H, et al: L-tryptophan supplementation does not improve running performance. Int J Sports Med 1992;13(6):481–485

32. Gatnau R, Zimmerman DR, Nissen SL, et al: Effect of excess dietary leucine and leucine catabolites on growth and immune response in weanling pigs. J Animal Sci 1995;73(1):159–165

33. Nissen SL, Fuller JC, Sell J, et al: The effect of β-hydroxy β-methylbutyrate on growth, mortality, and carcass qualities of broiler chickens. Poultry Sci 1994; 73(1): 137–155

34. Nissen SL, Morrical D, Fuller JC: The effects of the leucine catabolite β-hydroxy β-methylbutyrate on the growth and health of growing lambs. J Animal Sci 1992; 77(suppl 1):243

35. Ostaszewski P, Kostiuk S, Balasinska B, et al: The effect of the leucine metabolite β-hydroxy β-methylbutyrate (HMB) on muscle protein synthesis and protein breakdown in chick and rat muscle. J Animal Sci 1996;74(suppl):138

36. Van Koevering MT, Dolezal HG, Gill DR, et al: Effects of β-hydroxy β-methylbutyrate on performance and carcass quality of feedlot steers. J Anim Sci 1994;72(8): 1927–1935

37. Nissen SL, Sharp R, Ray M, et al: The effect of the leucine metabolite beta-hydroxy beta-methylbutyrate on muscle metabolism during resistance-exercise training. J Appl Physiol 1996;81(5):2095–2104

38. Nissen SL, Panton J, Wilhelm R, et al: The effect of beta-hydroxy beta-methylbutyrate (HMB) supplementation on strength and body composition of trained and untrained males undergoing intense resistance training. FASEB J 1996;10(3): A287

39. Hardman JG, Limdird LE (eds): Goodman and Gillman's The Pharmacologic Basis of Therapeutics, ed 9. New York City, McGraw-Hill, 1996, p 1413

40. Morales AJ, Nolan JJ, Nelson JC, et al: Effects of replacement dose dehydroepiandrosterone in men and women of advancing age. J Clin Endocrinol Metab 1994; 78(6):1360–1367

41. Yen SS, Morales AJ, Khorram O: Replacement of DHEA in aging men and women: potential remedial effects. Ann NY Acad Sci 1995;774(Dec 29):128–142

42. Abramowicz M (ed): Dehydroepiandrosterone (DHEA). The Medical Letter On Drugs and Therapeutics 1996;38(985):91–92

43. Abramowicz M (ed): Melatonin. The Medical Letter On Drugs and Therapeutics 1995;37(962):111–112

44. Benson MT (ed): NCAA Sports Medicine Handbook 1994–95, ed 7. Overland Park, Kansas, National Collegiate Athletic Association, 1994, p 30

Dr. Armsey is a clinical instructor and sports medicine fellow, and Dr. Green is a clinical associate professor in the Department of Family Medicine at the University of California, Los Angeles, Medical Center. Address correspondence to Gary A. Green, MD, University of California, Los Angeles, Medical Center, Box 951683, Los Angeles, CA 90095-1683; e-mail to *ggreen@fammed.medsch.ucla. edu.*

soy: Health Claims for Soy Protein, Questions About Other Components

By John Henkel

Vegetarians and health enthusiasts have known for years that foods rich in soy protein offer a good alternative to meat, poultry, and other animal-based products. As consumers have pursued healthier lifestyles in recent years, consumption of soy foods has risen steadily, bolstered by scientific studies showing health benefits from these products. Last October, the Food and Drug Administration gave food manufacturers permission to put labels on products high in soy protein indicating that these foods may help lower heart disease risk.

As with health claims for oat bran and other foods before it, this health claim provides consumers with solid scientific information about the benefits of soy protein and helps them make informed choices to create a "heart healthy" diet. Health claims encourage food manufacturers to make more healthful products. With soy, food manufacturers have responded with a cornucopia of soy-based wares. (See box, "The Soy Health Claim.")

No sooner had FDA proposed the health claim regulation, however, than concerns arose about certain components in soy products, particularly isoflavones. Resulting questions have engulfed the regulation in controversy.

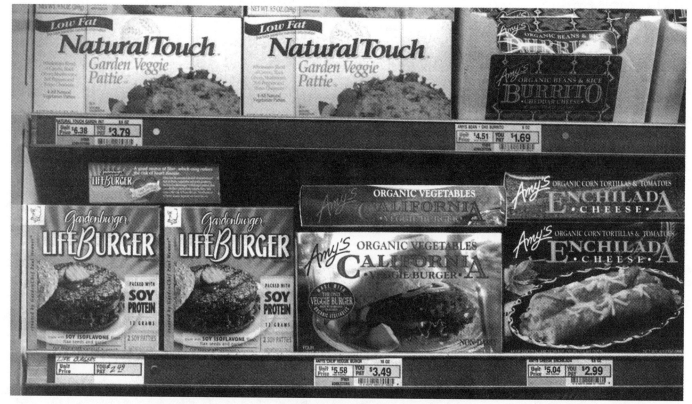

PHOTOGRAPHS BY NORMAN WATKINS

Mainstream grocery stores now offer soy foods such as "burgers" alongside meat or dairy-based products, making it convenient to find foods with soy protein.

From *FDA Consumer,* May/June 2000, pp.13-17. Reprinted by permission of *FDA Consumer,* the magazine of the U.S. Food and Drug Administration.

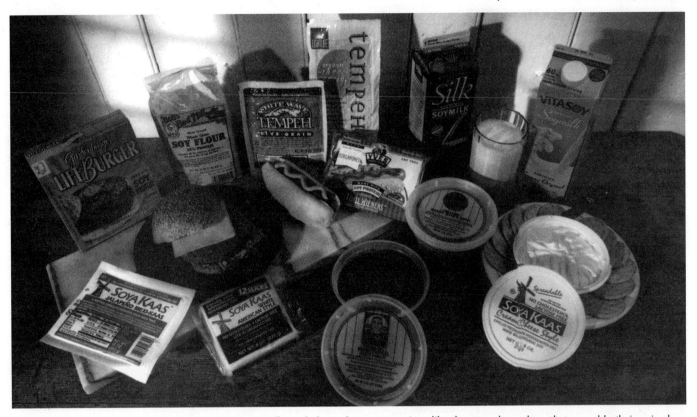

Many traditional foods such as hamburgers, hot dogs, milk, and cheese have soy versions like the ones shown here that resemble their animal-based counterparts in appearance and taste. Most of these foods qualify to carry the FDA-approved health claim for soy.

This came as no surprise to Elizabeth A. Yetley, Ph.D., lead scientist for nutrition at FDA's Center for Food Safety and Applied Nutrition (CFSAN). "Every dietary health claim that has ever been published has had controversy," she says, "even the relationship of saturated fat to a healthy diet."

While the controversy may seem confusing to the consumer giving it casual consideration, a careful review of the science behind the rule reveals a strict divide between what FDA allows as a health claim based on solid scientific research and related issues that go well beyond the approved statements about health benefits of soy protein.

What's known is that all foods, including soy, are complex collections of chemicals that can be beneficial for many people in many situations, but can be harmful to some people when used inappropriately. In that simple fact lies much of the scientific dilemma—when do data show a food is safe and when do they show there could be problems?

Scientists agree that foods rich in soy protein can have considerable value

Many traditional foods such as hamburgers, hot dogs, milk, and cheese have soy versions like the ones shown here that resemble their animal-based counterparts in appearance and taste. Most of these foods qualify to carry the FDA-approved health claim for soy.

to heart health, a fact backed by dozens of controlled clinical studies. A year-long review of the available human studies in 1999 prompted FDA to allow a health claim on food labels stating that a daily diet containing 25 grams

of soy protein, also low in saturated fat and cholesterol, may reduce the risk of heart disease.

"Soy by itself is not a magic food," says Christine Lewis, acting director of CFSAN's Office of Nutritional Products, Labeling and Dietary Supplements. "But rather it is an example of the different kinds of foods that together in a complete diet can have a positive effect on health."

Much of the research to date has examined dietary soy in the form of whole foods such as tofu, "soymilk," or as soy protein added to foods, and the public health community mostly concurs that these whole foods can be worthwhile additions to a healthy diet. The recently raised concerns, however, focus on specific components of soy, such as the soy isoflavones daidzein and genistein, not the whole food or intact soy protein. These chemicals, available over the counter in pills and powders, are often advertised as dietary supplements for use by women to help lessen menopausal symptoms such as hot flashes.

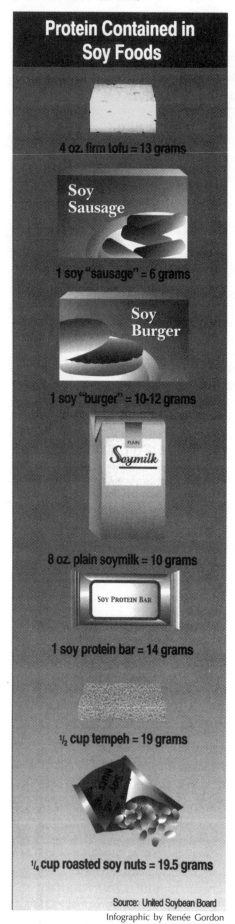

Protein Contained in Soy Foods

4 oz. firm tofu = 13 grams

Soy Sausage

1 soy "sausage" = 6 grams

Soy Burger

1 soy "burger" = 10-12 grams

PLAIN Soymilk

8 oz. plain soymilk = 10 grams

SOY PROTEIN BAR

1 soy protein bar = 14 grams

½ cup tempeh = 19 grams

¼ cup roasted soy nuts = 19.5 grams

Source: United Soybean Board

Infographic by Renée Gordon

The problem, researchers say, is that isoflavones are phytoestrogens, a weak form of estrogen that could have a drug-like effect in the body. This may be pronounced in postmenopausal women, and some studies suggest that high isoflavone levels might increase the risk of cancer, particularly breast cancer. Research data, however, are far from conclusive, and some studies show just the opposite—that under some conditions, soy may help *prevent* breast cancer. It is this scientific conundrum, where evidence simultaneously points to benefits and possible risks, that is causing some researchers to urge caution.

Unlike the controversy surrounding soy isoflavones, available evidence on soy protein benefits is much clearer. That's why FDA limited its health claim to foods containing intact soy protein. The claim does not extend to isolated substances from soy protein such as the isoflavones genistein and daidzein.

"The story's not all in yet," says Margo Woods, D.Sc., associate professor of medicine at Tufts University, who has studied soy's effects in post-menopausal women. "There's a lot of emerging data and it's confusing. In the meantime, we should be cautious." She says her concerns are centered mainly on isoflavone supplements and that she's "much more comfortable" recommending soy as a whole food. "There are probably hundreds of protective compounds in soy [foods]. It's just too big a leap to assume that a pill could do the same thing."

Daniel Sheehan, Ph.D., director of the Estrogen Knowledge Base Program at FDA's National Center for Toxicological Research, also urges caution in consumption of soy isoflavones. In formal comments submitted to the public record of his own agency while FDA was reviewing the health claim, Sheehan, along with colleague Daniel Doerge, Ph.D., wrote, "While isoflavones may have beneficial effects at some ages or circumstances, this cannot be assumed to be true at all ages. Isoflavones are like other estrogens in that they are two-

edged swords, conferring both benefits and risks."

As a science-based agency, FDA recognizes that research information evolves with time and that some of the existing confusion will be resolved as new studies are completed. "We continue to monitor the ongoing science," Yetley says. "As new data warrants, we make adjustments in our position and the advice we give to the public. We take this responsibility very seriously."

Soy Benefits

Soy protein products can be good substitutes for animal products because, unlike some other beans, soy offers a "complete" protein profile. Soybeans contain all the amino acids essential to human nutrition, which must be supplied in the diet because they cannot be synthesized by the human body. Soy protein products can replace animal-based foods—which also have complete proteins but tend to contain more fat, especially saturated fat—without requiring major adjustments elsewhere in the diet.

While foreign cultures, especially Asians, have used soy extensively for centuries, mainstream America has been slow to move dietary soy beyond a niche market status. In the United States, soybean is a huge cash crop, but the product is used largely as livestock feed.

With the increased emphasis on healthy diets, that may be changing. Sales of soy products are up and are projected to increase, due in part, say industry officials, to the FDA-approved health claim. "We've seen this before with other claims FDA has approved," says Brian Sansoni, senior manager for public policy at the Grocery Manufacturers of America. "It brings attention to products; there are newspaper and TV stories and information on the Internet."

To qualify for the health claim, foods must contain at least 6.25 grams of soy protein per serving and fit other criteria, such as being low in fat, cholesterol, and sodium. The claim is similar to others the agency

Adding *Soy Protein* To The Diet

For consumers interested in increasing soy protein consumption to help reduce their risk of heart disease, health experts say they need not completely eliminate animal-based products such as meat, poultry, and dairy foods to reap soy's benefits. While soy protein's direct effects on cholesterol levels are well documented, replacing some animal protein with soy protein is a valuable way to lower fat intake. "If individuals begin to substitute soy products, for example, soy burgers, for foods high in saturated fat, such as hamburgers, there would be the added advantage of replacing saturated fat and cholesterol [in] the diet," says Alice Lichtenstein, D.Sc., professor of nutrition at Tufts University. Whole soy foods also are a good source of fiber, B vitamins, calcium, and omega-3 essential fatty acids, all important food components.

The American Heart Association recommends that soy products be used in a diet that includes fruits, vegetables, whole grains, low-fat dairy products, poultry, fish, and lean meats. The AHA also emphasizes that a diet to effectively lower cholesterol should consist of no more than 30 percent of total daily calories from fat and no more than 10 percent of calories from saturated fat.

Nowadays, a huge variety of soy foods is on shelves not only in health food stores, but increasingly in mainstream grocery stores. As the number of soy-based products grows, it becomes increasingly easy for consumers to add enough soy to their daily diets to meet the 25-gram amount that FDA says is beneficial to heart health. According to soybean industry figures, the numbers add up quickly when you look at the protein contained in typical soy foods. For example:

- Four ounces of firm tofu contains 13 grams of soy protein.
- One soy "sausage" link provides 6 grams of protein.
- One soy "burger" includes 10 to 12 grams of protein.
- An 8-ounce glass of plain soymilk contains 10 grams of protein.
- One soy protein bar delivers 14 grams of protein.
- One-half cup of tempeh provides 19 grams of protein.
- And a quarter cup of roasted soy nuts contains 19.5 grams of soy protein.

Though some consumers may try soy products here and there, it takes a sustained effort to eat enough to reach the beneficial daily intake. This is especially true for those who have elevated cholesterol levels. "Dietary interventions that can lower cholesterol are important tools for physicians," says Antonio Gotto, M.D., professor of medicine at Cornell University, "particularly since diet is usually prescribed before medication and is continued after drug therapy is begun." He emphasizes

that in order to succeed, such diets must have enough variety that patients don't get bored and lapse back into old eating habits. He says his experience with patients suggests that it's important to learn how to "sneak" soy into the diet painlessly.

"People think it's challenging to get a high concentration of soy into your diet," says chef and cookbook author Dana Jacobi. "But it's actually easy to consume 25 grams [of soy protein], once you realize what a wide range of soy products is available." For those new to soy, she recommends what she calls "good-tasting" soy foods such as smoothies, muffins made with soy flour, protein bars, and soy nuts.

The American Dietetic Association recommends introducing soy slowly by adding small amounts to the daily diet or mixing into existing foods. Then, once the taste and texture have become familiar, add more.

Because some soy products have a mild or even neutral flavor, it's possible to add soy to dishes and barely know it's there. Soy flour can be used to thicken sauces and gravies. Soymilk can be added to baked goods and desserts. And tofu takes on the flavor of whatever it is cooked in, making it suitable for stews and stir-fries. "Cook it with strong flavors such as garlic, crushed red pepper, or ginger," says Amy Lanou, a New York-based nutritionist. "One of my favorites is tofu sautéed with a spicy barbecue sauce." She also suggests commercial forms of baked tofu, which she says has a "cheese-like texture and a mild, but delicious, flavor." For soy "newbies," she also recommends trying a high-quality restaurant that really knows how to prepare soy dishes—just to see how professionals handle soy.

Soy chefs and nutritionists suggest the following further possibilities for adding soy to the diet:

- Include soy-based beverages, muffins, sausages, yogurt, or cream cheese at breakfast.
- Use soy deli meats, soy nut butter (similar to peanut butter), or soy cheese to make sandwiches.
- Top pizzas with soy cheese, pepperoni, sausages, or "crumbles" (similar to ground beef).
- Grill soy hot dogs, burgers, marinated tempeh, and baked tofu.
- Cube and stir fry tofu or tempeh and add to a salad.
- Pour soymilk on cereal and use it in cooking or to make "smoothies."
- Order soy-based dishes such as spicy bean curd and miso soup at Asian restaurants.
- Eat roasted soy nuts or a soy protein bar for a snack.

—J.H.

has approved in recent years to indicate heart benefits, including claims for the cholesterol-lowering effects of soluble fiber in oat bran and psyllium seeds.

FDA determined that diets with four daily soy servings can reduce levels of low-density lipoproteins (LDLs), the so-called "bad cholesterol" that builds up in blood vessels, by as much as 10 percent. This number is significant because heart experts generally agree that a 1 percent drop in total cholesterol can equal a 2 percent drop in heart disease risk. Heart disease kills more Americans than any other illness. Disorders of the heart and blood vessels, including

stroke, cause nearly 1 million deaths yearly.

FDA allowed the health claim for soy protein in response to a petition by Protein Technologies International Inc., a leading soy producer that tracks its origins to soybean studies sponsored by Henry Ford in the early 1930s. The company was acquired by

E.I. du Pont de Nemours & Company (DuPont) in 1997. In considering the petition, FDA reviewed data from 27 clinical studies submitted in the petition, as well as comments submitted to the public record and studies identified by FDA. The available research consistently showed that regular soy protein consumption lowered cholesterol to varying degrees.

One of the studies, conducted over nine weeks at Wake Forest University Baptist Medical Center and reported in the *Archives of Internal Medicine* in 1999, found that soy protein can reduce plasma concentrations of total and LDL cholesterol but does not adversely affect levels of HDL, or "good" cholesterol, which at high levels has been associated with a reduction in heart disease risk. Another often-quoted study, published in the *New England Journal of Medicine* in 1995, examined 38 separate studies and concluded that soy protein can prompt "significant reductions" not only in total and LDL cholesterol, but also in triglycerides, another fat linked to health problems when present at elevated levels.

Other studies hint that soy may have benefits beyond fostering a healthy heart. At the Third International Symposium on the Role of Soy in Preventing and Treating Chronic Disease, held in late 1999, researchers presented data linking soy consumption to a reduced risk of several illnesses. Disorders as diverse as osteoporosis, prostate cancer, and colon cancer are under investigation.

Soy's Many Faces

Though soy may seem like a new and different kind of food for many Americans, it actually is found in a number of products already widely consumed. For example, soybean oil accounts for 79 percent of the edible fats used annually in the United States, according to the United Soybean Board. A glance at the ingredients for commercial mayonnaises, margarines, salad dressings, or vegetable shortenings often reveals soybean oil high on the list.

The *Soy* Health Claim

In October 1999, FDA approved a health claim that can be used on labels of soy-based foods to tout their heart-healthy benefits. The agency reviewed research from 27 studies that showed soy protein's value in lowering levels of total cholesterol and low-density lipoprotein (LDL, or "bad" cholesterol).

Food marketers can now use the following claim, or a reasonable variation, on their products: "Diets low in saturated fat and cholesterol that include 25 grams of soy protein a day may reduce the risk of heart disease. One serving of (name of food) provides __ grams of soy protein." To qualify for the claim foods must contain per serving:

- 6.25 grams of soy protein
- low fat (less than 3 grams)
- low saturated fat (less than 1 gram)
- low cholesterol (less than 20 milligrams)
- sodium value of less than 480 milligrams for individual foods, less than 720 milligrams if considered a main dish, and less than 960 milligrams if considered a meal.

Foods made with the whole soybean, such as tofu, may qualify for the claim if they have no fat other than that naturally present in the whole bean. —*J.H.*

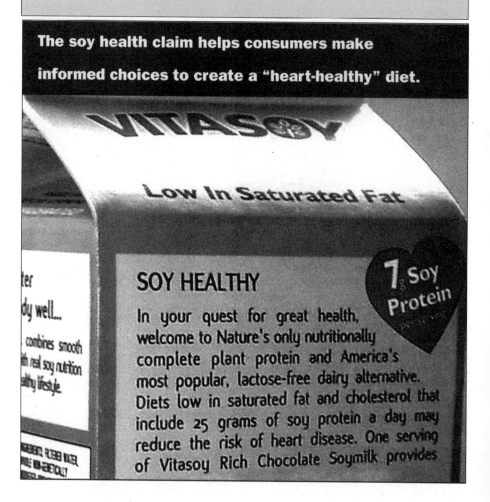

The soy health claim helps consumers make informed choices to create a "heart-healthy" diet.

But the health claim only covers the form that includes soy protein. This form can be incorporated into the diet in a variety of ways to help reach the daily intake of 25 grams of soy protein considered beneficial.

While not every form of the following foods will qualify for the health claim, these are some of the most common sources of soy protein:

Tofu is made from cooked puréed soybeans processed into a custard-like cake. It has a neutral flavor and can be stir-fried, mixed into "smoothies," or blended into a cream cheese texture for use in dips or as a cheese substitute. It comes in firm, soft and silken textures.

Isoflavones are a weak form of estrogen that could have a drug-like effect in the body.

"Soymilk," the name some marketers use for a soy beverage, is produced by grinding dehulled soybeans and mixing them with water to form a milk-like liquid. It can be consumed as a beverage or used in recipes as a substitute for cow's milk. Soymilk, sometimes fortified with calcium, comes plain or in flavors such as vanilla, chocolate and coffee. For lactose-intolerant individuals, it can be a good replacement for dairy products.

Soy flour is created by grinding roasted soybeans into a fine powder. The flour adds protein to baked goods, and, because it adds moisture, it can be used as an egg substitute in these products. It also can be found in cereals, pancake mixes, frozen desserts, and other common foods.

Textured soy protein is made from defatted soy flour, which is compressed and dehydrated. It can be used as a meat substitute or as filler in dishes such as meatloaf.

Tempeh is made from whole, cooked soybeans formed into a chewy cake and used as a meat substitute.

Miso is a fermented soybean paste used for seasoning and in soup stock.

Soy protein also is found in many "meat analog" products, such as soy sausages, burgers, franks, and cold cuts, as well as soy yogurts and cheese, all of which are intended as substitutes for their animal-based counterparts.

Since not all foods that contain soy ingredients will meet the required conditions for the health claim, consumers should check the labels of products to identify those most appro-

Soy For More Information

These organizations have further background on soybean products, as well as recipes and dietary tips:

American Soybean Association
Suite 100
12125 Woodcrest Executive Drive
St. Louis, MO 63141
1-800-688-7692
http://www.amsoy.org/

Soyfoods Association of North America
1723 U St., N.W.
Washington, DC 20009
(202) 986-5600

United Soybean Board
424 Second Ave. West
Seattle, WA 98119
1-800-TALK-SOY
(1-800-825-5769)
http://www.talksoy.com/
http://www.soyfoods.com/

priate for a heart-healthy diet. Make sure the products contain enough soy protein to make a meaningful contribution to the total daily diet without being high in saturated fat and other unhealthy substances.

Are Consumers Warming Up to Soy?

Although it's clear that Americans are increasing their consumption of soy products, the soybean has a long way to go before it becomes a staple in the average pantry. According to a 1999 survey by the United Soybean Board, two-thirds of consumers surveyed believe soy products are "healthy," up from 59 percent in 1997. While the public may think it's good for them, only 15 percent eat a soy product once a week.

The reason for the disparity appears to be a problem of perception. "Americans are not prepared to make massive lifestyle changes in order to

get healthy foods into their diet," says chef and soy cookbook author Dana Jacobi. "Many people have negative attitudes toward soy products due to their misconception of, or their experiences with, taste and texture. But in fact, there are so many ways to work soy into your diet."(See box, "Adding Soy Protein to the Diet.")

Industry figures show that in some cases, the popularity of soy foods is increasing dramatically. For example, in 1998, sales of soymilk grew 53 percent in mainstream supermarkets and 24 percent in health food stores over the previous year, according to data from Spence Information Services, a San Francisco sales tracking firm. Another research firm, HealthFocus, reports that 10 percent of shoppers in 1998, versus 3 percent in 1996, said they are eating more soy specifically because they believe it will reduce their risk of disease.

Soybeans contain amino acids that must be supplied in the diet because they cannot be synthesized by the human body.

According to the Soyfoods Association of North America, three factors are responsible for driving soy's upward trend:

- Baby boomers are more enlightened about, and more interested in, longevity and good health than previous generations.

- The double-digit growth in Asian populations in the United States has fueled demand for traditional soy foods. Americans also are eating more Asian foods, which often include soy.

- Young people are choosing more plant-based foods. A food industry survey found that 97 percent of colleges and universities now offer meatless entrées on their menus.

Mainstream grocery stores also have been prominently displaying soy products amid traditional foods. Soy-based burgers and sausages are often found in the freezer case next to other meats. Some stores offer refrigerated soymilk alongside cow's milk products. And it's not unusual to see tofu, along with soy cheese and cold cuts, in a store's fresh fruit and veggie department. "We expanded our line of soy products in the produce section even before [FDA approved] the health claim," says Paulette Thompson, nutritionist for Giant Food, a large East Coast grocery chain. "But soy is still rather mysterious to many consumers, so it's important to educate them." She says her company is offering information about soy in its Sunday newspaper supplements and its quarterly consumer magazine. It also plans a special "healthy products" promotion that will trumpet the benefits of soy and other diet components.

For consumers reluctant to try soy foods because they fear a bad taste, food manufacturers are creating new lines of soy-based products that contain enough soy to meet the claim requirement but are developed specifically to taste good. "Soy's major stumbling block has been its taste, real or perceived," says Meghan Parkhurst, spokeswoman for Kellogg Co. She says the company plans to introduce in several western states a granola-like soy cereal that got high marks for taste in consumer trials.

Examining the Controversy

While the existing scientific data strongly support the value of increasing soy protein as described in the health claim, questions have been raised about individual components of soy, especially when consumed as concentrated supplements by some segments of the population.

"FDA continues to monitor the debates about the relative safety of these individual soy components, and

Recent concerns focus on specific soy components such as isoflavones, not whole foods.

the scientific research that will eventually resolve them," says the Center for Food Safety and Applied Nutrition's Lewis. "If new results suggest an increased risk, the agency will modify or refine its policies in light of the new information."

A number of studies already are under way or in the planning stages now. In one study, Barry Delclos, Ph.D., a researcher at FDA's National Center for Toxicological Research (NCTR), is overseeing a long-term, multigeneration study in rats of the soy component genistein. Early data using rats suggest that genistein alone may prompt undesirable effects such as the growth of breast tissue in males. The study will analyze the relationship between dosage and any adverse outcomes.

The National Institutes of Health is sponsoring a long-term follow-up study on the safety of soy infant formula. The study is a "longitudinal retrospective epidemiological" assessment, in which young adults who consumed soy formula as infants will be compared with young adults who consumed milk-based formulas as infants. They will be evaluated for any adverse effects from infancy into their childbearing years.

NCTR's Sheehan says research is needed in this area because an earlier study, published in 1997 in the medical journal *The Lancet,* showed that infants consuming soy formula had five to 10 times higher levels of isoflavones in their blood serum than women receiving soy supplements who show menstrual cycle disturbances. He says these levels may cause toxicological effects. "Infants receive higher doses of soy and isoflavones than anybody because it is their only food and they are consuming it all the time." The American Academy

of Pediatrics, however, has published guidelines showing that in some cases, soy protein-based formulas "are appropriate for use in infants" when cow's milk cannot be tolerated.

Sheehan also expresses concern about the effects soy may have on the function of the thyroid gland. Animal study results, some of which date back to 1959, link soy isoflavones to possible thyroid disorders, such as goiter. A 1997 study in *Biochemical Pharmacology* identified genistein and daidzein as inhibitors of thyroid peroxidase, which data suggest may prompt goiter and autoimmune disorders of the thyroid. Critics of these studies suggest that iodine deficiency may be a factor that needs to be considered when evaluating study results.

Though the research community has varying degrees of concern about a possible "dark side" to soy consumption, one thread runs consistently through its messages: the need for more research for new uses of soy components. The health claim, however, focuses on uses of soy protein that are generally accepted among health professionals as useful for heart-healthy diets.

Sales of soy foods probably will continue to rise steadily for the foreseeable future, says Sansoni of the Grocery Manufacturers of America. "We're seeing a 'buzz' with soy products that intrigues people and they want to try them," he says. "But I don't believe soy is a fad. It's a continuing trend that's here for the long haul."

With the rising interest, the health claim for soy protein appears to have succeeded. It has provided specific guidelines to help the public improve the heart-healthiness of its diet and has stimulated the industry to produce new food products high in soy protein. These trends, in the end, should be good for those trying to lower their risk of heart disease.

John Henkel is a member of FDA's public affairs staff.

Food for Thought about Dietary Supplements

The surge of public interest in nutrition supplements has been fired by the recently enacted federal regulations governing health claims, which permits the health food industry to make claims about the function of nutrients not permitted for food products. This article provides healthy skepticism about the common rationales for the use of supplements.

PAUL R. THOMAS, Ed.D. R.D..

Paul Thomas, currently a Fellow at the Georgetown Center for Food and Nutrition Policy, Georgetown University, previously served as a staff scientist for the Food and Nutrition Board, Institute of Medicine, National Academy of Sciences. He is a registered dietitian who received an Ed.D. degree in nutrition education from Columbia University. He is an author and editor of several books on contemporary nutrition issues. Correspondence can be directed to him at the Georgetown Center for Food and Nutrition Policy, 3240 Prospect Street, N.W., Washington, DC 20007.

The dietary supplements industry is very healthy. Sales of vitamins, minerals, and other food concentrates are roughly $4 billion per year. Although at least one quarter of American adults swallow these pills, powders, and potions daily,[1] probably the majority of us take them at least occasionally. What are we getting in return?

I've asked myself this question since the 1960s when, as a teenager, I began taking dozens of supplements after reading about their magical powers in *Prevention* and *Let's Live* magazines, and books by

> **The Food and Nutrition Board recommends that those who choose supplements limit the dose to levels of the RDA or less.**

Adelle Davis. Surely they would help cure my adolescent acne; I just needed to find the right combination. But my pizza face only improved when I took tetracycline and topical retinoic acid (the drug, not the vitamin) prescribed by a dermatologist. Growing out of adolescence also helped.

My education about dietary supplements became more comprehensive when I discovered the medical library during my college education as a biology ("pre-med") major. I learned that the hype surrounding

them in the popular press was rarely supported by studies in the journals. Dietary supplements have benefited me in that they developed my interest in nutrition to the point where I chose to make a career in this discipline. But over time, and despite the growing popularity of supplements even among nutrition professionals, I have gone from being an enthusiastic vitamin promoter to a skeptic.

Most of us would agree that it's best to meet our nutritional needs with food, which means that everyone should eat a healthy, balanced diet. I believe that, short of that, dietary supplements are at best a poor and inadequate substitute. Supplements are appropriate for some people for specific purposes. But should they be taken every day, by everybody? I don't think so, and I make my case with the following eight points.

POINT 1: NO EXPERT BODY OF NUTRITION EXPERTS RECOMMENDS THE ROUTINE USE OF SUPPLEMENTS

A small number of nutritionists support regular supplement use. But no scientific body of nutrition experts recommends that everyone take supplements on a routine basis as dietary insurance or for optimal health. Expert bodies are by nature conservative and unlikely to recommend a practice until the evidence is convincing and perhaps even overwhelming. That's the point, since dietary guidance for most people should be based on strong evidence.

In 1989, the Food and Nutrition Board of the National Academy of Sciences issued a comprehensive review of the relationships between diet and health.[2] The report stated that dietary supplements should be avoided at levels above the Recommended Dietary Allowances (RDAs). Finally, however, a group of nutrition experts was not warning people to stay away from supplements with pronouncements of dire risks from their use. The recommendation was not to stay away from supplements, but to take them in no more than RDA amounts. The Food and Nutrition Board acknowledged that the long-term potential risks and benefits of supplements had not been adequately studied and called for more research.

> ## Some proponents feel that supplements are "magic bullets" for cancer, heart disease, and other maladies.

The latest pronouncements on supplements are found in the new (4th) edition of *Dietary Guidelines for Americans,* which was released in January.[3] The report states that "diets that meet RDAs are almost certain to ensure intake of enough essential nutrients by most healthy people," and that people with average requirements are likely to have adequate diets even if they don't meet RDAs.

About supplements, the report states: "Daily vitamin and mineral supplements at or below the Recommended Dietary Allowances are considered safe, but are usually not needed by people who eat the variety of foods depicted in the Food Guide Pyramid." It acknowledged, however, that some people might benefit from supplements. These include older people and others with little exposure to sunlight who may need extra vitamin D. Women of childbearing age might reduce the risk of neural-tube defects in their infants with folate-rich foods or folic acid supplements. Pregnant women usually benefit from iron supplements. And vegans, who avoid animal products, might need some nutrients in pill form. The report urges the public not to rely on supplements.

Surveys show that most supplementers take a one-a-day multiple-vitamin-mineral product. But some take large doses of single nutrients or nutrient combinations as self-prescribed medication for disease or to try to reach a more optimal state of health, the latter fueled most recently by the enthusiasm for antioxidants. The practices of these aggressive supplementers merit some concern.

POINT 2: NUTRITION IS ONLY ONE FACTOR THAT INFLUENCES HEALTH, WELL-BEING, AND RESISTANCE TO DISEASE

The major chronic diseases that prematurely maim and kill most Americans have multiple causes. However, just as the advent of antibiotics and vaccines led many to think that the cure of diseases awaited specific "magic bullets," some proponents of supplements seem to think that these products are nutritional magic bullets for cancer, heart disease, and other maladies.

Health reporter Jane Brody calls us "a nation hungry for simple nutritional solutions to complex health problems."[4] Edward Golub, in his recent book, *The Limits of Medicine,* warns us against "thinking in penicillin mode."[5] It can be easy to do in

> ## Supplements are not the answer to health and disease for the vast majority of people.

nutrition because the first identified nutrient-related diseases (*eg,* scurvy and beriberi) were caused by dietary deficiencies. Anyone who doesn't get enough of the proper nutrient will eventually succumb to the relevant deficiency disease. No matter how much you exercise, who your parents are, or whether or not you smoke, you will become scorbutic without sufficient vitamin C.

Unfortunately, there is no such simple cause-effect relationship for diseases such as cardiovascular disease, cancer, stroke, and diabetes. Large doses of vitamin E, for example, may or may not influence the risk of developing heart disease. For some people, it may potentially be important. For most, however, it is at best one factor, and probably not a major one.

A primary contributor to chronic disease risk is our genetic heritage. Nutritionist Elizabeth Hiser writes, "Genes have a powerful influence over body size and disease risk, and though diet helps temper unwanted tendencies, *who* you are is often more important than *what* you eat. . . . Because of genetics, diet helps some people a lot, some people a little, and a very few people not at all."[6] Genetic endowment accounts in large measure for why some people get heart disease when young, for example, no matter how well they care for themselves, and why others live long lives even when they violate many of the commandments of healthy living.

Chronic disease risk is also affected by whether or not we exercise, refrain from smoking, avoid drinking to excess, limit exposure to unproductive stressors, and have sufficient rest, relaxation, and fun—and, of course, eating a diet that meets dietary guidelines and the

RDAs. In our enthusiasm for supplements, however, we run the risk of reducing the importance of these factors.

One example of "thinking in penicillin mode" is linking calcium with the treatment, and especially prevention, of osteoporosis. However, bone health is influenced by many factors, including smoking, alcohol consumption, exercise, and intake of nutrients such as phosphorus, protein, and boron that affect calcium absorption, utilization, and excretion. In fact, osteoporosis is uncommon in several countries with relatively low calcium intakes.

Even, when and if, phytochemicals are reliably found in supplements, it will never be appropriate to take them in that form rather than from foods that contain them.

Social commentator H. L. Mencken said, "For every complicated problem there is a simple solution—and it is wrong."[7] Supplements are not the answer to health and disease for the vast majority of people. Who our parents are, how we live our lives, and the food we put into our mouths several times a day affect our health more profoundly.

POINT 3: FOOD IS MORE THAN THE SUM OF ITS NUTRIENTS

Nutritionists used to think that macro- and micronutrients made a food nutritious and good for health. Other food constituents, such as fiber, were seen as nonessential, and therefore unimportant, since death is not directly associated with fiber deficiency. However, we have learned that, while fiber is not essential in the traditional sense, its presence in the diet makes it much easier to defecate and influences blood cholesterol levels and risk of diseases such as diverticulosis and certain cancers.

Many compounds in food that are not classical nutrients can apparently influence health and risk of disease. Several hundred studies show that heavy fruit and vegetable eaters have approximately half the risk of cancer compared with those who don't eat these foods, but the results are not consistently related to one or several nutrients. New biologically active constituents found mostly in plant foods—phytochemicals (or "phytomins" as *Prevention* magazine calls them)—are being discovered regularly. They include flavonoids, monoterpenes, phenolics, indoles, allylic sulfides, and isothiocyanates. Phytochemicals became a "hot item" in 1994 when they were the subject of a cover story in Newsweek that April.[8] The title: "Better than Vitamins: The Search for the Magic Pill." (There's that word too often linked with supplements: magic! So is "miracle.")

Whole natural foods, to quote *Newsweek*, "harbor a whole ratatouille of compounds that have never seen the inside of a vitamin bottle for the simple reason that scientists have not, until very recently, even known they existed, let alone brewed them into pills." Even when phytochemicals can reliably be found in supplements, it will never be appropriate to swallow pills (or consume specially fortified processed foods) instead of eating recommended amounts of the foods that contain them, such as vegetables, fruits, whole grains, and legumes. To do so would be to inappropriately rely on preliminary science, when the future will bring the discovery of new phytochemicals that have always been available from today's natural foods. Determining whether and how isolated food constituents with biological activity may improve health, treat disease, or extend life is a daunting task that will occupy researchers for decades or longer.

Scientists continue to learn more about the complexity of foods and the myriad of biologically active constituents they contain that can influence health and disease risk. How ironic, then, that the calls this research generates for renewed efforts to persuade people to eat healthier diets—the tried and true—often seems to be drowned out by the acclaim for dietary supplements.

POINT 4: DEVELOPING RDAs AND OPTIMAL NUTRIENT RECOMMENDATIONS IS VERY DIFFICULT

As a staff scientist with the Food and Nutrition Board, I worked with the subcommittee that developed the most recent (10th) edition of the RDAs. I was surprised to learn that the research base for the RDAs is quite limited. There are not as many studies as one would like to determine minimum and average nutrient requirements for each age-sex group, estimate the population variability in need, and to feel more comfortable about the judgments made to derive nutrient allowances. Setting RDAs is tough work!

Developing recommendations for optimal nutrient intakes will be many times more complex than developing RDAs.

Now there is substantial discussion about so-called optimal intakes of nutrients, levels of intake that might allow people to be healthy and fit for a longer time. Some nutrition scientists believe optimal nutrient intakes will typically exceed RDA levels and may require supplements in some cases to achieve. Still, no one doubts that developing optimal nutrient intakes will be orders of magnitude more complex than developing RDAs.

The optimal intake of any nutrient will probably vary substantially among individuals and even throughout the person's life from infancy to old age. It will probably also depend on the parameter of interest. For ex-

---

Clinical studies help identify cause-and-effect relationships, whereas epidemiologic studies can only identify whether variables are related.

---

ample, an optimal intake of a nutrient to reduce the risk of heart disease might not be optimal to decrease cancer risk and might actually increase it. Defining, understanding, and assessing optimal nutrition is becoming one of the most exciting challenges for investigators in the nutrition and food sciences.

POINT 5: TAKING SUPPLEMENTS OF SINGLE NUTRIENTS IN LARGE DOSES MAY HAVE DETRIMENTAL EFFECTS ON NUTRITIONAL STATUS AND HEALTH

On April 14, 1994, the *New England Journal of Medicine* published the infamous Finnish study.[9] In this clinical trial, 29,000 male smokers in Finland were randomly divided into four groups, receiving either a placebo, 20 mg beta-carotene (approximately four to five times the amount in five servings of fruits and vegetables), 50 IU of vitamin E (about three to four times average dietary intakes, but still a small dose as a supplement), or both the beta-carotene and vitamin E. After 5 to 8 years, the beta-carotene takers had an 18% *higher* incidence of lung cancer, with hints that this carotenoid might also have raised their risk of heart disease. Vitamin E seemed to reduce the risk of prostate cancer but increased the risk of hemorrhagic stroke.

This study is noteworthy, both because of its surprising findings and the fact that it is one of the few large clinical trials on supplements and disease risk. The majority of studies investigating this relationship are epidemiologic in nature. Clinical trials in which subjects are randomly assigned to treatment or control groups help to identify cause-and-effect relationships. Epidemiologic studies, in contrast, can only identify whether the variables under study are related in some way.

The Finnish study showed that antioxidant nutrients might harm rather than help male smokers, so it has been scrutinized intensely. Blumberg, for example, noted that those with the highest plasma concentrations of vitamin E and beta-carotene at the start of the study had the lowest risk of developing lung cancer[10]; therefore, these nutrients may have provided some protection to some smokers. But for those who would suggest that the subjects should not have expected any benefits from supplements, given their deadly habit, two points should be made. First, several epidemiologic studies show that fruit and vegetable consumption reduces the risk of lung cancer in smokers— again, foods (containing beta-carotene and many other carotenoids and phytochemicals), not supplements. Second, dietary supplements are often promoted to smokers and those who are not eating or taking care of themselves as well as they should with claims that the products protect health.

A major concern with supplements is potential toxicity.

The Center for Science in the Public Interest, a consumer advocacy group that had recommended antioxidants to its readers, changed its position after the Finnish study.[11] "Shelve the beta-carotene," it said,

or take no more than about 3 mg per day, the amount found in many multivitamins. It also advised people to "reconsider taking vitamin E." *New York Times* medical writer Nicholas Wade, commenting on the Finnish study, said: "The vitamin supplement industry . . . would like everyone to believe the issue of benefits is settled. . . . For all who assumed the answer was already known, the Finnish trial offers two lessons. One is that science can't be rushed. The

---

Large doses of one nutrient can adversely affect nutritional status in relation to another nutrient.

---

other is not to put all your bets on those convenient little bottles: back to broccoli and bicycles."[12]

Time shows the wisdom of Wade's advice. Two large clinical trials were completed in January of this year that further debunk beta-carotene as a magic bullet. After 12 years of taking either 50 mg beta-carotene or a placebo every other day, 22,071 physicians learned that the phytochemical provided no protection against cancer or heart disease. In the second trial, 18,314 men and women at risk for lung cancer due to smoking or exposure to asbestos were given supplements of beta-carotene (30 mg/day), vitamin A (25,000 IU/day), or a placebo. Those receiving the supplements had a *higher* rate of death from lung cancer and heart disease; although the results were not statistically significant, the study was halted. Dr. Richard Klausner, the director of the National Cancer Institute, which financed both trials, concluded, "With clearly no benefit and even a hint of possible harm, I can see no reason that an individual should take beta-carotene."

A major concern with supplements is potential toxicity. Fat-soluble vitamins like A and D, which are stored in the body, are obviously harmful in excess, but so are some water-soluble nutrients. Large doses of vitamin B6, for example, can produce neuropathy in the arms and legs, leading to partial paralysis. Some people taking tryptophan have developed and died from eosinophilia-myalgia syndrome, a connective tissues disease characterized by high levels of eosinophils, severe muscle pain, and skin and neuromuscular problems. (It is not yet certain whether the syndrome was caused by the tryptophan itself, by a contaminant produced in the manufacturing process, or by the two in combination.) High-dose niacin supplements, especially in the time-released form, have caused liver damage. Large amounts of beta-carotene can be dangerous to alcoholics with liver disorders. And antioxidant nutrients can act as prooxidants under certain conditions, generating cell-damaging free radicals.[13]

Another concern with supplements is the possibility of adverse nutrient interactions. Calcium, for example, affects the absorption of iron and vice versa. Various amino acids compete with each other for absorption from the small intestine and to cross the blood-brain barrier. Large doses of one nutrient or phytochemical can adversely affect nutritional status in relation to another. In one study, for example, very large doses of beta-carotene, 100 mg/day given for 6 days, decreased the concentration of another important carotenoid, lycopene, in the low-density lipoproteins by 12 to 25%.[14] Beta carotene is not the only carotenoid of benefit to health, or perhaps even the most important one. I am reminded of Walter Mertz, the renowned nutrition and trace mineral expert, who was asked if he took beta-carotene as a supplement. He replied he would be "afraid" to take it, not knowing how extra beta-carotene would affect the balance of all the other carotenoids in his body that he obtained from food.

Little information is available to demonstrate that the long-term and possibly lifetime intake of large doses of nutrients is completely safe. Studies on the consequences of large nutrient intakes in humans rarely have a large sample size and go beyond several months. If high levels of iron in the body, for example, really increase the risk of heart disease, as at least one study suggests,[15] the chances are remote that a physician will think that a patient who died of a heart attack possibly did so because of supplemental iron. In other words, nutrient toxicity may be a cause of more illness and death than suspected, because the problems will not be linked (or even thought to have a possible link) to use of supplements.

POINT 6: DIETARY SUPPLEMENTS VARY SUBSTANTIALLY IN QUALITY

Few federal manufacturing and formulation standards exist for supplements, in part because they fall into a regulatory gray area between food and drugs.[16] A decade ago, investigators discovered that many calcium supplements did not disintegrate or dissolve in the digestive tract; the calcium was simply excreted. These results prompted the development of disintegration and dissolution standards for some types of supplements by the US Pharmacopoeia, the scientific organization that establishes drug standards. . . .

Garlic supplements provide an example of not necessarily getting what you think you paid for. They have become popular because several studies suggest that garlic may help to lower blood cholesterol and reduce the risk of cancers of the breast, colon, and other organs. Attention has focused on two compounds that may be responsible for these effects: allicin and s-allyl cysteine. The Center for Science in the Public Interest analyzed garlic powder and various garlic pills and found major differences by brand in their content of these two com-

pounds.[17] Plain garlic powder was best and least expensive, whereas the most popular brand of garlic supplement contained no allicin (Table 1). Similarly, Consumers Union recently found that ginseng products varied greatly in their content of ginsenosides, the root's supposed active ingredients.[18]

It is difficult to find a comprehensive, one-a-day type of supplement that supplies nutrients at RDA levels. Most products are not well balanced. They contain, for example, many times the recommended amount of inexpensive B vitamins like thiamin and riboflavin but only small amounts of calcium and magnesium, because recommended amounts of these minerals can add substantially to the size of the pill. Some supplements contain superfluous ingredients such as bee pollen, hesperidin complex, and PABA, which do little more than boost the price (see Refs. 19 and 20 for good advice on choosing a supplement).

POINT 7: SUPPLEMENTS ARE PROMOTED BY COMMERCIAL AND OTHER FORCES ON THE BASIS OF INCOMPLETE OR PRELIMINARY SCIENCE

I stated earlier that the bulk of evidence linking supplements to reduced risks of heart disease, cancer, and other diseases is epidemiologic in nature, or based on *in vitro*, mechanistic, or biochemical studies. They show correlations and indicate the possibility of protective effects, but do not prove cause and effect. So we do not know whether most of these suggestive data are of practical importance to people over the long run as they eat good or bad diets, smoke or refrain from smoking, live in polluted or clean environments, and are either exercisers or couch potatoes.

The scientific community tends to blame journalists for distorted reporting about nutrition. True, there are both good and mediocre reporters on the subject. And too often the

Table 1

Comparison of Garlic Supplements

Name of Supplement	Cost per Tablet* (cents)	Allicin (µg)†	SAC (µg)‡
McCormick Garlic Powder§	6	5,600	590
KAL Beyond Garlic	18	4,800	270
Garlique	33	3,840	130
Garlicin	18	2,165	145
Nature's Way	8	1,530	140
Kwai	11	815	60
Quintessence	9	535	185
Natural Brand (GNC)	10	300	45
P. Leiner (private label)‖	5	115	45
Kyolic¶	11	0	255

© 1995, CSPI. Adapted from *Nutricion Action Healthletter* (1875 Connecticut Ave., N.W., Suite 300, Washington DC 20009-5728. $24.00 for 10 issues).
* Based on list price when available or average price paid.
† One large clove of fresh garlic supplies about 5,000 µg allicin.
‡ S-allyl cysteine.
§ One-third teaspoon.
‖ Product usually carries the name of the drugstore or other chain where it is sold.
¶ The best-selling garlic supplement.

reporting is bad, incomplete, prepared from press releases, or focused on one study without placing it in perspective—a poor foundation for people to make intelligent decisions.

A recent study illustrates this point, Houn and colleagues examined popular press coverage of research on the association between alcohol consumption and breast cancer.[21] Of the 58 published journal papers on this topic over 7 years, only 11 were cited by the press. Three studies published in the *New England Journal of Medicine* and the *Journal of the Medical Association* were featured in more than three quarters of the news stories. And almost two thirds of the stories gave recommendations to women on alcohol consumption based on one study. Reporters ignored the published review articles and editorials that would have provided a better basis for advice. This highlighting of a few studies, which seems to occur in many other nutrition areas, tends to confuse people and lead them to think that a new study will undoubtedly contradict the findings of the previous one. It's the new math of media nutrition coverage: $1 + 1 = 0$. As syndicated columnist Ellen Goodman puts it, "Fresh research has a sell-by date that is shorter than the one on the cereal box."[22]

Responsibility for distorted reporting of nutrition does not rest with the media alone. Increasingly, it involves nutrition scientists. Although they tend not to make exaggerated claims when reporting their work at scientific meetings, some are more bold when they speak to reporters or the public. Sometimes their institution's press office encourages this boldness. As research funds become harder to secure, scientists and their employers are

> *Responsibility for distorted reporting of nutrition rests as much with some nutritional scientists as with the media; many major journals reach reporters before medical professionals.*

learning that being in the news raises their visibility, which can help to raise money.

Now, major journals like the *New England Journal of Medicine* and *Journal of the American Medical Association* reach reporters before they reach biomedical professionals. And because a growing amount of research is financed by industry, a company might seek publicity about a new finding to enhance the value of its stock or draw attention to itself. A good book on the changing nature of reporting scientific advances is *Selling Science,* by sociologist Dorothy Nelkin.[23]

The dietary supplements industry is busy making bold claims for its products on the labels, in advertising, and in product literature using preliminary science. The 1990 Nutrition Labeling and Education Act, which resulted in the new nutrition labels on packaged foods, allows supplement manufacturers to present the same health claims that are allowed on foods—claims supported by "significant scientific agreement" and preapproved by FDA. Two of the authorized health claims are relevant to supplements: the links between calcium and osteoporosis and between folate and neural tube defects.

However, the Dietary Supplement Health and Education Act passed in 1994 allows the industry to make claims pertaining to the structure and function of a nutrient. For example, a supplement could not claim that it helps cure AIDS, but it might be possible to state that the product "boosts the immune system." The legal basis for a claim is that (1) some substantiation exists, (2) FDA be notified of the claim within 30 days of its presence on the label, and (3) two additional sentences be added to such claims: "This statement has not been evaluated by FDA. This product is not in-

---

Dietary supplements provide a false sense of security.

---

tended to diagnose, treat, cure, or prevent any disease." Along with these so-called "structure-function" claims, a retailer may now provide literature on supplements, although it is supposed to be balanced scientifically and not be misleading. Some members of the dietary supplements industry are fighting even these limitations, arguing that their absolute freedom of speech to provide whatever information they think is appropriate is being threatened.

An advertisement in *Time* magazine last October for Bayer Corporation's One-A-Day Brand Vitamins suggests the growing boldness of claims for even mainstream dietary supplements. The copy states: "It's been all over the news. Findings on folic acid studies were announced recently at a medical conference in Bar Harbor, Maine, suggesting that adequate intake of folic acid may significantly lower elevated homocysteine levels, one of the risk factors for heart attacks and strokes in men. One-A-Day Men's Formula

contains 100% of the US RDA of folic acid. Why not start taking your One-A-Day today?"

Public health may benefit from the promotion of supplements by increasing the public's awareness of nutrient, diet, and disease relationships. But I fear the risks outweigh the benefits. The promotional copy typically fails to give information on food-related alternatives to supplements. In addition, the public rarely has the expertise to evaluate the information in the promotion. Furthermore, consumers' expectations of a product's effectiveness may be heightened by the hype and lead to irrational use of the product.

There can be a great difference between *a* truth and *the* truth. A truthful statement may inevitably be misleading. This lesson was made clear in the plethora of ridiculous health claims on foods back in the late 80s and early 90s. Some high-fat products, for example, were truthfully labeled as being cholesterol free, because manufacturers knew many people would think the product was more healthful.

Concentrating anything in the food chain, be it vitamin C, beta-carotene, salt, or fat, increases the likelihood of mistakes.

Supplements supplying nutrients at levels beyond what can reasonably by obtained from food should be viewed as nonprescription drugs. High-potency products should not be used without careful thought and perhaps expert help.

POINT 8: FOCUSING ON NUTRIENTS AND SUPPLEMENTS CAN TAKE ATTENTION AND CONVICTION AWAY FROM IMPROVING ONE'S LIFESTYLE

Nationally representative surveys of American adults show that approxi-

mately one third are interested in nutrition and think they are on the right track to healthy eating. In contrast, another third couldn't care less about meeting dietary guidelines. Those in the middle third claim they are trying to eat better, but find it difficult.

So, the good news is that two thirds of adult Americans say they care about their nutrition. But the bad news is that perhaps only 5 to 10% of the US population meets dietary recommendations regularly, such as eating five or more servings of fruits and vegetables per day and limiting fat to no more than 30% of calories. Furthermore, obesity is a growing epidemic in this country, now affecting one third of adults and one quarter of children. The irony is that people who eat well are most likely to take supplements, whereas those most likely to benefit from higher nutrient intakes are least likely to take them.

My greatest concern about dietary supplements is the false sense of security it provides some people, those who use supplements to an extent as substitutes for a good diet. It is natural for us to want an easier way or, ideally, some magic bullet, to achieve health short of being vigilant or saintly all the time. We're especially likely to cut corners when we are short of time and feeling stressed, such as by choosing foods on the basis of convenience and ease of preparation and by not exercising. Taking a basic supplement as one small part of a health-promoting lifestyle may be reasonable and perhaps even prudent. But taking supplements is a problem for people, probably the majority, who are not making the lifestyle changes they know they should. A recent advertisement by Hoffman-La Roche, Inc. for vitamin E states . . . "Many doctors . . . believe taking supplements or eating fortified foods containing vitamins and minerals is a sound health measure, particularly for people who don't eat a good diet. . . ." Unfortunately, some people use supplements as a deliberate or unconscious excuse for not trying to improve their diets and lifestyles.

A reporter called me some time ago to ask how people could use vitamins to stay healthy. I replied that people should pay more attention to their diets. He told me to be realistic and used himself as an example. He said he leads a very busy life, has little time to shop for food and prepare it, and there are few places near work that serve nutritious lunches. So what supplements would help him cope more productively with his situation? Here is an example where supplements may harm more than help, by being used as a surrogate for tackling the hard things that would really improve his nutritional status, such as preparing lunches the night before, convincing nearby restaurants to offer more nutritious fare, and making sure he eats a very nutritious breakfast and dinner. This reporter was looking for what he acknowledged to be a second-best solution, but taking a supplement will make him even less likely to attempt the best but more difficult solution.

CONCLUDING THOUGHTS

. . . Those who recommend that healthy people supplement their diets with extra vitamins and minerals often call it a form of dietary insurance, as essential to have as car or home insurance. I disagree. When you purchase insurance, the benefits and costs of the policy are detailed and you choose a specific level of protection. The terms of a dietary insurance policy, though, can never be known, much less specified. Taking supplements without a clear need is more analogous to playing the lottery. You hope to win some money, and ideally the jackpot, by buying lottery tickets. You won't hurt yourself unless you buy more tickets over time than you can afford, but you are not likely to win anything either, especially the big prize.

Even comprehensive dietary supplements are, at best, poor substitutes for nutrient-rich foods. Foods, about which we know little, are more than the sum of their parts, about which we have some knowledge. Furthermore, it's harder to hurt yourself with foods than with supplements. Concentrating anything in the food chain—be it vitamin C, beta-carotene, salt, or fat—increases the likelihood of mistakes. Nutrients and other nonnutrient substances relevant to health are readily available in familiar and attractive packages called fruits, vegetables, legumes, grains, and animal products. And they come in concentrations and in combinations with which humans have had long cultural familiarity.[29] . . .

REFERENCES

1. Slesinski MJ, Subar AF, Kahle LL. Trends in use of vitamin and mineral supplements in the United States: The 1987 and 1992 National Health Interview Surveys. *J Am Diet Assoc* 1995; 95: 921–3.
2. National Research Council. *Diet and Health: Implications for Reducing Chronic Disease Risk.* Washington, DC: National Academy Press, 1989.
3. US Department of Agriculture, Department of Health and Human Services. *Nutrition and Your Health: Dietary Guidelines for Americans,* 4th ed. Washington, DC: Government Printing Office, 1995.
4. Brody J. Personal health: Sorting out the benefits of taking extra vitamin E. *New York Times,* July 26, 1995: C8.
5. Golub E. *The Limits of Medicine: How Science Shapes Our Hope for the Cure.* New York: Times Books, 1994.
6. Hiser E. Getting into your genes. *Eating Well* 1995; 6 (1): 48–9.
7. Herbert V, Kasdan TS. Misleading nutrition claims and their gurus. *Nutr Today* 29 (3): 28–35, 1994.
8. Begley S. Beyond vitamins: The search for the magic pill. *Newsweek,* April 25, 1994: 45–9.
9. The Alpha-Tocopherol, Beta-Carotene Cancer Prevention Study Group. The effect of vitamin E and beta carotene on the incidence of lung cancer and other cancers in male smokers. *N Engl J Med* 1994; 330: 1029–35.
10. Blumberg JB. Considerations of the scientific substantiation for antioxidant vitamins and B-carotene in disease prevention. *Am J Clin Nutr* 1995; 62: 1521S–1526S.
11. Liebman B. Antioxidants: Surprise, surprise. *Nutr Action Healthletter* 1994; 21 (5): 4.
12. Wade N. Method and madness: Believing in vitamins. *New York Times Magazine,* May 22, 1994: 20.
13. Herbert V. The antioxidant supplement myth. *Am J Clin Nutr* 1994; 60: 157–8.
14. Graziano JM, Johnson EJ, Russell RM, Manson JE, Stampfer MJ, Ridker PM, Frei B, Hennekens CH, Krinsky NI. Discrimination in absorption or transport of B-carotene isomers after oral supplementation with either all-*trans*- or 9-*cis*-β-carotene. *Am J Clin Nutr* 1995; 61: 1248–52.
15. McCord JM. Free radicals and prooxidants in health and nutrition. *Food Tech* 1994; 48 (5): 106–11.
16. Anon. Buying vitamins: what's worth the price? *Consumer Rep* 1994; 59: 565–9.
17. Schardt, D. Schmidt S. Garlic: Clove at first sight? *Nutr Action Healthletter* 1995; 22(6): 3–5.
18. Anon. Herbal roulette. *Consumer Rep* 1995; 60: 698–705.
19. Anon. A 9-point guide to choosing the right supplement. *Tufts Univ Diet & Nutr Letter* 1993; 11(7): 3–6.
20. Liebman, B, Schardt D. Vitamin smarts. *Nutr Action Healthletter* 1995; 22(9): 1, 6–10.
21. Houn F, Bober MA, Huerta EE, Hursting SD, Lemon S, Weed DL. The association between alcohol and breast cancer: Popular press coverage of research. *Am J Publ Health* 1995; 85: 1082–6.
22. Goodman E. To swallow or not to swallow. *Liberal Opinion Week,* April 24, 1994.
23. Nelkin D. *Selling Science: How the Press Covers Science and Technology,* revised edition. New York: WH Freeman and Company, 1995.
24. Anon. Many shoppers not yet aware of nutrition facts label. *Food Labeling News* 1995; 3(32): 21–3.
25. Gussow JD. *A Word on Behalf of Food.* Presentation at the Alumni Advances Conference of the dietetic internship program at Oregon Health Sciences University, Portland, OR, May 1995.
26. Shepherd SK. Nutrition and the consumer: Meeting the challenge of nutrition education in the 1990s. *Food & Consumer News* 1990;62 (1): 1–3.
27. Goodman E. Food literacy. *Liberal Opinion Week,* December 14, 1992.
28. Stacey M. *Consumer: Why Americans Love, Hate, and Fear Food.* New York: Touchstone Books, 1994.
29. Gussow JD, Thomas PR. *The Nutrition Debate: Sorting Out Some Answers.* Palo Alto, CA: Bull Publishing Co., 1986.

The views expressed in this article are those of the author and do not reflect the position of the Center for Food and Nutrition Policy.

Are Health Food Stores Better Bets Than Traditional Supermarkets?

THE DOOR SWINGS OPEN, and over a terra-cotta tile floor you step, passing between two rows of lush, fragrant flowers at the peak of their bloom. Straight ahead, extending the color scheme found in the fragrant blossoms, lie red and green apples, artfully arranged next to smooth, round oranges and lovely-looking vegetables.

No, you haven't happened onto a Martha Stewart set. You've entered a supermarket-size natural foods store owned by Austin, Texas-based Whole Foods Market, which operates almost 100 outlets in more than 20 states. In Boston, it's called Bread & Circus, although depending on where you live, you may know it as Whole Foods, Fresh Foods, Wellspring Group, Bread of Life, or Merchant of Vino.

Whatever name it goes by, it's the present-day version of a health food store, specializing in organic fruits and vegetables, nutrition supplements, and myriad grains, beans, rice, and granola sold in bulk. And it's not alone. A company called Wild Oats owns 59 stores in 16 states and Canada with names like Alfalfa's, Capers, and Uptown Whole Foods. And many

areas have local health food supermarkets of their own.

Make no mistake. These are not the crunchy-granola counterculture hangouts of yore. They're big business supermarketing, with collective sales in the billions of dollars a year.

The question for the consumer, of course, is whether picking up your groceries in them means eating more healthfully than if you go to a traditional supermarket. To find out, we did some comparison shopping.

Organically terrific

Organically grown fruits and vegetables, farmed without pesticides, herbicides, and fungicides, have not been shown to be more nutritious than other produce. No matter what methods are used to raise crops, they will have the same abundance of vitamins, minerals, fiber, and other phytochemicals important to good health.

But organic fruits and vegetables are definitely better for the planet—keeping toxic chemicals out of ground water supplies, stemming soil deterioration via crop rotation, and safeguarding farm workers and livestock from potentially harmful com-

pounds. If those issues are a concern for you and you want to take a stand through your food purchases, today's health food markets offer a much greater variety of organic foods than traditional supermarkets.

Not only can you buy everything from beautiful-looking organic Romaine lettuce and asparagus to organic oranges and apples, you can also purchase tomato sauce made only with organically grown ingredients, organic applesauce, organic olive oil, and the list goes on.

Meat, fish, and poultry are "organic" in these stores, too. Granted, as markets like Bread & Circus plainly point out, the U.S. Department of Agriculture presently does not recognize the term "organic" in relation to meat production, but meats offered in health food markets are raised on organic feed. The meat is also produced without the use of drugs such as growth hormones and antibiotics.

Cutting back on the routine use of antibiotics in animals can help stem the development of super-strength bacteria that then prove resistant to the antibiotics used to treat infections in humans. Consider that more than 40

From the *Tufts University Health & Nutrition Letter,* May 1999, pp. 4-5. © 1999 by Tufts University Health & Nutrition Letter. Reprinted by permission.

percent of the antibiotics produced in this country are used in animals, and many of them are the same as or similar to antibiotics used in humans. The more that various bacteria are exposed to antibiotics, the greater the chance they will mutate to forms that make them immune to the drugs' effects. The upshot: the drugs lose their effectiveness.

Of course, meat produced without antibiotics, as well as other foods made with the environment in mind, all come with a price. And it's a hefty one. A 25-ounce jar of Whole Foods organic applesauce costs $2.99, while a 23-ounce jar of Mott's, housed on the same shelf for the faint of pocketbook, retails for $1.49. (In a regular supermarket, we found the same-size jar of Mott's for just $1.29.)

Similarly, a 10-ounce package of Organic Cascadian Farm Chopped Spinach costs $2.39, while a 10-ounce package of Birds Eye Spinach in the same freezer case goes for 99 cents (67 cents in the regular store). And a pound of bottom round rump roast: a rather astounding $4.59 (as compared to $2.39 in the traditional market).

Supplementally disappointing

If the availability of organic foods is the high (albeit expensive) point of natural foods markets, their large supplement sections are the low point. Mixed in with the multivitamins and other potentially helpful tables are some of the most bogus products making some of the most outlandish claims we've ever seen.

The label on the bottle of Hot Flash tables we found at Bread & Circus, for instance, promises that the supplement "helps reduce hot flash frequency." We doubt it. Yes, it contains a small amount of soy concentrate, which preliminary research suggests might help reduce the symptoms of menopause. But the $9.99 bottle (which contains only 15 days' worth of tables) is basically an unproven concoction of ingredients that includes licorice root extract and dong quai. Neither of those sub-

stances have been scientifically proven to help quell hot flashes.

Another health food store we visited, Wild Harvest, offers KidCalm, a "St. John's Wort Complex for your child's emotional well-being and nervous system function" (we don't even know all the science relating to St. John's wort in adults). It also contains more than 2,000 percent of the recommended level of vitamin B_6 for children four to eight years old, with 50 milligrams of kava root and 100 milligrams of valerian root extract mixed in. How those substances in those proportions can be good for a child is a mystery. Scientists are only now beginning to take a rigorous look at herbs like kava and valerian.

In the same section appears Fat Defense, "an effective natural formula for weight management" with ingredients like garcinia cambogia extract and gymnema sylvestre powder (benefits unproven). The cost: $14.79 for 10 to 20 days' worth of tablets, or up to about $500 a year—enough to join a health club and lose weight via a *proven* method.

We inquired about the training of the "nutrition manager" at Wild Harvest, whose store position was printed on his name tag. His response was that he had been doing it for six years. "It," it turned out, was working at other stores that sell supplements, such as GNC. He also told us he learned about nutrition from vendors who supply the products— that is, people who stand to make money off the sale of supplements.

Mixed messages

Scorecard so far: for the environmentally concerned consumer who wants a wide selection of organic foods, a plus. But a big minus for the minefield of scientifically unproven potions.

On some issues, however, the takeaway points are less obvious, and they often occur in the aisles with packaged goods. Consider, for instance, that in the "National Selections" section of Wild Harvest, a pound of Davinci spaghetti imported from Italy is 99 cents. Yet just across

the aisle in "Traditional Groceries," *two* pounds of Ronzoni spaghetti (made in the U.S.) cost $1.19.

Other than in price, we couldn't see any difference between the two products. The wheat used to produce the Italian spaghetti was not organic. In fact, the ingredients on the Italian and American packages were identical. Both listed semolina wheat and the same five nutrients added for enrichment. The extra cost for the Italian spaghetti, it seemed, could be chalked up solely to its cachet as a European product and the fact that it had to be shipped thousands of miles over the Atlantic Ocean.

Consider, too, that a health food supermarket might stock ruby red, fresh, organic raspberries in early April, which is great for people who want to eat the widest variety possible of delicious produce. But a placard above some raspberries that we saw in one store indicated that they had been shipped from Chile, which seemed to go against the store's own commitment to the environment. A company with a deep concern for ecologically sound food practices might prefer to ask people to wait until summer, when raspberries can be grown locally (and therefore don't have to use up fuel resources in being shipped thousands of miles), or to choose frozen raspberries grown closer to home.

Other products also have the aura of being produced with the planet in mind but come with a compromise that isn't necessarily apparent at first glance. For instance, health food supermarkets make it easy to buy many items in bulk, which allows you not only to buy just the amount you need but also cuts down on wasteful packaging that clutters landfills. But they also sell products like 15-ounce packages of frozen split pea soup that contain just two servings. Granted, the soup is organic, but it seems to us that any store that professes to help safeguard the environment would not sell two servings of a product that's so easy to package in large quantities.

In addition, there's the "all natural" burst printed on many products in health food stores. It *sounds* better for you, but it doesn't necessarily signify any extra health benefits. All Natural Born Free Vanilla Pecan Chip Cookies, for example, are made with "no refined sugar." But the so-called raw sugar they contain (and the sugar used in the chocolate chips) is nutritionally equivalent to refined table sugar: all have 16 calories a teaspoon and virtually no other nutrients. Similarly, while the "frosted crisps and puffs of brown rice" in Rice Twice Cereal come "naturally," the rice is glazed with honey—again, the nutritional equivalent of sugar.

Making it particularly difficult to see all sides of products in health food emporiums is the fact that the stores are so undeniably pleasant to shop in. In fact, for sheer entertainment value, they're matchless. As mentioned earlier, they're beautiful, with wide aisles and attractive displays. And the employees in these markets tend to act less like store clerks and more like wait staff at a restaurant that prides itself on service. Furthermore, at least at the Bread & Circus we visited, there were lots of delicious free samples of food—baby carrots with pepper Parmesan dip in the produce section; tortilla chips with parsley, scallion and red pepper hummus in the takeout section; cookie pieces in the bakery section, and so on. You could leave literally stuffed without spending a cent.

But while these stores are a feast for both the stomach and the senses (even wandering past the glistening displays of fresh striped bass, rainbow trout, salmon fillets, and monkfish in the seafood section is entertaining), the bottom line is that you have to read labels carefully, just like you would in a traditional supermarket. And, if the health of the planet is on your mind and you're looking at two servings of organic, packaged, frozen soup, it pays to think past the "organic/all natural" burst on the front and decide whether, for $2.99, you're being as good to Mother Earth—and to yourself—as the box suggests.

Unit 7

Unit Selections

Key Points to Consider

❖ How extensive is global malnutrition and infection?

❖ What are some of the causes of global malnutrition?

❖ To what extent can agricultural development alleviate poverty and malnutrition?

❖ What sort of role will genetically modified food have in the future in feeding people in developing countries?

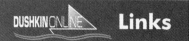 **Links**   **www.dushkin.com/online/**

These sites are annotated on pages 4 and 5.

The cause of malnutrition worldwide is poverty. The United Nations Food and Agriculture Organization (FAO) determined that a body mass index (BMI) (body weight divided by the square root of height) of 18.5 is indicative of chronic energy deficit in adults. Approximately 840 million people are malnourished in the developing world: Asia has the largest number of them and children under 5 years of age are the most susceptible. Infectious disease kills approximately 10 million children each year. Thus, the director general of FAO launched, in 1994, a special Programme for Food Security (SPFS) for low-income food-deficit countries (LIFDCs), which was endorsed by the World Food Summit held in Rome in 1996. They pledged to increase food production and access to food in LIFDCs so that the number of malnourished people would be reduced by half. They set goals to increase sustainable agricultural production within the cultural, political, and economic millieu of the country to improve access to food, to increase the role of trade, and to deal effectively with food emergencies.

Malnutrition is also the main culprit for lowered resistance to disease, infection, and death, especially in children. The malnutrition-infection combination results in stunted growth, lowered mental development in children, and lowered productivity and higher incidence of degenerative disease in adulthood. This directly affects the economies of developing countries.

According to Gro Harlem Brundtland, Director General of the World Health Organization, diet-related areas that we need to focus on to stop this vicious cycle between malnutrition and infection are vitamin A and iron deficiencies that occur simultaneously with protein-energy deficits. Nutrient deficiencies magnify the effect of disease and result in more severe symptoms and greater complications of the disease. For example, vitamin A deficiency leads to blindness in about 250,000–300,000 children annually, and exacerbates the symptoms of measles. Iron deficiency, which is widespread among pregnant women and those in the child-bearing years in developing countries, increases the risk of death from hemorrhage in their offspring and reduces physical productivity and learning capacity. Finally, iodine deficiency causes brain damage and mental retardation. It is estimated that 1.5 billion people are at risk for iodine deficiency disorders (IDD).

Malnutrition does not only affect children and adults in developing countries but is also prevalent in this country. Thirty million Americans, of whom 11 million are children, experience food insecurity and hunger. In a country where one-fifth of the food is wasted and 130 pounds of food per person is disposed of, it is unacceptable that Americans go hungry.

In a survey conducted by the U.S.D.A. in 1989, approximately 66 percent of low-income children did not consume the Recommended Dietary Allowance (RDA) for calories. The primary nutrient deficiencies in this country, as in developing countries, are iron deficiency anemia, common in infants, young children,

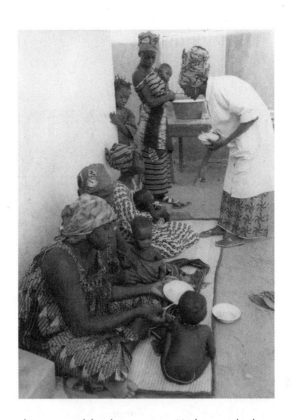

and teens, and lead poisoning. Undernourished pregnant women give birth to low-weight babies who suffer developmental delays and increases in mortality rate. Another group in the United States that experiences health problems due to hunger are the elderly. Articles about Food Assistance Programs that are available in the United States to combat hunger and new initiatives for policy changes that may eradicate hunger and ensure food security for all citizens are included in this unit.

Even though some developing countries have increased agricultural growth, it still has failed to benefit the poor. Environmental problems may slow down production in the future. Future strategies should focus on increasing agricultural growth without endangering the natural resources and on alleviating poverty equitably. Biotechnologists believe that genetically modified (GM) foods such as rice that is fortified with beta-carotene and iron may not only help feed the world, but also eradicate nutritional deficiencies. Additionally, GM foods may decrease damage to crops from pests, viruses, bacteria, and drought. Yet it seems too good to be true. If farmers cannot afford to grow GM crops or afford to buy the food, if the infrastructure for transport and distribution is not available, the same products may never reach the consumers. Since the safety of humans and the efficacy for the environment of GM crops has not been adequately studied, the Union of Concerned Scientists believes that genetic engineering is by no means the panacea for hunger. They propose that educating the farmer to increase production, limiting environmentally destructive practices, and promoting sustainable intensification of agricultural production will solve many of the problems connected to hunger and malnutrition.

HUNGER AND FOOD INSECURITY

KATHERINE L. CASON, Ph.D, R.D.
Associate Professor, Department of Family
and Youth Development
Clemson University

ABSTRACT

Approximately 30 million Americans, including 11 million children, currently experience hunger and food insecurity. Assistance programs and policies help alleviate poverty and food insecurity; however, the rate of hunger and malnutrition has increased. Recent welfare reform legislation decreases funding for assistance. Approaches are needed to achieve long-term food security in our communities. Family and consumer scientists can help through education, food-recovery programs, cost-effectiveness program assessments, and public issues education.

According to data released by the U.S. Census Bureau in September 1997, 36.5 million Americans, or 13.7% of the population, lived in poverty in 1996. Poverty is a high priority on the agendas of many economists and politicians; yet no one has been able to overcome the problems and obstacles associated with this social disease.

Living in poverty often means that individuals are victims of hunger (Clancy & Bowering, 1992). Living below the poverty line puts tremendous strains on a household budget, adversely affecting the ability to purchase a nutritionally adequate diet (Clancy & Bowering, 1992). Hunger and the broader issue of food security have been a public concern in the United States since our nation's inception. One of the earliest underlying goals of public policy (still in effect) is to assure an adequate supply of safe, nutritious food at reasonable cost (Voichick & Drake, 1994). Recent studies suggest at least 30 million Americans, including 11 million children, currently experience food insecurity (Wehler, Scott & Anderson, 1996).

Food security can be defined as access by all people at all times to enough food for an active, healthy life. Food security includes a ready availability of nutritionally adequate and safe foods and an ability to acquire acceptable foods in socially acceptable ways (Hamilton et al., 1997). The complex issues surrounding food insecurity encompass physiological, social, and economic dimensions. Food, or lack of it, is a determinant of human development, health, and behavior. Its absence affects a community's economy, taxes its resources, and influences its social policies (Breglio, 1992).

Those who experience food insecurity may try to avoid hunger by decreasing the size of meals, skipping meals, or not eating any food for one or more days. When food is severely limited, these methods for avoiding hunger are ineffective (Klein, 1996).

Lack of food, and the subsequent undernutrition, affects physiological functioning in every stage of the life cycle. Most adversely affected are the fetus, pregnant and lactating women, children, and older adults. According to the Community Childhood Hunger Identification Project (CCHIP), hungry children suffer from two to four times as many individual health problems as low-income children whose families do not experience food shortages. Only 44% of low-income children consumed at or above 100% of the Recommended Dietary Allowance (RDA) for calories (USDA, 1989).

Failure to grow over time is a consequence of undernutrition. Inadequate food intake limits the ability of children to learn about the world around them (Center on Hunger, Poverty and Nutrition Policy, 1993). When children are chronically undernourished, their bodies attempt to conserve energy by shutting down "nonessential" bodily functions, leaving energy available for vital organs and growth. If any energy remains, it can be used for social activity and cognitive development. When the body conserves energy, decreased activity levels and increased apathy soon follow. This in turn affects social interactions, inquisitiveness, and overall cognitive functioning. In comparison to nonhun-

Food Stamp Program

Anxiety, negative feelings about self-worth, and hostility toward the outside world can result from chronic hunger and food insecurity

gry children, hungry children are more than four times as likely to suffer from irritability; more than 12 times as likely to report dizziness; and almost three times as likely to suffer from concentration problems (Food Research and Action Center [FRAC], 1991).

In the United States, iron deficiency anemia is still common in infants and young children between 6 months and 3 years, and again during adolescence. About twice as many 4- to 5-year-old African American children have iron deficiency as Mexican American or Caucasian children. The most common causes of anemia in childhood are inadequate intakes of iron, infection, and lead poisoning. Among children 12 to 36 months of age with iron deficiency anemia, 20.6% were from low-income families (Fomon, 1993).

Pregnant women who are undernourished are more likely to experience low birth weight babies. These infants are more likely to suffer delays in their development and are more likely to experience behavior and learning problems later in life. The infant mortality rate is closely linked to inadequate quantity of quality in the diet of the infant's mother (U.S. Department of Health and Human Services [USDHHS], 1994).

Older adults are also at increased risk of suffering health consequences as a result of food insecurity and hunger. Older adults have a number of risk factors that place them at an increased risk for developing malnutrition. Among these risk factors are diseases such as chronic lung disease, heart disease, neurological diseases; disabilities, functional impairments; sensory losses; poor dental health; multiple medication use; therapeutic diets; and social isolation. Malnutrition in older adults can result in loss of muscle mass, which can lead to disabilities that affect levels of independence. Malnutrition can also compromise the immune function, increasing susceptibility to infections (Codispoti & Bartlett, 1994).

Insecurity about whether a family will be able to obtain enough food to avoid hunger also have an emotional impact on children and their parents. Anxiety, negative feelings about self-worth, and hostility toward the outside world can result from chronic hunger and food insecurity (World Hunger Year, 1994).

FOOD ASSISTANCE PROGRAMS

During the 1960s, food security became a high-priority issue at all levels of the government. Government officials and influential leaders, the media, and the general public could no longer ignore the issue of hunger (Egan, 1980).

Several programs were implemented in the 1960s and early 1970s, including the Food Stamp Program; the Special Supplemental Program for Women, Infants and Children (WIC); the Community Food and Nutrition Program; and the Expanded Food and Nutrition Education Program (EFNEP) within the Cooperative Extension Service Program. The media has labeled these years the "War on Hunger" (Voichick & Drake, 1994).

During the 1980s, hunger increased primarily due to a combination of economic factors and resulting cuts in federal assistance programs (FRAC, 1991). In the early 1990s, advocates were hopeful about the renewed interest among elected leaders in improving programs that feed people. The historic passage of the Mickey Leland Childhood Hunger Relief Act in August 1993 helped to improve benefits to food stamp families and improve access for those who had been unable to participate in the Food Stamp Program. The president and Congress committed to place the Special Supplemental Nutrition Program for Women, Infants, and Children (WIC) on track for full funding by 1996, and Congress made funding available to start and expand the School Breakfast and Summer Food Programs (Uvin, 1994).

The Food Stamp Program puts food on the table for some 9 million households and 22 million individuals each day. It provides low-income households with coupons or electronic benefits used like cash at most grocery stores to ensure access to a healthy diet. The current program structure was implemented in 1977 with a goal of alleviating hunger and malnutrition by permitting low-income households to obtain a more nutritious diet through normal channels of trade. It provided more than $19 billion in benefits in 1997 (FRAC, 1997).

The Food Stamp Program began as a federal assistance program designed to help farmers dispose of surplus food products. While assistance to farmers remains a part of the program, the current objective is to help low-income families increase their food purchasing power and achieve a nutritionally adequate diet (Social Security, 1996). However, CCHIP data and other sources indicate that food stamps are not used by millions of people who appear eligible to participate in them due to barriers to participation, lack of information about eligibility, and inadequate funding. Survey results consistently show food stamp benefits are not sufficient to protect many low-income families from experiencing hunger (FRAC, 1998). The *Third Report on Nutrition Monitoring in the United States (1995)* indicates that individuals receiving food stamps have less than adequate diets than those low-income individuals who do not receive food stamps. The report suggests that such risk factors as obesity, hypertension, and high serum cholesterol are major concerns for low-income individuals and place them at higher risk for developing chronic diseases due to inadequate diets. The lack of improvement in adequacy of the diets of food stamp recipients suggests that food stamp recipients would benefit from nutrition education; yet nutrition education is not a mandatory component of the program (Joy & Doisy, 1996).

Since 1986, USDA funds have been available for development and implementation of nutrition education programs; however, only 21 states have instituted such programs. Evaluation of the program is at the discretion of each state (Joy & Doisy, 1996).

National School Lunch Program (NSLP)

The National School Lunch Program was created by Congress 50 years ago as a measure of national security, to safeguard the health and well-being of the nation's children. The NSLP provided meals to 25.1 million children in 1997. Of the more than 26 million children participating in the lunch program, 14.6 million low-income children receive free or reduced price lunches daily (FRAC, 1997).

School Breakfast Program

The School Breakfast Program was established by Congress, initially as a temporary measure through the Child Nutrition Act of 1966 in areas where children had long bus rides to school and in areas where mothers were in the workforce. Permanent authorization in 1975 assisted schools in the provision of a nutritious morning meal to children. In 1997, more than 7 million children and 67,063 schools participated in the School Breakfast Program; 86% were from families with low incomes (FRAC, 1997).

Summer Food Service Program

The Summer Food Service Program was created by Congress in 1968. It is an entitlement program designed to provide funds for eligible sponsoring organizations to serve nutritious meals to low-income children when school is not in session. In the summer of 1996, the program served more than 2.2 million children at more than 28,000 sites operated by more than 3,400 sponsoring organizations nationwide (FRAC, 1997).

Child and Adult Care Feeding Program (CACFP)

The CACFP was founded in 1968 to provide federal funds for meals and snacks to licensed public and nonprofit child-care centers and family and group child-care homes for preschool children. Funds are also provided for meals and snacks served at after-school programs for school-age children, and to adult day-care centers serving chronically impaired adults or people over the age of 60. In 1966, CACFP served more than 2.6 million children daily, providing approximately 1.5 billion meals and snacks; and served more than 40,000 elderly persons in the Adult Day Care portion of the program (FRAC, 1997).

The Special Supplemental Program for Women, Infants, and Children (WIC)

WIC was established by Congress as a pilot program in 1972 and authorized as a national program in 1975. WIC is a federally funded, preventive nutrition program that provides nutritious foods, nutrition education, and access to health care to low-income pregnant women, new mothers, and infants and children at nutritional risk. The WIC program appropriation in fiscal year 1997 was $3.7 billion, which the USDA estimated would serve approximately 7.4 million participants (FRAC, 1997).

The Expanded Food and Nutrition Education Program (EFNEP)

EFNEP is administered by the Cooperative State Research Education and Extension Service of the U.S. Department of Agriculture, in cooperation with state Cooperative Extension Services in the 55 U.S. states and territories. In 1968, EFNEP was federally initiated by the USDA Extension Service with $10 million (from Section 32 of An Act to Amend the Agricultural Adjustment Act). In 1970, EFNEP received funding under the Smith-Lever Act; in 1977, under the Food and Agriculture Act; and in 1981, under the Agriculture and Food Act.

Since the program's inception, EFNEP paraprofessionals have taught limited-resource families how to improve dietary practices and become more effective managers of their available resources. The paraprofessionals provide intensive nutrition education to individuals and groups in a variety of nonformal education settings, including homes, community centers, housing complexes, WIC offices, and churches.

While EFNEP is not a food-assistance program, it is an effective educational program with a mission to reduce food insecurity. EFNEP teaching is tailored to the needs, interests, financial resources, age, ethnic backgrounds, and learning capabilities of participants.

EFNEP's objectives are to improve diets and nutritional welfare for the total family; to increase knowledge of the essentials of human nutrition; to increase the ability to select and buy food that satisfies nutritional needs; to improve practices in food production, storage, preparation, safety, and sanitation; to increase ability to manage food budgets and related resources such as food stamps.

Personal Responsibility and Work Opportunity Reconciliation Act of 1996

The Personal Responsibility and Work Opportunity Reconciliation Act of 1996 (PRWORA) is the most comprehensive welfare reform program since the Social Security Act of the 1930s. The PRWORA has far-reaching implications in a number of programs. The act fundamentally reforms the Food Stamp Program, Supplemental Security Income (SST) for children, the Child Support Enforcement Program, and benefits for legal immigrants. The act modifies the child nutrition programs and provides cuts in the Social Service Block Grants (SSBG).

The act features decreases in funding for programs for low-income children and families and requires structural changes in the Aid to Families with Dependent Children (AFDC) program. The act converts AFDC and Job Opportunities and Basic Skills (JOBS) into the Temporary Assistance to Needy Families (TANF) block grant. Family assistance is limited to 5 years, while granting states the option to limit assistance for a shorter time period.

The PRWORA significantly reduced funding for food assistance programs and represented a sharp reversal from

Hunger and the broader issue of food security have been a public concern in the United States since our nation's inception.

the trends of the early 1990s. This 1996 legislation contains numerous, significant structural changes to the Food Stamp Program, public assistance programs in general, to the Summer Food Program, and the Child and Adult Care Food Program. Start-up and expansion funds for the School Breakfast and Summer Food Programs were eliminated by this legislation. Entire classes of people have been eliminated from eligibility for the Food Stamp Program. For example, unemployed, childless individuals aged 18 to 50 years can receive food for only 3 of every 36 months.

strengthen the array of food assistance programs in place. The benefits of food assistance programs such as Food Stamps, WIC, School Breakfast Program, and the Summer Food Service Program have not been fully realized because a large percentage of eligible households are not participating. Barriers exist that prevent those needing and wanting assistance from receiving the services. Little research has been conducted that identifies the barriers and possible methods to reduce them. Extensive needs assessment, which includes addressing the social diagnosis phase

tion programs offered through the Food Stamp Program, EFNEP, and WIC need to be enhanced and adequately funded to meet the needs of all low-income families and youth. Family and consumer scientists have a direct role in the provision of innovative nutrition education targeted at health promotion and disease prevention. Professionals serve as advocates to provide support for public policy and legislation that promotes cost-effective food assistance programs that require nutrition education for participants.

Up to one fifth of America's food goes to waste each year, with an estimated 130 pounds of food per person ending up in landfills.

Cuts in food assistance programs are likely to cause an increase in hunger and food insecurity. State and local governments and private charities, enlisted to make up for federal cutbacks and budget restraints, are increasingly unable to shoulder the burden. Many states, in financial crisis, have previously made severe cuts in human services programs.

RECOMMENDATIONS AND IMPLICATIONS FOR FAMILY AND CONSUMER SCIENTISTS

The physical, psychological, social, and economic tolls of food insecurity are both interconnected and interdependent. While important work has been conducted to redefine and clarify terms related to hunger and food security, redefinition of the solution to food insecurity is needed.

Family and consumer scientists understand the complexity of food security issues and their interrelatedness with other social, economic, and environmental problems that affect the individual, the family, and society.

Strengthen the Safety Net

The most immediate and direct way to reduce hunger and food insecurity is to

of Green and Kreuter's PRECEDE-PROCEED planning framework (1991) is needed. Social diagnosis allows the researcher to determine the target population's perceptions of its own needs or quality of life through multiple information-gathering activities. There are only a few methodologies that allow the emic point of view emphasized in social diagnosis. The focus group method provides an ideal venue for eliciting emic data, and it is proven to be effective in collecting this type of information (Dignan, 1995). Family and consumer scientists can work to increase awareness, identify barriers through focus group techniques, and make recommendations to policy makers and program directors on ways to reduce barriers to participation.

Education

The importance of education in resolving the food security issue has been recognized by researchers as well as policy makers. Education is necessary to elicit changes in behavior that will lead to improved food security. While nutrition and family food economics education is provided by some states as a part of the food assistance programs, it is not a mandatory component of all of the available programs. The nutrition educa-

Food Recovery

Food recovery is a creative way to decrease hunger in America. It supplements the federal food assistance programs by making better use of a food source that already exists. Up to one fifth of America's food goes to waste each year, with an estimated 130 pounds of food per person ending up in landfills. The annual value of this wasted food is approximately $31 billion. It is estimated that about 49 million people could have been fed by these lost resources (USDA, 1996).

Food recovery is the collection of wholesome food for distribution to those who are hungry. Gleaning, the gathering of food after harvest, dates back to biblical times. Today the terms gleaning and food recovery cover a variety of different efforts. Gleaning refers to the collection of crops from farmers' fields that have been mechanically harvested or from fields where it is not economically profitable to harvest. Food rescue refers to the collection of perishable food from wholesale and retail stores, and prepared and processed food from the food processors and food service industry. Family and consumer scientists can actively support and participate in food recovery programs. They can assist diverse agencies and community-based groups to work together to establish local hunger programs, administer food-recovery programs, and coordinate gleaning efforts. Family and consumer scientists provide a national network of practical science-based knowledge; an important contribution may be education and training for recipients, staff, and volunteers working with food recovery. Information may be provided on food preparation and handling, nutrition, food preservation and safety, dietary guidance, and balanced meal planning.

Cost Effectiveness Analysis and Impact Assessment

The cost effectiveness of food assistance programs must be assessed so that program directors can modify the programs to best meet the needs of those receiving benefits. Family and consumer scientists are positioned to conduct or participate in research on the cost effectiveness of food assistance programs, to assist in the evaluation of nutrition education programs designed to alleviate food insecurity, and to monitor the effects of welfare reform in their communities.

The PRWORA is in its early stages of implementation, and scholars and policy makers have not assessed its impact on welfare recipients. Examination of how the PRWORA and subsequent changes in policies and programs affect food security is important research. Assessment of the impacts of PRWORA implementation on food security of families and children will provide a better understanding of program benefits as well as adverse effects on those in poverty. This information is crucial for program planning and management. These issues are very important in making public policy decisions that address the food security problems associated with poverty.

Public Issues Education

Public policy shapes and directs actions to achieve defined societal goals. It may be adopted and implemented formally through government action or adopted informally through common practice and assumptions. Public policy provides direction for personal and group behavior based on values and beliefs as well as government and economic systems. Public policy decisions affect food security and nutritional well-being of the population. There is a need for broad public participation in policy decisions that affect food security. Family and consumer scientists can assist communities in this process through building societal capacity to understand and address this critical issue. The democratic political process works when citizens believe that they have sufficient power to negotiate for their own rights and interests. As people develop their public leadership skills and gain access to information, they are better able to achieve food security for themselves and their communities. Family and consumer scientists can facilitate a greater awareness and understanding of the food security situation in communities throughout the nation.

SUMMARY

Despite all the programs implemented and legislation designed to reduce poverty and its consequences, hunger and food insecurity will continue to be critical issues in the next century. Hunger and food insecurity have serious, complex effects. Clearly, new approaches are necessary to achieve long-term food security in our communities.

Family and Consumer Science professionals can work for policy changes that would increase cost effectiveness and decrease barriers to participation in food assistance programs, provide intensified education about hunger, and help to shape public policy at the local, state, and national levels. Aggressive action is needed to bring an end to hunger and to achieve food security for all citizens.

References

Breglio, V. J. (1992). *Hunger in America: The voter's perspective.* Lanham, MD: Research/Strategy/Management (RMS).

Center for Hunger, Poverty and Nutrition Policy. (1993). *The link between nutrition and cognitive development in children.* Medford, MA: Tufts University.

Clancy, K. L., & Bowering, J. (1992). The need for emergency food: Poverty problems and policy responses. *J Nutr Ed., 24,* 12S–17S.

Codispoti, C. L., & Bartlett, B. J. (1994). *Food and nutrition for life: Malnutrition and older Americans.* Washington, DC: National Aging Information Center. (Publication No. NAIC–12).

Dignan, M. B. (1995). *Measurement and evaluation of health education.* Springfield, IL: C. C. Thomas Publisher.

Egan, M. (1980). Public health nutrition services: Issues today and tomorrow. *JADA, 77,* 423–427.

Federation of American Societies for Experiment Biology, Life Sciences Research Office. (1995). *Third Report on nutrition monitoring in the United States.* Washington, DC: U.S. Government Printing Office.

Fomon, S. J. (1993). *Normal nutrition of infants.* St. Louis, MO: Mosby.

Food Research and Action Center (FRAC). (1991). *Community Childhood Hunger Identification Project: A survey of childhood hunger in the United States.* Washington, DC.

Food Research and Action Center (FRAC). (1997). *Community Childhood Hunger Identification Project: A survey of childhood hunger in the United States.* Washington, DC.

Green, L. W., & Kreuter, M. W. (1991). *Health promotion planning: An educational and environmental approach* (2nd ed.). Mountain View, CA: Mayfield.

Hamilton, W. L., Cook, J. T., Thompson, W. W., Buron, L. F., Frongillo, E. A., Olson, D. M., & Wehler, C. A. (1997). *Household food security in the United States in 1995.* Washington, DC: U.S. Department of Agriculture Food and Consumer Service.

Joy, A. B., & Doisy, C. (1996). Food stamp nutrition education program: Assisting food stamp recipients to become self-sufficient. *J Nutr Ed., 28,* 123–126.

Klein, B. W. (1996). Food security and hunger measures: Promising future for state and local household surveys. *Family Econ Nutr Rev., 9,* 31–37.

U.S. Department of Agriculture. (1989). *Nationwide Food Consumption Survey, continuing survey of food intakes by individuals, low income women 19–50 years and their children, 1–5 years, 4 days.* (NFCF, CSFII Report 85-4). Hyattsville, MD: U.S. Government Printing Office.

U.S. Department of Agriculture. (1996). *A citizen's guide to food recovery.* Washington, DC: U.S. Government Printing Office.

U.S. Department of Health and Human Services. (1994). *Healthy People 2000 review 1993.* (DHHS Publication No. PHS 94-1232-1). Hyattsville, MD: U.S. Government Printing Office.

Uvin, P. (1994). The state of world hunger. *Nutr Rev., 52,* 151–1161.

Voichick, J., & Drake, L. T. (1994). Major stages of U.S. Food and Nutrition Policy Development Related to Food Security. *In: Food security in the United States: A guidebook for public issues education.* Washington, DC: USDA Cooperative Extension System.

Wehler, C. A., Scott, R. I., & Anderson, J. J. (1996). *The Community Childhood Hunger Identification Project: A survey of childhood hunger in the United States.* Washington, DC: Food Research and Action Center.

World Hunger Year. (1994). *Reinvesting in America: Hunger and poverty wheel.* New York: Reinvesting in America.

Nutrition and Infection: Malnutrition and Mortality in Public Health

Gro Harlem Brundtland, M.D., M.P.H.

Dr. Brundtland is the Director-General of the World Health Organization, CH-1211, Geneva, Switzerland. This paper was originally presented in a slightly different form as an address.

Earlier this century a number of eminent nutrition scientists recognized that nutrition deficiency, particularly with respect to vitamin A, was likely to be responsible for a large number of infectious conditions, but the biological mechanisms were entirely unknown. Thirty-one years ago, WHO published a historic monograph by Scrimshaw, Taylor, and Gorden that comprehensively reviewed the slowly mounting evidence of the interaction of nutrition and infection. This review marked a decisive turning point in research, epidemiologic investigation, and the management of malnutrition and infectious disease.

An important implication of this work is that, by working together—in science, in policy formulation and implementation, in nutrition and in infectious diseases, and in health and economic development—we are likely to raise the quality of life more than we do by working independently. In partnership, we can achieve more than we can separately.

In repeating this message today, I would like to give you a number of concrete examples, and look to a future where these partnerships must be routinely created because there is still much work to be done.

The combination of malnutrition and infectious disease is deadly. Separately, the effect of each is huge. Together, their impact is far greater than the sum of their parts. Both are conditions of poverty. They arise from poverty and they keep people in poverty, not just for one generation, but for many generations.

In a well-nourished child, a common infectious disease is usually a passing illness. In a malnourished child, the same disease can precipitate life-long disabilities such as blindness. A rapid sequence of common infection and malnutrition too often leads to death.

A slow sequence of disease followed by malnutrition leads to stunting and wasting, and affects mental development, decisively handicapping the affected millions that do not die. The survivors have special difficulties in terms of their cognitive and physical development. Their handicap, though invisible, is lasting. And when they reach adulthood, they are less productive and they earn less.

The malnutrition-infection complex is a drain on human resources. One condition aggravates the other. Infections lead to malnutrition, and malnutrition exacerbates infections, increasing their duration and severity. A look at the figures for each condition helps us to understand the true magnitude of this interaction.

Worldwide, infectious diseases kill approximately 10 million children each year before they reach the age of 5. Fifty percent of these deaths are associated with malnutrition. Seven of 10 of these deaths are due to diarrheal diseases, pneumonia, malaria, and measles, in combination with malnutrition. This is not counting tuberculosis, intestinal parasitic infestations, and HIV—which also comprise huge numbers in terms of ill-health and death—and are also associated with malnutrition.

Globally, children who are poorly nourished have up to 160 days of illness each year, with 3–4 episodes of diarrhea and 4–5 illnesses owing to severe respiratory infections. They often come from large poor families whose mothers are not well educated, who have, or will have, many dependent children, who themselves are not well nourished, and who produce low-birth-weight infants. Such women are themselves likely to have been born with low birth weight; their time and energy are stretched to the limit.

A large proportion of the world's population is affected by at least one of the several major forms of malnutrition. I am referring to low-birth-weight infants, wasted and stunted children, people who are brain-damaged from iodine deficiency, pre-schoolers who die or become blind from vitamin A deficiency and who are intellectually impaired as a result of iron deficiency, mothers who die in childbirth because of anemia, and the large numbers of malnourished elderly who are largely overlooked. This is how malnutrition kills, maims, cripples, blinds, and retards, thereby impairing human and national development on a massive scale.

Now, let us examine the interaction of malnutrition and infectious disease. Malnutrition magnifies the effect of disease. A malnourished person has more severe disease episodes, more complications, and spends more time ill for each episode.

Because they aggravate one another, we cannot partition deaths into those owing to malnutrition and those owing to infection. In any population, the impact of malnutrition depends on the prevalence of infection, and the impact on infection—in terms of severity and duration—depends upon the nutrition base. Both need to be vigorously tackled.

Historically, despite its magnitude and obvious importance for morality, the prevention and management of malnutrition took a back seat, both clinically and programmatically, to the prevention and management of infectious diseases. Clinicians in developing countries still find it much easier to deal with diarrhea, pneumonia, measles, or tuberculosis than to mange severe protein-energy malnutrition. In many health-care centers there is still a 30% mortality rate in children with severe malnutrition, compared with only 5% in those receiving proper management. Similarly, in developing countries, most national health services pour resources into combating communicable diseases, whereas relatively meager resources are fed into national nutrition programs. Yet, where malnutrition prevails, the incidence of infectious disease, and its associated mortality, remains high.

Death rates increase exponentially with the degree of malnutrition. We have consistently found this to be so in all countries for which data are available. Any deterioration in nutrition status carries with it an increased risk of death. Thus, a severely malnourished child is 11 times more likely to die than a well-nourished child, a moderately malnourished child is 3 times more at risk of death, and a mildly malnourished child is twice as likely to die than a well-nourished child.

This reality has serious policy implications. The volume of malnutrition globally is in the mild and moderate category. And as long as half or greater (45–83%) of all malnutrition-related deaths occur to children in the mild to moderate category, we need to focus on this group. We shall not be making a dent in mortality if our policies and programs focus only on the severely malnourished.

It is true that there are many children who are severely malnourished but we need to think on a still broader front. For every child that is severely malnourished, there are many more who are moderately or mildly malnourished. Indeed, this is precisely how all severely malnourished children started out! Severe malnutrition is but the tip of an exceedingly great iceberg. We need to pay attention to the base. And we can expect to achieve the greatest impact by tackling the base.

Poor nutrition, however, is not the whole story. The more infectious disease there is in a population, the higher the death rate at any level of malnutrition; the bigger the burden of disease, the bigger the iceberg. This has profound policy implications. It means that we can reduce deaths by improving nutrition and we can reduce deaths by reducing infection but the greatest impact is likely to be achieved by addressing both at the same time.

Malnutrition, however, should be regarded as not just a single disease, but a range of conditions, many life-threatening or irreversibly disabling, resulting from an imbalance in availability or use of nutrients. Poverty and lack of education, which are so often the effects of underdevelopment, are usually the primary causes of hunger and malnutrition. There are poor people in most societies who do not have adequate access to food, care, safe water and sanitation, health services, and education. All of these are basic requirements for proper nutrition, and they require both short-term and long-term sustainable solutions and strategies.

There are several critical strategic approaches of proven effectiveness for preventing, reducing, and eliminating malnutrition. Whereas not all approaches are the primary mandate, the health sector has the overall leadership role in combating malnutrition. This is most likely because of its unique diagnostic contribution in assessing, measuring, and monitoring the different forms of malnutrition and alerting other sectors to its magnitude, trends, consequences, and the population groups affected.

These strategies include incorporating nutrition objectives into national development policies and programs; ensuring household food security, including food and nutrition as a human right; preventing and managing infectious diseases; promoting breastfeeding; caring for the socioeconomically deprived and nutritionally vulnerable; preventing and eliminating micronutrient malnutrition; promoting healthful diets and lifestyles; and assessing, analyzing, and monitoring nutrition status. Not all of these are completely or primarily within the domain of the health sector. However, they all affect health and nutrition well-being. This means that we must look outside of our sector and into other sectors that affect our goals in order to make the difference.

There are three major areas on which I would focus. The first is pregnancy and early nutrition. The sequence that begins with fetal malnutrition and results in a low-birth-weight baby is well known. One-third of low-birth-weight babies are moderately and severely malnourished by 6 months of age, and half are malnourished by 1 year. The poorer the start babies have in life, the more likely they are to become sick and malnourished and to die.

The antecedent of the sick malnourished child is low birth weight. Low birth weight results from pregnancies that are too short, too close together, too many, or too long. Pregnancies that are too close together do the most damage, especially among teenage or young mothers. Births that are spaced too closely do not give time for mothers to recover. Those who have not recovered cannot provide adequate nutrition for their fetus and fetal growth is retarded.

To improve the nutrition status of children, we must give them a healthy start. We must increase birth spacing and the rate of exclusive early breastfeeding of infants. We must ensure that mothers are adequately nourished before and during pregnancy.

A special issue in pregnancy is anemia. The prevalence of anemia in pregnant women is high: 63% in Africa, 80% in South Asia, and 30% in Latin America. It is increased when the mother lives in a malaria-endemic area, and is pregnant for the first time. Severe anemia in pregnancy is a major obstetric problem in malaria-endemic areas and a primary cause of maternal morbidity and mortality. The risk for underweight babies is twice as high in a malaria-endemic area as for an area without malaria. Five hundred million people live in malaria-endemic areas. Stillbirths are more common there as is the risk for miscarriage. Half of the pregnant women who develop cerebral malaria die.

One of the most important factors in reducing child deaths and the vicious cycle between nutrition, infection, and poverty is female education and literacy. Female education determines infant (and child) health and is statistically more significant than rural-urban differentials, income differentials, or ethnic origin.

Malnutrition and infection in children is the outcome of poverty, ignorance, and, among other factors, high-risk pregnancies. The responsibility for improving them lies with those dealing with economic development, education, social affairs, and agriculture, as well as with health. We need to be able to convince those dealing with education and economic development that their efforts affect health outcomes. To do this we must be backed by evidence.

The evidence can only come from interventions that are undertaken on a large enough scale to measure impact and that are done well enough to be generally applicable. Armed with such convincing evidence, we need to ensure that food and nutrition objectives are adequately incorporated into national development policies and programs. We need to ensure that sustainable improvement of nutrition and health, particularly of the most deprived and vulnerable population groups, goes hand in hand with permanent reduction of poverty and sustainable national development.

The role of health in development has been underestimated. The role of economic development in health is also underestimated. Poverty, poor female education, and rapid birth spacing give babies a poor start in life. A healthy start makes good economic sense.

The second point is related to repairing immune function. One of the most important interventions in interrupting the link between malnutrition and infection is the use of vitamin A supplementation. Since the 1920s we knew that an important function of vitamin A is its ability to repair immune function, and that the body is unable to properly resist infection without this micronutrient. Vitamin A supplementation is therefore a crucial immediate intervention that can break the malnutrition-infection complex in areas where vitamin A deficiency is prevalent. By increasing resistance to infection, it reduces case fatality rates when the infection does occur, as in diarrheal disease and measles.

Large supplementation trials show that routine vitamin A supplements given between 6–72 months of age can reduce overall mortality by at least 23% where vitamin A deficiency exists in a population. The impact of this single supplementation on childhood mortality is therefore as great as, or greater than, that of any single vaccine and it only costs a couple of cents per dose. Given to breastfeeding mothers postpartum, it protects infants from vitamin A deficiency.

The combined approach to nutrition and infection has achieved more. In the last 3 years we established that a combination of the two most cost-effective tools, vitamin A supplementation and vaccines, achieves more than the sum of their benefits. An example of the power of this combined approach is the case of the measles vaccine and vitamin A.

The measles vaccine, developed in the 1960s, is safe and effective, and provides long lasting immunity to measles infection. The priority target group for protection against vitamin A deficiency and measles is the same: infants and young children of poor families living in overcrowded housing who are already at risk of malnutrition.

Measles infection claimed 7–8 million of these lives per year before the vaccine became available. Measles causes loss of vitamin A, frequently precipitating acute vitamin A deficiency and blindness. Of children who become blind, half die within one year. Measles also leads to long-term complications including deafness, chronic lung disease, poor growth, and recurrent infections. Given the measles vaccine at approximately 9 months of age with vitamin A enables infants to receive both interventions for the addition of only a few cents per child.

Today, approximately 900,000 infants die from measles each year. These deaths are preventable. When vitamin A is introduced as part of measles management, the case fatality rate can be reduced by greater than 50%.

Last year, of those countries classified by WHO as having clinical signs or severe, moderate, or mild subclinical symptoms of vitamin A deficiency, over 40 countries administered vitamin A with their National Immunization Day vaccines. Now, many other countries include vitamin A in their routine immunization services.

We must also be clear that the ultimate battle to reduce and eliminate vitamin A deficiency and effectively combat malnutrition will not and cannot be won simply through short-term interventions such as providing vitamin A supplements, nor through clinic and hospital-based improved management systems, even though these are important and effective for saving lives.

These short-term interventions must be backed up by long-term enduring sustainable solutions to vitamin A deficiency and malnutrition in general. These include food-based dietary approaches, breastfeeding, appropriate complementary feeding, and fortification of appropriate foods with vitamin A.

The third area in which we can make a difference is iron supplementation. The nutrition science community is no doubt aware of the importance placed upon rolling back malaria. The effect of this disease upon iron status was, until recently, unquantified. Iron deficiency is, of course, the most common nutrition disorder in the world, affecting more than 1 billion people, particularly reproductive women and preschool children in tropical areas. Uncorrected, it leads to severe anemia, reduced work capacity, diminished learning ability, increased susceptibility to infection, and increased risk of death associated with pregnancy and childbirth.

Because the adverse affects of iron deficiency are preventable, iron supplementation has been WHO's policy in all areas where there is iron deficiency, except in malaria-endemic areas. In areas where there is malaria, efforts were hampered by conflicting evidence on the effects of iron deficiency (some studies show that iron supplementation triggers latent malaria or increases severe malaria episodes). As a result of this controversy, which has prevented the 500 million people in malaria-endemic areas with iron deficiency anemia from obtaining iron supplementation, WHO funded a study to establish whether or not iron supplementation increased risk of malaria or protected against severe iron deficiency anemia.

These results are now well known. Iron supplementation protects a child who is at high risk of dying from severe anemia in the first 2 years of life. However, antimalarial prophylaxis protects against severe anemia much more. The work, published recently, has provided us with evidence that malaria is the single largest contributor to the etiology of severe iron deficiency anemia in malaria-endemic areas.

In short, in areas of intense malaria transmission, reducing malaria makes more of a difference than iron supplementation in preventing severe anemia. By rolling back malaria, a major cause of iron deficiency anemia will be removed.

There is so much more that could be said in examining the nutrition-infection relationship and exploring its implications for public health policy. The World Health Organization is committed to reducing the mortality caused by malnutrition and infectious diseases. The impact we are likely to achieve to give children a healthy nutrition start in life is not likely to be made through the health sector alone. Solid evidence of strategies that are as good for health as for development is needed, as are the price tag and the impact.

We have a greater chance of making a difference, of getting programs implemented, when the benefits and costs are apparent to all the stakeholders. We depend upon evidence not only on the nutrition and health cost/benefit relationship of a program, but projections of these calculations into broader benefits for the economy. Making every child a wanted child, a healthier child, a more productive child and adult, through female education and better birth spacing, has implications for human development as well as for economic growth.

I count on the scientific community to join forces with the World Health Organization in this task, so that together we can make a difference.

Linking Environment and Health:
Malnutrition

Poverty—not insufficient global food production—is the root cause of malnutrition. Poor families lack the economic, environmental, or social resources to purchase or produce enough food. In rural areas, land scarcity and degradation, water salinity due to overirrigation, soil erosion, droughts, and flooding can all undermine a family's ability to grow enough food. In urban areas, low wages, lack of work and underemployment, and rapid changes in food prices often place food supplies out of the reach of poor households. War and civil strife almost always cause upheaval in the food system and often result in widespread famine, as with the civil wars in Rwanda and Somalia.

Although overall trends are positive, with the proportion of people with malnutrition declining, many remain at risk, and some regions are hit especially hard. Between 1990 and 1992, approximately 841 million people—or 1 out of every 5 people in the developing world—did not have access to enough food for healthy living.[1]

The health consequences of inadequate nutrition are enormous. According to one estimate, malnutrition contributed to roughly 12 percent of all deaths in 1990.[2] Although much of this toll stems from underconsumption of protein and energy, deficiencies in key micronutrients such as iodine, vitamin A, and iron also undermine health.[3]

When poverty limits an adequate and varied diet, deficiencies of iron, iodine, and vitamin A often occur simultaneously with protein-energy malnutrition. Geography and soil characteristics also influence the amount of these nutrients commonly found in food. Mountainous areas are often deficient in iodine; the most severely deficient regions are the Himalayas, Andes, European alps, and mountains of China.[4] Areas with arid, infertile land or heavy rainfall and humidity may be deficient in vitamin A.[5] Africa, the Andean region of South America, and many parts of Asia are at risk from not only protein energy malnutrition, but also from all three main micronutrient deficiencies because of both poverty and environmental factors.

Iron deficiency is the most common micronutrient disorder. In developing countries, 40 percent of nonpregnant women and 50 percent of pregnant women are anemic, and 3.6 billion people suffer from iron deficiencies.[6] The problem is most severe in India, where 88 percent of pregnant women are anemic. Anemia increases the risk of death from hemorrhage in childbirth. Iron deficiencies can also reduce physical productivity and affect a child's capacity to learn.[7]

Globally, some 42 million children under age 6 have mild to moderate vitamin A deficiency. In its severe form, vitamin A deficiency can cause blindness; indeed, it is the single most important cause of childhood blindness in developing countries. About 250,000 to 300,000 children go blind annually, and 50 to 80 percent of those die within 1 year.[8] Up to 3 million more children suffer lesser but still serious effects, such as loss of night vision. An estimated 254 million children of preschool age are at risk of vitamin A deficiency.[9]

Iodine deficiency is the world's leading single cause of preventable brain damage and mental retardation. In 1990, some 26 million people suffered from brain damage associated with iodine deficiency.[10] An estimated 1.5 billion people are at risk of iodine deficiency disorders (IDD), and 655 million people are affected by goiter, which is the enlargement of the thyroid gland, an indicator of IDD.[11] Where this deficiency is endemic, the entire population may be affected, with different symptoms appearing in different age groups. In pregnant women, for instance, iodine deficiency may cause irreversible brain damage in the developing fetus.[12]

The combination of malnutrition and infectious disease can be particularly pernicious. Protein-energy malnutrition can impair the immune system, leaving malnourished children less able to battle common diseases such as measles, diarrhea, respiratory infections, tuberculosis, pertussis, and malaria. Vitamin A deficiencies are often worsened by infectious disease; and reciprocally, poor vitamin A status is likely to prolong or exacerbate the course of an illness such as measles.[13] Similarly, malaria parasites, which require iron in order to multiply in blood, can cause or exacerbate anemia.[14] Malnutrition can also heighten the adverse impacts of toxic substances. Deficiencies of pro-

Fron World Resources Institute Washington. D.C. 1998–1999. Reprinted by permission.

tein and some minerals, for example, can significantly influence the absorption of lead and cadmium into the body.[15,16]

The consequences of food and nutrition shortfalls are enormous. Africa and Southeast Asia confront problems of both malnutrition and such diseases as diarrhea, malaria, and measles—a combination that is likely to increase the toll that either problem would take alone. In rapidly industrializing cities with high levels of malnutrition as well as disease and growing industrial pollution, residents may confront a triple burden of malnutrition, infection, and toxic pollution.

References and Notes

1. Food and Agriculture Organization of the United Nations (FAO), *The Sixth World Food Survey* (FAO, Rome, 1996), pp. v–vi.
2. Christopher J.L. Murray and Alan D. Lopez, eds. *The Global Burden of Disease: Volume 1* (World Health Organization, Harvard School of Public Health, and The World Bank, Geneva, 1996), p. 311.
3. The World Bank, *World Development Report 1993: Investing in Health* (The World Bank, Washington, D.C., 1993), p. 75.
4. World Health Organization (WHO), United Nations Children's Fund (UNICEF), and the International Council for the Control of Iodine Deficiency Disorders, "Global Prevalence of Iodine Deficiency Disorders," Micronutrient Deficiency Information System Working Paper No. 1 (WHO, Geneva, 1993), p. 7.
5. World Health Organization (WHO) and the United Nations Children's Fund (UNICEF), "Global Prevalence of Vitamin A Deficiency," Micronutrient Deficiency Information System Working Paper No. 2 (WHO, Geneva, 1995), p. 5.
6. World Health Organization (WHO), *The World Health Report 1997: Conquering Suffering, Enriching Humanity* (WHO, Geneva, 1997), p. 51.
7. Op. cit. 3.
8. Henry M. Levin *et al.*, "Micronutrient Deficiency Disorders," in *Disease Control Priorities in Developing Countries*, Dean T. Jamison *et al.*, eds. (Oxford University Press, New York, 1993), p. 424.
9. *Op. cit.* 5, pp. ix, 16.
10. *Op. cit.* 4, pp. 5, 8.
11. *Op. cit.* 4, p. 5.
12. *Op. cit.* 4, p. 5.
13. Andrew Tomkins and Fiona Watson, *Malnutrition and Infection: A Review* (United Nations Administrative Committee on Coordination/Subcommittee on Nutrition, WHO, Geneva, 1989), pp. 5–6.
14. *Ibid.*, p. 7.
15. Howard Hu, Sudha Kotha, and Troyen Brennan, "The Role of Nutrition in Mitigating Environmental Insults: Policy and Ethical Issues," *Environmental Health Perspectives*, Vol. 103, Supplement No. 6 (1995), p. 186.
16. Kathryn R. Mahaffey, "Nutrition and Lead: Strategies for Public Health," *Environmental Health Perspectives*, Vol. 103, Supplement No. 6 (1995), p. 193.

AGRICULTURAL GROWTH, POVERTY ALLEVIATION, AND ENVIRONMENTAL SUSTAINABILITY: Having It All

by Peter Hazell

Many developing countries have achieved impressive growth rates in agriculture in recent decades. Asia, for example, was threatened by hunger and mass starvation in the 1960s but is now self-sufficient in staple foods, even though its population has more than doubled. Despite this success, serious concerns remain for the future. Hunger and malnutrition persist in many countries, often because past patterns of agricultural growth were insufficient or failed to adequately benefit the poor. Expected increases in agricultural demand associated with population growth and rising per capita incomes will require continuing increases in agricultural productivity, although evidence indicates that yield growth is slowing and prospects for further expansion of cropped and irrigated areas are limited. And environmental problems associated with agriculture could, if not checked, threaten future levels of agricultural productivity and impose severe health and environmental costs at the national and international levels.

Continued agricultural growth is a necessity, not an option, for most developing countries. But this growth must not jeopardize the underlying natural resource base or impose costly externalities on others. It must also be equitable if it is to help alleviate poverty and food insecurity. These three goals—agricultural growth, poverty alleviation, and environmental sustainability—are not necessarily complementary, and achieving all three simultaneously cannot be taken for granted. Although much depends on the specific social, economic, and agroecological circumstances, a high degree of complementarity is more likely to be achieved when agricultural development is (1) broadly based and involves small- and medium-sized farms, (2) market driven, (3) participatory and decentralized, and (4) driven by technological change that enhances factor productivity but does not degrade the resource base. Such growth can reduce food prices while increasing farm incomes; is employment intensive; and increases the effective demand for nonfood goods and services, particularly in small towns and market centers. By reducing poverty and promoting economic diversification in rural areas, it also relieves livelihood demands on the natural resource base.

THE FIVE I'S FOR AGRICULTURAL GROWTH

The requirements for broad-based agricultural development are reasonably well understood and should not be forgotten in the contemporary quest for environmental sustainability. Since they are so important, they are briefly reviewed here.

Back in the 1950s and 1960s, policymakers and agricultural development experts were primarily interested in growth, and the lessons that emerged from that experience can be summarized as the five I's for agricultural growth.

Innovation. Strong national agricultural research and extension systems (both public and private) to generate and disseminate productivity-enhancing technologies.

Infrastructure, particularly good road and transport systems.

Inputs. Efficient delivery systems for agricultural services, especially for modern farm inputs, agroprocessing, irrigation water, and credit.

Institutions. Efficient, liberalized markets that provide farmers with ready access to domestic and international markets and effective public institutions to provide key services where these cannot be developed to the private sector.

Incentives. Conducive macro, trade, and sector policies that do not penalize agriculture.

EQUITY MODIFIERS: HOW AGRICULTURAL DEVELOPMENT CAN REDUCE POVERTY

In the 1970s and 1980s, policymakers and development experts began to focus on ways of using agricultural development to reduce poverty and food security as well as contribute to growth. The lessons that emerged from that era can be summed up in six "equity modifiers" to agricultural growth:

1. Promote broad-based agricultural development. There are few economies of scale in agricultural production in developing countries (unlike processing and marketing). Hence, targeting family farms is attractive on both equity and efficiency grounds. But small- and medium-sized farms must receive priority in publicly funded agricultural research and extension and in marketing, credit, and input supplies.

2. Undertake land reforms, where necessary. Such reforms, particularly market-assisted redistribution programs, may be needed where productive land is too narrowly concentrated among large farms.

3. Invest in human capital, such as rural education, clean water, health, family planning, and nutrition programs, to improve the productivity of poor people and increase their opportunities for gainful employment.

4. Ensure that agricultural extension and education, as well as credit and small business assistance programs, reach rural women, since women play a key role in farming and ancillary activities.

5. Let all rural stakeholders (not just the rich and powerful) participate in setting priorities for public investments that they expect to benefit from or to help finance.

6. Actively encourage the rural nonfarm economy. It is not only an important

From *Brief 59,* March 1999: © International Food Policy Research Institute. Reprinted by permission.

source of income and employment in rural areas, especially for the poor, but it benefits from powerful income and employment multipliers when agriculture grows. In many countries, these potential multiplier effects are constrained by investment codes and related legislation that discriminate against small, rural nonfarm firms.

ENVIRONMENTAL MODIFIERS FOR SUSTAINABLE AGRICULTURAL DEVELOPMENT

The new priority of environmental sustainability that has emerged in the 1990s does not negate the need for agriculture to continue to contribute to growth, poverty alleviation, and increased food security; it is just that agriculture is now required to accomplish all of these in ways that do not degrade the environment. In addition to the five I's and the six equity modifiers (there are no shortcuts here), eight environmental modifiers are now required for sustainable agricultural development. These modifiers have yet to be fully worked out and tested through development experience. In many ways the process is still at the research and design stage.

1. Give higher priority to backward regions in agricultural development, even though many of these may be resource poor. Considering the rapid population growth and limited nonfarm opportunities, agricultural growth is the only viable means of meeting the food and livelihood needs of growing populations in many backward areas for the next few decades. Failure to do so will lead to excessive outmigration, which will add to the problems of already overloaded urban slums. It will also lead to worsening poverty and further degradation of hillsides, forests, and soils. The development of backward regions will require additional re-

sources for agricultural development, not diversion of resources from favorably endowed agricultural regions, where productivity increases are still important.
2. Pay more attention in agricultural research to sustainability features of recommended technologies, to broader aspects of natural resource management at the watershed and landscape levels, and to the problems of resource-poor areas.
3. Ensure that farmers have secure property rights over their resources. This does not necessarily imply that governments should invest in ambitious land registration programs. In many cases (in Sub-Saharan Africa, for example), the indigenous tenure systems still work surprisingly well. They are better able to meet equity needs and to recognize the rights of multiple users than are fully privatized property rights systems.
4. Privatize common property resources, or where this is not desirable (because of externality benefits or for equity reasons), strengthen community management systems.
5. Resolve externality problems through optimal taxes on polluters and degraders, regulation, empowerment of local organizations, or appropriate changes in property rights. But note that free market prices are not always the best; externalities may require optimal tax or subsidy interventions.
6. Improve the performance of relevant public institutions that manage and regulate natural resources (such as irrigation and forestry departments). Devolve management decisions to resource users, or groups of users, wherever possible. This also requires transfer of secure property or use rights.
7. Correct price distortions that encourage excessive use of modern inputs in intensive agriculture. That is, remove subsidies on fertilizers and pesticides and charge the full costs of irrigation water and electricity. It may still be necessary

to subsidize fertilizer in backward regions where current use is low and soil fertility is being mined.
8. Establish resource monitoring systems to track changes in the condition of key resources, educate farmers about the environment effects of their actions, and delineate and protect sites of particular environmental value.

CONCLUSIONS

Past patterns of agricultural growth have sometimes harmed the environment and exacerbated poverty and food insecurity among rural people, even as agriculture has met national food needs and contributed to export earnings. But poverty and environmental degradation are not an inevitable outcome of agricultural growth. Rather, these negative effects reflect inappropriate economic incentives for managing modern inputs in intensive farming systems, insufficient investment in many heavily populated backward areas, inadequate social and poverty concerns, and political systems that are often biased against rural people. With appropriate government policies and investments, institutional development, and agricultural research, there is no reason why agricultural development cannot simultaneously contribute to growth, poverty alleviation, and environmental sustainability.

For more information, see Peter Hazell and Ernst Lutz, "Integrating Environmental and Sustainability Concerns into Rural Development Policies," in *Agriculture and the Environment: Perspectives on Sustainable Rural Development,* ed. Ernst Lutz, with the assistance of Hans Binswanger, Peter Hazell, and Alexander McCalla (Washington, D.C.: World Bank, 1998).

Peter Hazell is director of the Environment and Production Technology Division at the International Food Policy Research Institute.

WILL FRANKENFOOD
FEED THE WORLD?

Genetically modified food has met fierce opposition among well-fed Europeans, but it's the poor and the hungry who need it most

BY BILL GATES

Bill Gates is chairman and chief software architect of Microsoft and co-founder of the Bill and Melinda Gates Foundation

If you want to spark a heated debate at a dinner party, bring up the topic of genetically modified foods. For many people, the concept of genetically altered, high-tech crop production raises all kinds of environmental, health, safety and ethical questions. Particularly in countries with long agrarian traditions—and vocal green lobbies—the idea seems against nature.

In fact, genetically modified foods are already very much a part of our lives. A third of the corn and more than half the soybeans and cotton grown in the U.S. last year were the product of biotechnology, according to the Department of Agriculture. More than 65 million acres of genetically modified crops will be planted in the U.S. this year. The genetic genie is out of the bottle.

Yet there are clearly some very real issues that need to be resolved. Like any new product entering the food chain, genetically modified foods must be subjected to rigorous testing. In wealthy countries, the debate about biotech is tempered by the fact that we have a rich array of foods to choose from—and a supply that far exceeds our needs. In developing countries desperate to feed fast-growing and underfed populations, the issue is simpler and much more urgent: Do the benefits of biotech outweigh the risks?

The statistics on population growth and hunger are disturbing. Last year the world's population reached 6 billion. And by 2050, the U.N. estimates, it will probably near 9 billion. Almost all that growth will occur in developing countries. At the same time, the world's available cultivable land per person is declining. Arable land has declined steadily since 1960 and will decrease by half over the next 50 years, according to the International Service for the Acquisition of Agri-Biotech Applications (ISAAA).

The U.N. estimates that nearly 800 million people around the world are undernourished. The effects are devastating. About 400 million women of childbearing age are iron deficient, which means their babies are exposed to various birth defects. As many as 100 million children suffer from vitamin A deficiency, a leading cause of blindness. Tens of millions of people suffer from other major ailments and nutritional deficiencies caused by lack of food.

How can biotech help? Biotechnologists have developed genetically modified rice that is fortified with beta-carotene—which the body converts into vitamin A—and additional iron, and they are working on other kinds of nutritionally improved crops. Biotech can also improve farming productivity in places where food shortages are caused by crop damage attributable to pests, drought, poor soil and crop viruses, bacteria or fungi.

Damage caused by pests is incredible. The European corn borer, for example, destroys 40 million tons of the world's corn crop annually, about 7% of the total. Incorporating pest-resistant genes into seeds can help restore the balance. In trials of pest-resistant cotton in Africa, yields have increased significantly. So far, fears that genetically modified, pest-resistant crops might kill good insects as well as bad appear unfounded.

Viruses often cause massive failure in staple crops in developing countries. Two years ago, Africa lost more than half its cassava crop—a key source of calories—to the mosaic virus. Genetically modified, virus-resistant crops can reduce that damage, as can drought-tolerant seeds in regions where water shortages limit the amount of land under cultivation. Biotech can also help solve the problem of soil that contains excess aluminum, which can damage roots and cause many staple-crop failures. A gene that helps neutralize aluminum toxicity in rice has been identified.

Many scientists believe biotech could raise overall crop productivity in developing countries as much as 25% and help prevent the loss of those crops after they are harvested.

Yet for all that promise, biotech is far from being the whole answer. In developing countries, lost crops are only one cause of hunger. Poverty plays the largest role. Today more than 1 billion people around the globe live on less than $1 a day. Making genetically modified crops available will not reduce hunger if farmers cannot afford to grow them or if the local population cannot afford to buy the food those farmers produce.

Nor can biotech overcome the challenge of distributing food in developing countries. Taken as a whole, the world produces enough food to feed everyone—but much of it is simply in the wrong place. Especially in countries with undeveloped transport infrastructures, geography restricts food availability as dramatically as genetics promises to improve it.

Biotech has its own "distribution" problems. Private-sector biotech companies in the rich countries carry out much of the leading-edge research on genetically modified crops. Their products are often too costly for poor farmers in the developing world, and many of those products won't even reach the regions where they are most needed. Biotech firms have a strong financial incentive to target rich markets first in order to help them rapidly recoup the high costs of product development. But some of these companies are responding to the needs of poor countries. A London-based company, for example, has announced that it will share with developing countries technology needed to produce vitamin-enriched "golden rice."

More and more biotech research is being carried out in developing countries. But to increase the impact of genetic research on the food production of those countries, there is a need for better collaboration between government agencies—both local and in developed countries—and private biotech firms. The ISAAA, for example, is successfully partnering with the U.S. Agency for International Development, local researchers and private biotech companies to find and deliver biotech solutions for farmers in developing countries.

Will "Frankenfoods" feed the world? Biotech is not a panacea, but it does promise to transform agriculture in many developing countries. If that promise is not fulfilled, the real losers will be their people, who could suffer for years to come.

Biotechnology and the World Food Supply

Today, in a world with abundant food, more than 700 million people are chronically undernourished. Over the next 20 years, the world's population will probably double. The global food supply would need to double just to stay even, but to triple for the larger population to be fed adequately. Meanwhile, we are approaching limits in arable land and productivity and are employing practices that are destroying the soil's capacity to produce food.

Some see biotechnology as the answer to the problem of enabling this much larger population to feed itself. But biotechnology, if by this we mean crops engineered to contain new genes, is not *essential*. It could play a minor and useful role in developing new agricultural products, but other factors—including other kinds of breeding technologies—will be much more important than transgenic crops in determining whether we meet this challenge. It would be a tragedy if other necessary actions were not taken because of a mistaken belief that genetic engineering is some sort of a panacea for hunger. Some of the reasons biotechnology should not be relied on to enable the world to feed itself are outlined below.

More productive crops are only part of the solution to the world's food crisis.

There are many reasons for the current and projected food crisis. Among the most important are lack of income to buy food, lack of infrastructure like roads to get products to market, trade policies that disadvantage farmers in the developing world, lack of inputs such as fertilizer, lack of information, and low-yield farming practices. More productive crops will do little to alleviate hunger if

deficiencies in those areas are not addressed as well.

Where more productive crops are needed, there is little reason to believe that genetic engineering will be better than other technologies—in particular, sophisticated traditional breeding—at producing higher yielding crops.

Many technologies can increase the yields of crops. These include traditional breeding, production of hybrids, so-called marker-assisted breeding (a sophisticated way of enhancing traditional breeding by knowing which plant cultivars carry which trait), and tissue culture methods for propagating virus-free root stocks. All of these could help improve the productivity of crops in the developing world, but currently only limited resources are available for applying them there.

So far, there no reason to believe that genetic engineering would be markedly better than these more traditional technologies in improving crops. Early "gene dreams" were of nitrogen-fixing crops, higher intrinsic yield, and drought tolerance. But so far none of these seems realistic because most involve complex multigene traits. For the most part, genetically engineered crops are limited to one or two gene transfers and have relative few applications of use to hungry people. Those that are of use, such as insect resistance and virus tolerance, do not increase intrinsic yield and vary in effectiveness. In addition, they appear to be short lived due to the almost certain evolution of resistant pests.

Currently, there is no reason to believe that the limited resources for agricultural development would be better

spent on producing genetically engineered crops rather than on applying breeding technologies.

For the most part, genetic engineering techniques are being applied to crops important to the industrialized world, not crops on which the world's hungry depend.

Most genetic engineering in agriculture is being done by large transnational corporations that need to sell their products at premium prices to cover the cost of research. These companies are developing products for farmers in rich countries who can afford to pay high prices for seed. Such farmers are interested in field crops like corn, soybeans, and cotton and fruits like tomatoes and cantaloupes. And that is what the agricultural biotechnology industry is providing. In many cases, genetically engineered fruits are sold at premium prices and seeds are sold with an added technology fee to cover the costs of research. These products are of virtually no value to hungry farmers in Africa, who cannot afford the products of traditional technology, much less these expensive genetically engineered products. In addition, these products are often inappropriate for the developing world because, among other things, they require large amounts of fertilizers, pesticides, and water.

In sum, more productive crops are only part of the solution to the world hunger problem and transgenic crops are not uniquely capable of increasing food production. While some genetically engineered crops will undoubtedly prove useful, there is no reason at this time to invest huge sums in them, especially at the expense of traditional breeding.

What can be done to increase the food supply, particularly for the poor?

Many, many things. At bottom, we need more and better targeted agricultural research. Unlike the past, research can no longer concentrate exclusively on increased production—it must find ways to minimize the soil erosion, degradation of lakes and rivers, and groundwater pollution that can result from industrial agricultural practices. Growing appreciation of environmentally destructive impacts has led to a renewed interest in agroforestry, intercropping, mixed crop-livestock operations as systems that can increase production with minimal chemical fertilizers and pesticides and a high degree of environmental protection.

Much can be done to promote the sustainable intensification of agricultural production. Most of it should be done in developing countries to enable people to feed themselves so that they do not become dependent on commodities from abroad. All of it depends on local climates, cultures, and economic conditions. Rice farmers in Southeast Asia, for example, are in a far different situation from farmers living at the edge of the Sahara desert. Among the many research areas important for increasing production are the efficient use of irrigation water, crop improvement through traditional plant breeding, and new ways to manage crop-pest interactions, such as integrated pest management.

There is every reason to expect that research along these lines will lead to increased yields. Recently, agricultural scientists working in the Philippines announced that they had used sophisticated traditional breeding techniques to develop a rice variety that increased the proportion of the plant devoted to rice grains in ways that improved rice yields by 20 percent, a stunning achievement considering the importance of rice in the human diet. (Interestingly, the announcement was not accompanied by headlines like "Traditional Crop Breeding Can Feed the World!")

Improvements in other parts of the agricultural system are also essential. These include building and maintaining roads so that farmers can get their crops to market, organizing cooperatives so that farmers can purchase equipment and fertilizer, and reducing post-harvest losses of crops.

Finally, meeting the world food crisis will require changes outside of agriculture like improving the incomes of the poor through microenterprises and shifting the diet of the rich away from excessive dependence on grain-fed livestock. Growing corn to feed cows and chickens is a much less efficient use of limited arable land than growing corn for humans to eat directly.

Glossary

Absorption The process by which digestive products pass from the gastrointestinal tract into the blood.

Acid/base balance The relationship between acidity and alkalinity in the body fluids.

Amino acids The structural units that make up proteins.

Amylase An enzyme that breaks down starches; a component of saliva.

Amylopectin A component of starch, consisting of many glucose units joined in branching patterns.

Amylose A component of starch, consisting of many glucose units joined in a straight chain, without branching.

Anabolism The synthesis of new materials for cellular growth, maintenance, or repair in the body.

Anemia A deficiency of oxygen-carrying material in the blood.

Anorexia nervosa A disorder in which a person refuses food and loses weight to the point of emaciation and even death.

Antioxidant A substance that prevents or delays the breakdown of other substances by oxygen; often added to food to retard deterioration and rancidity.

Arachidonic acid An essential polyunsaturated fatty acid.

Arteriosclerosis Condition characterized by a thickening and hardening of the walls of the arteries and a resultant loss of elasticity.

Ascorbic acid Vitamin C.

Atherosclerosis A type of arteriosclerosis in which lipids, especially cholesterol, accumulate in the arteries and obstruct blood flow.

Avidin A substance in raw egg white that acts as an antagonist of biotin, one of the B vitamins.

Basal metabolic rate (BMR) The rate at which the body uses energy for maintaining involuntary functions such as cellular activity, respiration, and heartbeat when at rest.

Basic four The food plan outlining the milk, meat, fruits and vegetables, and breads and cereals needed in the daily diet to provide the necessary nutrients.

Beriberi A disease resulting from inadequate thiamin in the diet.

Beta-carotene Yellow pigment that is converted to vitamin A in the body.

Biotin One of the B vitamins.

Bomb calorimeter An instrument that oxidizes food samples to measure their energy content.

Buffer A substance that can neutralize both acids and bases to minimize change in the pH of a solution.

Calorie The energy required to raise the temperature of one gram of water one degree Celsius.

Carbohydrate An organic compound composed of carbon, hydrogen, and oxygen in a ratio of 1:2:1.

Carcinogen A cancer-causing substance.

Catabolism The breakdown of complex substances into simpler ones.

Celiac disease A syndrome resulting from intestinal sensitivity to gluten, a protein substance of wheat flour especially and of other grains.

Cellulose An indigestible polysaccharide made of many glucose molecules.

Cheilosis Cracks at the corners of the mouth, due primarily to a deficiency of riboflavin in the diet.

Cholesterol A fat-like substance found only in animal products; important in many body functions but also implicated in heart disease.

Choline A substance that prevents the development of a fatty liver; frequently considered one of the B-complex vitamins.

Chylomicron A very small emulsified lipoprotein that transports fat in the blood.

Cobalamin One of the B vitamins (B12).

Coenzyme A component of an enzyme system that facilitates the working of the enzyme.

Collagen Principal protein of connective tissue.

Colostrum The yellowish fluid that precedes breast milk, produced in the first few days of lactation.

Cretinism The physical and mental retardation of a child resulting from severe iodine or thyroid deficiency in the mother during pregnancy.

Dehydration Excessive loss of water from the body.

Dextrin Any of various small soluble polysaccharides found in the leaves of starch-forming plants and in the human alimentary canal as a product of starch digestion.

Diabetes (diabetes mellitus) A metabolic disorder characterized by excess blood sugar and urine sugar.

Digestion The breakdown of ingested foods into particles of a size and chemical composition that can be absorbed by the body.

Diglyceride A lipid containing glycerol and two fatty acids.

Disaccharide A sugar made up of two chemically combined monosaccharides, or simple sugars.

Diuretics Substances that stimulate urination.

Diverticulosis A condition in which the wall of the large intestine weakens and balloons out, forming pouches where fecal matter can be entrapped.

Edema The presence of an abnormally high amount of fluid in the tissues.

Emulsifier A substance that promotes the mixing of foods, such as oil and water in a salad dressing.

Enrichment The addition of nutrients to foods, often to restore what has been lost in processing.

Enzyme A protein that speeds up chemical reactions in the cell.

Epidemiology The study of the factors that contribute to the occurrence of a disease in a population.

Essential amino acid Any of the nine amino acids that the human body cannot manufacture and that must be supplied by the diet, as they are necessary for growth and maintenance.

Essential fatty acid A fatty acid that the human body cannot manufacture and that must be supplied by the diet, as it is necessary for growth and maintenance.

Fat An organic compound whose molecules contain glycerol and fatty acids; fat insulates the body, protects organs, carries fat-soluble vitamins, is a constituent of cell membranes, and makes food taste good.

Fatty acid A simple lipid—containing only carbon, hydrogen, and oxygen—that is a constituent of fat.

Ferritin A substance in which iron, in combination with protein, is stored in the liver, spleen, and bone marrow.

Fiber Indigestible carbohydrate found primarily in plant foods; high fiber intake is useful in regulating bowel movements, and may lower the incidence of certain types of cancer and other diseases.

Flavoprotein Protein containing riboflavin.

Folic acid (folacin) One of the B vitamins.

Fortification The addition of nutrients to foods to enhance their nutritional values.

Fructose A six-carbon monosaccharide found in many fruits as well as honey and plant saps; one of two monosaccharides forming sucrose, or table sugar.

Galactose A six-carbon monosaccharide, one of the two that make up lactose, or milk sugar.

Gallstones An abnormal formation of gravel or stones, composed of cholesterol and bile salts and sometimes bile pigments, in the gallbladder; they result when substances that normally dissolve in bile precipitate out.

Gastritis Inflammation of the stomach.

Glucagon A hormone produced by the pancreas that works to increase blood glucose concentration.

Glucose A six-carbon monosaccharide found in sucrose, honey, and many fruits and vegetables; the major carbohydrate found in the body.

Glucose tolerance factor (GTF) A hormone-like substance containing chromium, niacin, and protein that helps the body to use glucose.

Glyceride A simple lipid composed of fatty acids and glycerol.

Glycogen The storage form of carbohydrates in the body; composed of glucose molecules.

Goiter Enlargement of the thyroid gland as a result of iodine deficiency.

Goitrogens Substances that induce goiter, often by interfering with the body's utilization of iodine.

Heme A complex iron–containing compound that is a component of hemoglobin.

Hemicellulose Any of various indigestible plant polysaccharides.

Hemochromatosis A disorder of iron metabolism.

Hemoglobin The iron-containing protein in red blood cells that carries oxygen to the tissues.

High-density lipoprotein (HDL) A lipoprotein that acts as a cholesterol carrier in the blood; referred to as "good" cholesterol because relatively high levels of it appear to protect against atherosclerosis.

Hormones Compounds secreted by the endocrine glands that influence the functioning of various organs.

Humectants Substances added to foods to help them maintain moistness.

Hydrogenation The chemical process by which hydrogen is added to unsaturated fatty acids, which saturates them and converts them from a liquid to a solid form.

Hydrolyze To split a chemical compound into smaller molecules by adding water.

Hydroxyapatite The hard mineral portion (the major constituent) of bone, composed of calcium and phosphate.

Hypercalcemia A high level of calcium in the blood.

Hyperglycemia A high level of "sugar" (glucose) in the blood.

Hypocalcemia A low level of calcium in the blood.

Hypoglycemia A low level of "sugar" (glucose) in the blood.

Incomplete protein A protein lacking or deficient in one or more of the essential amino acids.

Inorganic Describes a substance not containing carbon.

Insensible loss Fluid loss, through the skin and from the lungs, that an individual is unaware of.

Insulin A hormone produced by the pancreas that regulates the body's use of glucose.

Intrinsic factor A protein produced by the stomach that makes absorption of B$_{12}$ possible; lack of this protein results in pernicious anemia.

Joule A unit of energy preferred by some professionals instead of the heat energy measurements of the calorie system for calculating food energy; sometimes referred to as "kilojoule."

Keratinization Formation of a protein called keratin, which, in vitamin A deficiency, occurs instead of mucus formation; leads to a drying and hardening of epithelial tissue.

Ketogenic Describes substances that can be converted to ketone bodies during metabolism, such as fatty acids and some amino acids.

Ketone bodies The three chemicals—acetone, acetoacetic acid, and betahydroxybutyrie—that are normally involved in lipid metabolism and accumulate in blood and urine in abnormal amounts in conditions of impaired metabolism (such as diabetes).

Ketosis A condition resulting when fats are the major source of energy and are incompletely oxidized, causing ketone bodies to build up in the bloodstream.

Kilocalorie One thousand calories, or the energy required to raise the temperature of one kilogram of water one degree Celsius; the preferred unit of measurement for food energy.

Kilojoule *See* Joule.

Kwashiorkor A form of malnutrition resulting from a diet severely deficient in protein but high in carbohydrates.

Lactase A digestive enzyme produced by the small intestine that breaks down lactose.

Lactation Milk production/secretion.

Lacto-ovo-vegetarian A person who does not eat meat, poultry, or fish but does eat milk products and eggs.

Lactose A disaccharide composed of glucose and galactose and found in milk.

Lactose intolerance The inability to digest lactose due to a lack of the enzyme lactase in the intestine.

Lacto-vegetarian A person who does not eat meat, poultry, fish, or eggs but does drink milk and eat milk products.

Laxatives Food or drugs that stimulate bowel movements.

Lignins Certain forms of indigestible carbohydrate in plant foods.

Linoleic acid An essential polyunsaturated fatty acid.

Lipase An enzyme that digests fats.

Lipid Any of various substances in the body or in food that are insoluble in water; a fat or fat-like substance.

Lipoprotein Compound composed of a lipid (fat) and a protein that transports both in the bloodstream.

Low-density lipoprotein (LDL) A lipoprotein that acts as a cholesterol carrier in the blood; referred to as "bad" cholesterol because relatively high levels of it appear to enhance atherosclerosis.

Macrocytic anemia A form of anemia characterized by the presence of abnormally large blood cells.

Macroelements (also macronutrient elements) Those elements present in the body in amounts exceeding 0.005 percent of body weight and required in the diet in amounts exceeding 100 mg/day; include sodium, potassium, calcium, and phosphorus.

Malnutrition A poor state of health resulting from a lack, excess, or imbalance of the nutrients needed by the body.

Maltose A disaccharide whose units are each composed of two glucose molecules, produced by the digestion of starch.

Marasmus Condition resulting from a deficiency of calories and nearly all essential nutrients.

Melanin A dark pigment in the skin, hair, and eyes.

Metabolism The sum of all chemical reactions that take place within the body.

Microelements (also micronutrient elements; trace elements) Those elements present in the body in amounts under 0.005 percent of body weight and required in the diet in amounts under 100 mg/day.

Monoglyceride A lipid containing glycerol and only one fatty acid.

Monosaccharide A single sugar molecule, the simplest form of carbohydrate; examples are glucose, fructose, and galactose.

Monosodium glutamate (MSG) An amino acid used in flavoring foods, which causes allergic reactions in some people.

Monounsaturated fatty acid A fatty acid containing one double bond.

Mutagen A mutation-causing agent.

Negative nitrogen balance Nitrogen output exceeds nitrogen intake.

Niacin (nicotinic acid) One of the B vitamins.

Nitrogen equilibrium (zero nitrogen balance) Nitrogen output equals nitrogen intake.

Nonessential amino acid Any of the 13 amino acids that the body can manufacture in adequate amounts, but which are nonetheless required in the diet in an amount relative to the amount of essential amino acids.

Nutrients Nourishing substances in food that can be digested, absorbed, and metabolized by the body; needed for growth, maintenance, and reproduction.

Nutrition (1) The sum of the processes by which an organism obtains, assimilates, and utilizes food. (2) The scientific study of these processes.

Obesity Condition of being 15 to 20 percent above one's ideal body weight.

Oleic acid A monounsaturated fatty acid.

Organic foods Those foods, especially fruits and vegetables, grown without the use of pesticides, synthetic fertilizers, etc.

Osmosis Passage of a solvent through a semipermeable membrane from an area of higher concentration to an area of lower concentration until the concentration is equal on both sides of the membrane.

Osteomalacia Condition in which a loss of bone mineral leads to a softening of the bones; adult counterpart of rickets.

Osteoporosis Disorder in which the bones degenerate due to a loss of bone mineral, producing porosity and fragility; normally found in older women.

Overweight Body weight exceeding an accepted norm by 10 or 15 percent.

Ovo-vegetarian A person who does not eat meat, poultry, fish, milk, or milk products but does eat eggs.

Oxidation The process by which a substrate takes up oxygen or loses hydrogen; the loss of electrons.

Palmitic acid A saturated fatty acid.

Pantothenic acid One of the B vitamins.

Pellagra Niacin deficiency syndrome, characterized by dementia, diarrhea, and dermatitis.

Pepsin A protein-digesting enzyme produced by the stomach.

Peptic ulcer An open sore or erosion in the lining of the digestive tract, especially in the stomach and duodenum.

Peptide A compound composed of amino acids that are joined together.

Peristalsis Motions of the digestive tract that propel food through the tract.

Pernicious anemia One form of anemia caused by an inability to absorb vitamin B_{12}, owing to the absence of intrinsic factor.

pH A measure of the acidity of a solution, based on a scale from 0 to 14: a pH of 7 is neutral; greater than 7 is alkaline; less than 7 is acidic.

Phenylketonuria (PKU) A genetic disease in which phenylalanine, an essential amino acid, is not properly metabolized, thus accumulating in the blood and causing early brain damage.

Phospholipid A fat containing phosphorus, glycerol, two fatty acids, and any of several other chemical substances.

Polypeptide A molecular chain of amino acids.

Polysaccharide A carbohydrate containing many monosaccharide subunits.

Polyunsaturated fatty acids A fatty acid in which two or more carbon atoms have formed double bonds, with each holding only one hydrogen atom.

Positive nitrogen balance Condition in which nitrogen intake exceeds nitrogen output in the body.

Protein Any of the organic compounds composed of amino acids and containing nitrogen; found in the cells of all living organisms.

Provitamins Precursors of vitamins that can be converted to vitamins in the body (e.g., beta-carotene, from which the body can make vitamin A).

Pyridoxine One of the B vitamins (B_6).

Pull date Date after which food should no longer be sold but still may be edible for several days.

Recommended Daily Allowances (RDAs) Standards for daily intake of specific nutrients established by the Food and Nutrition Board of the National Academy of Sciences; they are the levels thought to be adequate to maintain the good health of most people.

Rhodopsin The visual pigment in the retinal rods of the eyes which allows one to see at night; its formation requires vitamin A.

Riboflavin One of the B vitamins (B_2).

Ribosome The cellular structure in which protein synthesis occurs.

Rickets The vitamin D deficiency disease in children characterized by bone softening and deformities.

Saliva Fluid produced in the mouth that helps food digestion.

Salmonella A bacterium that can cause food poisoning.

Saturated fatty acid A fatty acid in which carbon is joined with four other atoms; i.e., all carbon atoms are bound to the maximum possible number of hydrogen atoms.

Scurvy A disease characterized by bleeding gums, pain in joints, lethargy, and other problems; caused by a deficiency of vitamin C (ascorbic acid).

Standard of identity A list of specifications for the manufacture of certain foods that stipulates their required contents.

Starch A polysaccharide composed of glucose molecules; the major form in which energy is stored in plants.

Stearic acid A saturated fatty acid.

Sucrose A disaccharide composed of glucose and fructose, often called "table sugar."

Sulfites Agents used as preservatives in foods to eliminate bacteria, preserve freshness, prevent browning, and increase storage life; can cause acute asthma attacks, and even death, in people who are sensitive to them.

Teratogen An agent with the potential of causing birth defects.

Thiamin One of the B vitamins (B_1).

Thyroxine Hormone containing iodine that is secreted by the thyroid gland.

Toxemia A complication of pregnancy characterized by high blood pressure, edema, vomiting, presence of protein in the urine, and other symptoms.

Transferrin A protein compound, the form in which iron is transported in the blood.

Triglyceride A lipid containing glycerol and three fatty acids.

Trypsin A digestive enzyme, produced in the pancreas, that breaks down protein.

Underweight Body weight below an accepted norm by more than 10 percent.

United States Recommended Daily Allowance (USRDA) The highest level of recommended intakes for population groups (except pregnant and lactating women); derived from the RDAs and used in food labeling.

Urea The main nitrogenous component of urine, resulting from the breakdown of amino acids.

Uremia A disease in which urea accumulates in the blood.

Vegan A person who eats nothing derived from an animal; the strictest type of vegetarian.

Vitamin Organic substance required by the body in small amounts to perform numerous functions.

Vitamin B complex All known water-soluble vitamins except C; includes thiamin (B_1), riboflavin (B_2), pyridoxine (B_6), niacin, folic acid, cobalamin (B_{12}), pantothenic acid, and biotin.

Xerophthalmia A disease of the eye resulting from vitamin A deficiency.

Test Your Knowledge Form

We encourage you to photocopy and use this page as a tool to assess how the articles in **Annual Editions** expand on the information in your textbook. By reflecting on the articles you will gain enhanced text information. You can also access this useful form on a product's book support Web site at **http://www.dushkin.com/online/.**

NAME: DATE:

_____

TITLE AND NUMBER OF ARTICLE:

_____

BRIEFLY STATE THE MAIN IDEA OF THIS ARTICLE:

_____

LIST THREE IMPORTANT FACTS THAT THE AUTHOR USES TO SUPPORT THE MAIN IDEA:

_____

WHAT INFORMATION OR IDEAS DISCUSSED IN THIS ARTICLE ARE ALSO DISCUSSED IN YOUR TEXTBOOK OR OTHER READINGS THAT YOU HAVE DONE? LIST THE TEXTBOOK CHAPTERS AND PAGE NUMBERS:

_____

LIST ANY EXAMPLES OF BIAS OR FAULTY REASONING THAT YOU FOUND IN THE ARTICLE:

_____

LIST ANY NEW TERMS/CONCEPTS THAT WERE DISCUSSED IN THE ARTICLE, AND WRITE A SHORT DEFINITION:

_____

ANNUAL EDITIONS revisions depend on two major opinion sources: one is our Advisory Board, listed in the front of this volume, which works with us in scanning the thousands of articles published in the public press each year; the other is you—the person actually using the book. Please help us and the users of the next edition by completing the prepaid article rating form on this page and returning it to us. Thank you for your help!

ANNUAL EDITIONS: Nutrition 01/02

ARTICLE RATING FORM

Here is an opportunity for you to have direct input into the next revision of this volume. We would like you to rate each of the 57 articles listed below, using the following scale:

1. **Excellent: should definitely be retained**
2. **Above average: should probably be retained**
3. **Below average: should probably be deleted**
4. **Poor: should definitely be deleted**

Your ratings will play a vital part in the next revision. So please mail this prepaid form to us just as soon as you complete it. Thanks for your help!

RATING

ARTICLE

1. The Changing American Diet
2. Healthy Lifestyles for Healthy Americans: Report on USDA's Year 2000 Behavioral Nutrition Roundtable
3. Nutrient Requirements Get a Makeover: The Evolution of the Recommended Dietary Allowances
4. Picture This! Communicating Nutrition Around the World
5. Food Portions and Servings: How Do They Differ?
6. A Reality Check for the Lunch-On-the-Run Crowd
7. The 100 Healthiest Foods
8. Supermarket Psych-Out
9. Should You Be Eating *More* Fat and *Fewer* Carbohydrates?
10. Fats: The Good, the Bad, the Trans
11. National Academy of Sciences Introduces New Calcium Recommendations
12. Vitamin Deficiencies in North America in the 20th Century
13. Can Taking Vitamins Protect Your Brain?
14. When (and How) to Take Your Vitamin and Mineral Supplements
15. The Best D-Fense
16. Folate May Offer Protection
17. Nutrient-Drug Interactions and Food
18. Solving the Diet-and-Disease Puzzle
19. Food as Disease-Fighter
20. Guess Who's Coming to Dinner?
21. Homocysteine: "The New Cholesterol"?
22. Soy: Cause for Joy?
23. Questions and Answers About Cancer, Diet and Fats
24. Micronutrient Shortfalls in Young Children's Diets: Common, and Owing to Inadequate Intakes Both at Home and at Child Care Centers
25. A Focus on Nutrition for the Elderly: It's Time to Take a Closer Look
26. Physical Activity and Nutrition: A Winning Combination for Health
27. Halting the Obesity Epidemic: A Public Health Policy Approach

RATING

ARTICLE

28. NIH Guidelines: An Evaluation
29. Why We Get Fat
30. The Great Weight Debate
31. Simplifying the Advice for Slimming Down
32. Weight Loss Diets and Books
33. Americans Ignore Importance of Food Portion Size
34. Dieting Disorder
35. The Effects of Starvation on Behavior: Implications for Dieting and Eating Disorders
36. America's Dietary Guideline on Food Safety: A Plus, or a Minus?
37. Don't Mess With Food Safety Myths!
38. Bacterial Food-Borne Illness
39. About Food Safety and Spoilage
40. Avoiding Cross-Contamination in the Home
41. Campylobacter: Low-Profile Bug Is Food Poisoning Leader
42. *E. Coli* 0157:H7—How Dangerous Has It Become?
43. Is It Safe to Eat?
44. Nutrition Quackery
45. Yet Another Study—Should You Pay Attention?
46. The Mouse That Roared: Health Scares on the Internet
47. Herbals for Health?
48. Nutrition Supplements: Science vs Hype
49. Soy: Health Claims for Soy Protein, Questions About Other Components
50. Food for Thought About Dietary Supplements
51. Are Health Food Stores Better Bets Than Traditional Supermarkets?
52. Hunger and Food Insecurity
53. Nutrition and Infection: Malnutrition and Mortality in Public Health
54. Linking Environment and Health: Malnutrition
55. Agricultural Growth, Poverty Alleviation, and Environmental Sustainability: Having It All
56. Will Frankenfood Feed the World?
57. Biotechnology and the World Food Supply

(Continued on next page)

We Want Your Advice

ANNUAL EDITIONS: NUTRITION 01/02

BUSINESS REPLY MAIL
FIRST-CLASS MAIL PERMIT NO. 84 GUILFORD CT

POSTAGE WILL BE PAID BY ADDRESSEE

McGraw-Hill/Dushkin
530 Old Whitfield Street
Guilford, CT 06437-9989

ABOUT YOU

Name _____ Date _____

Are you a teacher? ☐ A student? ☐
Your school's name _____

Department _____

Address _____ City _____ State ___ Zip ___

School telephone # _____

YOUR COMMENTS ARE IMPORTANT TO US !

Please fill in the following information:
For which course did you use this book?
_____

Did you use a text with this *ANNUAL EDITION*? ☐ yes ☐ no
What was the title of the text?
_____

What are your general reactions to the *Annual Editions* concept?
_____

Have you read any particular articles recently that you think should be included in the next edition?
_____

Are there any articles you feel should be replaced in the next edition? Why?
_____

Are there any World Wide Web sites you feel should be included in the next edition? Please annotate.
_____

May we contact you for editorial input? ☐ yes ☐ no
May we quote your comments? ☐ yes ☐ no